YOUNGER
by the DAY

YOUNGER
by the DAY

---

*365 Ways to Rejuvenate Your Body
and Revitalize Your Spirit*

Victoria Moran

HarperSanFrancisco
A Division of HarperCollins*Publishers*

This book is written as a source of information only. The information contained in this book should by no means be considered a substitute for the advice of a qualified medical professional, who should always be consulted before beginning any new diet, exercise, or other health program.

All efforts have been made to ensure the accuracy of the information contained in this book as of the date published. The author and the publisher expressly disclaim responsibility for any adverse effects arising from the use or application of the information contained herein.

Jennifer Raymond, recipes from *The Peaceful Palate*. Copyright © 1992, 1996 by the author. Used by permission of Jennifer Raymond.

Joan Price, M.A., with Lawrence Kassman, MD, F.A.C.E.P., excerpt from *The Anytime, Anywhere Exercise Book*. Copyright © 2003 by Joan Price. Used by permission of Joan Price.

From *Eat to Beat Cancer* by J. Robert Hatherill, PhD. Copyright © 1998 by the author and reprinted by permission of St. Martin's Press, LLC.

Hal A. Lingerman, excerpt from *The Healing Energies of Music*. Copyright © 1983, 1995 by the author. Used by permission of The Theosophical Publishing House, Wheaton, Illinois.

Kit Chow and Ione Kramer, excerpt from *All the Tea in China*. Copyright © 1990, 1998 by the authors. Used by permission of China Books & Periodicals, Inc., San Francisco.

FIRST EDITION

Designed by Kris Tobiassen
Illustrations by Lydia Hess

Library of Congress Cataloging-in-Publication Data is available on request.

ISBN 0–06–073062–5 (hardcover)

04 05 06 07 08 ❖/RRD(H) 10 9 8 7 6 5 4 3 2

To Frankie, in Memoriam

You made life a grand adventure and middle age downright stunning

Contents

Acknowledgments

To my agent Linda Chester, editor Renee Sedliar, and foreign rights agent Linda Michaels: thank you for believing in this book and in me. You carried me through. To William: thank you for standing by me more than any wife could expect and reminding me that all that matters is how I see myself. To Adair: thank you for bearing with me through yet another book, for invaluable research assistance, bright ideas, and steady encouragement.

Appreciation is also due everyone at HarperSanFrancisco and HarperCollins who has had a hand in this book, including Stephen Hanselman, Margery Buchanan, Claudia Boutote, Miki Terasawa, Mark Tauber, Lisa Zuniga, Kris Tobiassen, cover designer Jim Warner, Lydia Hess, and all the other miracle workers. Thanks to copyeditor Kathy Reigstad, freelance editor Caroline Pincus, and Ms. Chester's assistant, Gary Jaffe, for making many potential difficulties easy.

Thanks also go to my mother, Gladys Marshall, for modeling so exquisitely the next phase of life; my stepdaughter, Siân Melton, for her eye to fashion that transcends generations; my mother-in-law, Betty Melton, for lessons in wit and gratitude; and idea merchants, mentors, and moral supporters Barbara Barrington, LCH, LCPH; Tess Brubeck; Kris Carlson; Richard Carlson, PhD;

Rosemary Cathcart; Elizabeth Cutting; Scott Gerson, MD; Suzanne Hatlestad; Terry Jordan; Crystal Leaman; Jean Lebedun; Leslie Levine; Lane Lynn; Ian McGrady; Rev. Chris Michaels; Jay Mulvaney; Ellen Politis; Erin Reese; Alysia Reiner; Linda Ruocco; Deborah Shouse; Elizabeth Simons; and Carol Wiesner.

I am indebted to Jennifer Raymond for the recipes from her cookbook *The Peaceful Palate*; and to all the people who generously gave of their time to be interviewed: Nathaniel Altman; Irene Angster; Darrick Antell, MD; Neal Barnard, MD; Barbara Biziou; Patti Breitman; Pauline Canelias, DC; Mary Cordaro; Lisa Everett, RPh, CCN; Lorna Flamer-Caldera, DDS; Necia Gamby, LMT; Marsha Lynn Gordon, MD; Marc Grossman, OD; Pam Grout; Michael Halpern; Mari Lyn Henry; Suzanne Havala Hobbs, DrPH, RD; Kevin Kelly; Charla Krupp; Cheryl Morgan, PhD; Stephen Parker; Lynn Robinson; Karen Rowinsky; Denise Ruidant; Judith Sachs; Rev. Fran Sherwood; Jane Thebo, AuD; Tim Trader, ND; Barbara Unell; Fern Korman Werman; and Kelyang Yeshe.

Thanks, too, for input and assistance to Penny Drue Baird, Barbara Bartocci, Carolyn Bell, Terry Berenson, Diane Bliss, Teri Conti, Amanda Coppola, Laurel Donnellan, Emily Eldridge, Linda Flake, Melanie Frey, Judy Goldstein, MD, Gail Grasso, Vilborg Halldórsdóttir, Hildur Hermóðsdóttir, Sam Horn, Thora Sigrur Ingólfsdóttir, Martha Kemp, Jennifer Louden, Gail McMeekin, Abbie Miller, Nava Namdar, Jackie Roberts, Róósa Traustadóóttir, Lynda Turan, and Sallyan Windt. And to the wonderful women of the *Younger by the Day* focus group: Omkari Williams Benzinger, Nancy Brickley, Joy Brakke, Lani Gerity, Karen Johnson, Nancy Long, Sandi Moran, Jan Mueller, June Pardoe, Mary Beth Reutter, Deanna Seiler, Letitia Suk, Rena Tucker, and Angie Ware. You brought this book to life.

Finally, I wish to acknowledge all those who provided testimonials for *Younger by the Day* and Baba for continual inspiration.

Introduction

Younger by the Day is a daily guide to turning back the clock for you, for real. If you heed its practical instructions, and allow the more inspirational aspects to take root within you, you *will* look and feel younger. And you will be less concerned about the passage of time. This is because *Younger by the Day* is concerned not only with your physical body and its conscientious care, but with the deep layers of your being: your mind, your emotions, and—especially—your spirit.

These principles will work for you at whatever point you are on your life journey. I write from the vantage point of a woman in her fifties, because it was the simultaneous arrival of menopause and my fiftieth birthday that made aging an issue in my life for the first time. I'd heard about "the change," but I never expected changes so noticeable—or so rapid. My body changed shape overnight: I went to bed with a flat tummy and round bottom and woke up with a protruding stomach and a washboard butt. It was *Invasion of the Body Snatchers* in my own bedroom.

My hair got thinner. "It's not the cut, honey," the stylist chided. "You just don't have as much hair as you used to." (Too bad nobody told my chin that growing hair was such a challenge.) My hands got freckles. Oh, shoot, they weren't freckles. Freckles are those cute things that go with sunsuits and pigtails. These were age spots, "liver spots," the plague addressed by tiny ads in the backs of magazines, right there between "Our Psychics Know *Your* Future" and "Top Recording Artists Are Waiting for *Your* Songs." My waistline vanished. My jowls sagged. My breasts drooped. My triceps jiggled. I was tired, and watching way too much "television for women." Even my brain was missing beats: I'd say the wrong word or dial the wrong number. "It's midlife brain fog," I heard from the similarly afflicted.

I felt powerless against too much stress and too few hormones. On the outside, I could see my body paying for every late night and crash diet, grief and heartbreak, sunburn and surgery I had ever experienced. And in the inner reaches of my physical self, in places I didn't know or understand, legions of psychopathic molecules were busily oxidizing to make me age, the way the flesh of a cut apple exposed to the air discolors and turns soft and unappealing.

I tried to be philosophical: everybody said fifty was the new forty, so I'd gotten ten good years for free. Still, I was angry. Sometimes I blamed myself: "I should have exercised more. . . . I should have rested more. . . . I should have saved up for cosmetic surgery. . . ." Other times I blamed God and life and nature: "I've done (almost) everything right. This shouldn't be happening. It's just not fair."

I found myself at a familiar juncture, where accepting the present facts was imperative for changing the future. I'd been here at thirty-three, when a lifelong struggle with food and weight had either to end or be the end of me. In that case, I had to get out of the food business and turn the whole thing over to a Power who could do what I couldn't. The weight came off and I've been free these twenty years. I was there again at forty-six when, single for nearly a decade, I vowed to replace the longing for a partner with contentment around all I did have. Once that happened—and so quickly it still astounds me—I met the man who is now my husband.

In both these incidences, and in countless smaller ones along the way, I had learned to accept what was, do my part, and leave the outcome to forces wiser than I. It hadn't been easy and I didn't want to have to take this leap of faith again, but there was nowhere else to go. Once I was willing to do it, however, principles that had changed my life in other phases were on hand to change it again.

More help came, as it usually does for me, from other people: women who lived long without growing old. They taught me what they knew: "Live simply but passionately." "Laugh a lot." "Never stop dancing." "Lighten up—except about your health: there you can't be too careful." "Believe that you're young and beautiful now; in thirty years you'll know you were."

Also put in my path was Ayurvedic physician Dr. Scott Gerson. I'd dabbled in Ayurvedic medicine, the ancient Indian health-care system that translates as "the science of long life," back when dabbling was sufficient. Dr. Gerson took me from curious to committed. I did what I was told and things got better. In addition, through the thriving live foods community (proponents of fresh fruits, raw vegetables, sprouts, and juices) in New York City, I learned that vitality is contagious and that foods bursting with life lead to cells bursting with health, regardless of the age of the person those cells comprise. With the guidance of my various mentors—and a renewed trust in my own instincts—life started to sparkle again. So did I. I'm fifty-four now, a postmenopausal woman subject to the physical realities of that state, and yet younger in a great many visible and viable ways than when I started this process. That's why I wrote this book—so, whatever your age, you can be younger, too.

Here is how to use *Younger by the Day* to your best advantage:

- *The daily readings.* I suggest you consider reading the book through once—just a read, no action necessary. Then start with the current day and work through the year.

- *The monthly keynote.* The first day of every month focuses on a keynote, an idea or attitude to hold in mind that month. It requires minimal effort, just a willingness to let more of its essence into your life.

- *"Rejuvenate yourself with action."* At the end of many of the readings you'll see, "Rejuvenate yourself with action," an invitation to do something on your own behalf. Either do this exercise the day you read it or make a note on your calendar to do it at your first opportunity. When the action step asks one or more questions, you can answer them in your head or, ideally, write your thoughts about them in your journal.

- *"Revitalize your life with words."* Instead of closing with a call to action, some entries end with "Revitalize your life with words," followed by an affirmation to help program your mind with a life-affirming, self-approving idea. Work with this thought throughout the day, reciting it and writing it down. (There is more detail on how to do this in the January 4 reading.)

- *Play days.* For many people, payday comes on the fifteenth and the thirtieth of the month. For growing younger by the day, these will be *play* days. Use them either to play in earnest, or to play catch-up—getting back to an essay you didn't read, a participation exercise you missed, or something you think needs more attention.

As you progress through these pages, you will be altering both habits and attitudes, the way you treat yourself and the way you see yourself. As you do this, you will look younger to other people and feel younger in your own skin. It will start as soon as you do. By this time next year, you'll be amazed.

January

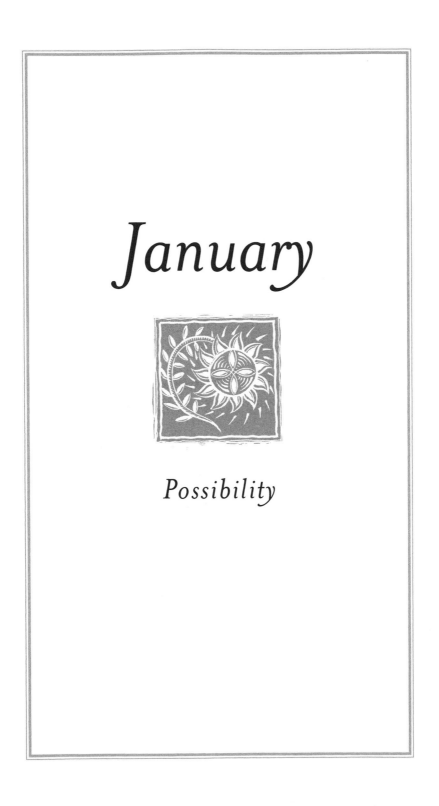

Possibility

Amazing Things Are Possible

Having a fresh year stretched out ahead of you like untracked snow speaks of boundless possibility. As you embark on this year of becoming younger by the day, let *possibility* be the keynote. It is fully possible for you to look and feel younger this time next year than you do right now. It is absolutely possible that you can come to love the age you are, and the ages you'll be in the future, even if that seems like a stretch today. It is completely possible that as you go through this year, you'll come to see midlife and later through your own unbiased eyes, without society's often skewed opinions clouding your vision.

All these things, and what you yourself want from this year, are possible. You can't force them to come about, but you can think and act in a way that allows them access to your life. Today, all you have to do is have a holiday. Eat black-eyed peas—good luck for the New Year according to Southern tradition, and a way to get some fiber and disease-preventing phytochemicals while you're at it. If making New Year's resolutions is a tradition for you, make them, but consider altering the process a little. Call them "possibilities" instead of "resolutions"—that takes the pressure off. Write them in the present tense as statements of fact dated January 1, *Next Year*. This way, instead of the standard "I will work out every day," you'll write "I am fitter and healthier than I've been in years"—a statement of possibility fulfilled.

REJUVENATE YOURSELF WITH ACTION: *Keep in mind through the month of January that all manner of wondrous things are possible, and that you are open to all possibilities.*

Seeing Your Age in a Bright New Light

One day while walking our dog, my daughter Adair met a woman who told her that, as a child, she had had a similar dog. "His name was Brownie," the woman said. "Let's see, I'm ninety-five now, so that must have been ninety years ago." Adair is not quite twenty. This may have been the oldest person she'd ever met. She was in awe. To someone her age, I'm old, too, just not the cool kind of old.

It's a funny thing: all your life practically everybody is older than you and then one day most people are younger. It's like crossing the International Date Line, but it's an age line instead. On one side of the line there's you, along with the people your age and older. On the other side is everybody who thinks you're old. To see your age in a new light, it is necessary to stop thinking of anybody as old. Think of everyone, yourself included, as ageless—eternal even.

If you believe in the soul, you know this already. If your soul is indeed who you are, your body is simply its vehicle. Some souls are buzzing around town in jazzy new sports cars. Others are in vintage sedans. In the big picture, your current chassis is pretty much irrelevant. Souls don't have VIN numbers, or birthdays. When you make a point of seeing everyone as a soul living in a body, the age of the body means a great deal less and the quality of the soul a great deal more.

The longer you do this, the easier it is to see that you and I are not beings bound by chronology. We are splendid creations with noble purpose. We're here to walk our dogs and love our children and talk to ninety-five-year-olds so that advanced age, when we get there, won't be such a strange country after all.

REJUVENATE YOURSELF WITH ACTION: *Practice being ageless today. Do what makes you feel good. Wear whatever strikes your fancy. You can be playful like a child, as wise as your own grandmother, or both—a day is long enough.*

Start Your Rejuvenation Journal

There is a singular reality to ink on paper. If you're not keeping a diary at the moment, treat yourself to a pretty blank journal or a thrifty spiral notebook to accompany you on your growing-younger journey. Use it as a workbook for plotting your strategies, writing your affirmations, and taking the action steps that call for writing, as well as for recording your insights and wrestling with the thoughts and feelings that can arise when you're facing head-on the reality of the passage of time. If you already do journal writing, you can incorporate all this into your current journal. (With lipsticks a notable exception, duplication complicates life when having one would do just as well.)

Writing your thoughts and feelings clears your head and helps you make wise choices. It also puts you in touch with inner wisdom and intuitive glimmerings you might not have accessed otherwise. If you're stressed, writing can ease the tension, or if you're ecstatic, recording that mood will allow you to revisit it later: "October 16—I am ecstatic." If you're angry, you can write instead of yelling. If you're sad, you can write instead of crying, or you can write *and* cry—double catharsis. You can use your journal for writing letters to people you're mad at, to people who are no longer living, or even to God. Some of the best letters are not meant for a mailbox, postal or electronic.

For the purposes of growing younger, a journal documents your process while it supports your progress. When you feel discouraged, it provides documentation of how far you've come. When you write, "I ate two fruits and three vegetables today—I'm getting this," you know you are. If you find yourself writing that you've gone to bed with makeup on for the fourth night in a row, you *know* you need to wash your face right after dinner or when you come home from work. There's no denying it anymore because it's there in black and white.

Write about how you feel about yourself at this moment and what you hope to accomplish in the year ahead. Write your doubts and concerns as well. Often when you start to write your worries, you find yourself writing their antidote. The journal is a tool. Along with tomorrow's reading about speaking revitalizing words, and the next day's suggestion of doing this program with a group of friends, it gives you the framework for your process. Everything else is just growing younger.

REJUVENATE YOURSELF WITH ACTION: *Get yourself a notebook or blank book and initiate your rejuvenation journal. If you already keep a journal, introduce into it the notion that it will be doubling for rejuvenation, too.*

JANUARY 4

Revitalizing Words

Truth, with a capital T, is life as it should be. Facts are life as it is. The ideal state is when you fully accept the facts and yet reach for the Truth for yourself and others. One way to do this is by making statements of Truth often enough that they become a working part of your mind, changing the way you see yourself, your life, and the world.

This powerful technique is not new, and you may have worked with it before. It is vital in becoming younger, because you're trying to do something that you *may* not believe is possible and that people around you definitely don't. The tape is playing in all our heads: "Nobody gets younger. What a lot of poppycock! Time marches on and bodies fall apart. Everybody knows that." To evidence something different, even a little bit, you have to overcome both your own resistance and that of the culture in which you live. This is where affirmations come in.

When you come to an affirmation in *Younger by the Day*—it will be introduced with "Revitalize your life with words"—read it over several times, preferably aloud. Write it at least once in your journal—three times if you can spare the extra minute or two. If you read in the morning, it's nice to check in with the day's affirmation again at night, and give yourself the mental suggestion that it is taking hold and becoming part of the way you see things.

If you're working through this book at a reading-a-day pace, you won't be able to do detailed work with every affirmation, and you don't need to. When a particular one speaks to you, however, or when you know in your heart of hearts that it's something you especially need, choose this one for additional attention. Make it your "affirmation of the month" and give it a full thirty days to become a part of you. Say it aloud thirty times a day—fifteen in the morning and fifteen in the evening, or ten times with each meal. Write it thirty times as well. Copy it and post it places—on your desk, the fridge, the bathroom mirror, wherever you're likely to see it, read it, and soak it up. Your mind can easily accommodate a primary affirmation as well as the ones you'll come to during the month and deal with in a more cursory fashion.

The upshot of programming your mind with revitalizing statements is that your thinking changes, not only in the specific area to which that affirmation applies, but in every aspect of your life. As you get used to voicing affirmations, negative statements you make in conversation (or in conversations with yourself) will start to sound odd. You won't like them and you'll make them less often. Affirmations help you create a better life out of words and attitudes that hold fast to the best and the highest, states with which you deserve to become intimately familiar.

REJUVENATE YOURSELF WITH ACTION: *Review the ways you'll use the affirmations in this book. Most of them you'll (a) read over several times, preferably aloud, (b) write down in your journal one to three times, and (c) read over once again before bed. When a statement strikes you as particularly relevant, select it for a full thirty days' work: say it aloud thirty times a day for a month, and write it thirty times a day for a month as well. (If you come upon another affirmation that seems important while you're still working on this one, jot the new one down for later. Intense work with one at a time is plenty.)*

JANUARY 5

A Circle of Friends

You can get group support, deepen existing friendships, and see rejuvenation take place before your eyes by forming a *rejuvenation circle,* a group of women who all want to look and feel more youthful, while at the same time accepting and celebrating the gifts of the age at which they find themselves. When there are people around you doing what you're doing, you encourage one another. You can often see the advancements someone else makes when you can't yet see your own, and other group members can see yours and point them out to you.

In forming such a group, consider not only friends who are your exact age but a coworker your mom's age, and your little sister who, hard as it is to believe, is hearing the clock tick, too. Ask people you know and encourage them to invite people you don't know; you might even put up a sign somewhere that is apt to attract compatible people—perhaps a natural food store, a bookshop, or a yoga center.

Group members can meet in person every couple of weeks and keep in phone and e-mail contact. You can "bookend" the *Younger by the Day* participation exercises by committing to another group member what you intend to do and getting back with her after you've done it. You can also engage in some rejuvenation together, like meeting for power walks, or a stress-zapping, seriously funny movie and dinner at that place with the prettiest salads in town. You might join a gym with one of the women, make a weekly farmers' market trip with another, or book a monthly partner pedicure with a third. (A partner pedicure is when you sit next to your pal at the salon and chat while you get tantalizing toes. If this catches on, it could replace meeting for coffee.)

REJUVENATE YOURSELF WITH ACTION: *Ask some women you know to join you in becoming younger by the day. Assemble a group of five to ten and plan for the next year to meet every other week, keep in touch between face-to-face gatherings, and help one another accomplish incredible things.*

JANUARY 6

Conquering Invisibility

You hear women in midlife mention it sometimes: "I think I've become invisible." If you feel that you were overlooked in the queue at the coffee shop, or by the clerk at the store, it may not be your imagination. Middle-aged women *are* overlooked—by younger men in particular, younger people in general, and even men our own age who, with society's blessing, get by believing they're younger than we are.

People see what they're trained to see. If you're trained in art, for instance, you might lose yourself in a gallery, drinking in the details of color and shape, while someone else sees only pictures. Our culture as a whole is trained to see young women. There are proportionally far more of them on magazine covers, on TV, and in films than in the actual population. As a result, we have a citizenry taught to see the young and ignore the not-so-young. It isn't conscious; it's Pavlovian.

You can address invisibility by shouting "I was here first!" This will get you your latté or the key to the fitting room, but you are unlikely to leave the encounter feeling good about it. I have found it best to deal with invisibility on the level where it starts, the subconscious. I wish I'd known this when I was overweight (fat people can be invisible, too, even young ones), but I know it now: *It's all in how you see yourself.* You change how you see yourself by making your first conscious thought of the day a remembrance of who you truly are: one of a kind, extraordinary, a woman with a destiny. Remind yourself of this when you walk into a meeting or a shop, when you speak with your boss or your teenager, when you greet a gatekeeper of any sort. When you do, it's as if a red carpet is rolled out before you and a subliminal messenger announces your arrival.

Some people find this easier to do than others. My friend Lane is one of them. Once, when I was in New York on a book tour and staying at the Plaza Hotel, I made a date with her. I was looking forward to afternoon tea in the Palm Court, like a celebrity or Eloise. To my dismay, Lane, still in a cast with a broken leg, showed up placidly attired in sweats. My face fell: we couldn't have tea with the swells in sweats.

"Sure we can," Lane said. "Give me the phone." I listened in awe to her air of authority. "See here," she began. (It made me sit up straighter, and she wasn't even talking to me.) "I'm in room 1801 and my friend has a broken leg. You certainly wouldn't expect her to *dress* for tea, now would you?" "Oh, no Ma'am," came the voice on the other end. "We'll have a table ready for you immediately." When we arrived at the Palm Court, a substantial Saturday crowd was waiting for tables, but we were led right through, Lane with her sweats and her crutches, me looking as if I had just observed the parting of the Red Sea.

Lane has never been invisible, and the rest of us don't have to be either. Regardless of what the world is trained to see, you can be the exception. It's all in the way you see yourself.

REVITALIZE YOUR LIFE WITH WORDS: *I am one of a kind, extraordinary, a woman with a destiny.*

JANUARY 7

Eating for Life

Eating well is simple. It's nutrition that's complex. Getting mired in nutritional details will, in fact, drive you nuts long before it makes you younger. Instead of thinking about grams and ounces, protein and carbs, I'd like you to think first about the sensual pleasures of eating the foods nature has so generously provided. Bring to mind the way the juice from a thick chunk of watermelon feels when it runs down your chin. Think about peeling an orange and getting a burst of citrus spray like a tiny, fragrant geyser. Remember the sweet corn from your grandparents' garden that was so fresh each kernel tasted like candy, and the first time you stared at a crosswise apple slice and saw a perfect star. Nutrition charts will never be as motivating as stars and geysers.

Besides, researchers will always come up with some new chemical in arugula or kumquats that will, if you believe the headlines, save the day. When this happens, you may want to put some arugula in your salad and have a few kumquats when they're in season, but there is no need to base your life or your meals on what somebody came up with in a lab somewhere. We're dealing here with the basics, the big picture, with nature and the foods nature gives us. This is food that furnishes you not only with nutrients we know about, but with those we don't.

Fresh, whole, unprocessed foods are also repositories of the subtle life force the yogis call *prana*, or life energy. The young are full of it. We're always telling toddlers and puppies to get down, calm down, slow down, and "Sit!" while we ourselves are drinking coffee and eating energy bars in hopes of getting back some of the exuberance they have in spades. We can get it more reliably from whole, unprocessed foods that nourish every cell, support the body's self-healing propensity, and don't bog us down with excess calories or artificial chemicals our cells can't understand.

Know this: aging in reverse is an alchemical exercise. You're attempting to get a message to the very cells that comprise your body that they can back up a little, and then age more slowly than they had been. This is going to take life force aplenty. You get it in food the way nature grew it, a diet that emphasizes fresh vegetables and fruits, nuts, seeds, beans, and grains that haven't been processed to pieces. Let meals brimming with life force give you more life.

REJUVENATE YOURSELF WITH ACTION: *As you choose your food today and in the days that follow, think about how much life force it's giving you. Is it attractive? Colorful? Fresh? Carefully prepared and artfully presented? You deserve nothing less.*

JANUARY 8

Sure Signs of the Superbly Groomed

You know the preschool song "Heads and Shoulders, Knees and Toes"? We can chime in today with "Hands and Eyebrows, Legs and Toes." These are the punctuation marks of your visual impression. You've probably received a letter or clipping and been distracted from its content by errant commas and wild exclamation marks. Peeling polish, untamed brows, legs with stubbly hairs showing, and feet in sore need of a pedicure are like that, too.

It doesn't take long or cost much to tend to such things. Even so, superb grooming is relatively rare, because you have to stay on top of it. If you do, you'll look fresher, prettier, younger—and you'll feel that way. This is how you get your money's worth from a pedicure in the middle of winter when you're in boots all day, bunny slippers at night, and nobody sees your toes. *You* know they're ravishing, and that's enough.

When you give yourself a manicure or smooth your feet with an exfoliating scrub, you're nurturing yourself in hands-on fashion. If you get your fingernails or eyebrows done professionally, you're investing in your personal well-being. So much money goes to mundane expenses—taxes, mortgage, utility bills, home and car repairs—that spending a little of it on yourself is a treat even before the nail tech puts lotion on your hands or feet and starts that delicious massage.

You can go to an elegant salon and pay a lot. These establishments do offer perks; one of my favorites is being called "Madam." Most of the time, though, I patronize the storefront places that offer manicures, pedicures, and waxing for a song. Beauty schools are another cut-rate option.

Think today about being superbly groomed. Can you get your basic upkeep on a schedule so you're always ready for the unexpected? This way you can run into anybody on the street and know you look fine, or pack your sandals for an impromptu weekend away because you'll know your toes are presentable. Do some writing in your journal about what's realistic for you: hands and eyebrows, legs and toes, as well as haircuts, color touch-ups, tooth-whitening, and wardrobe maintenance. When your grooming essentials are in order, your life will seem more orderly and you will more often feel your best.

REVITALIZE YOUR LIFE WITH WORDS: *I treat myself as someone priceless, down to the smallest detail.*

JANUARY 9

The Power of the Present

When you take control of your time, you take control of your life. You also lengthen your life, since you're more aware of living it. To gain this control and benefit from this awareness, you sometimes have to stand up to time and call its bluff. Time will intimidate you if you give it a chance. It will try to convince you that there isn't enough of it and that it's racing past you at warp speed. You won't win by arguing. Just say, "Thanks for the information. I'm still going to sit here with this novel or notebook or newspaper and savor every minute."

When you trust yourself to use your discretionary time in ways that suit you, you join those women who never seem to rush, yet who are invariably on time and not panting. These are the women who either have the time to talk when you call them, or let their machine pick up. You don't hear them complaining or gossiping or justifying themselves. They tend to age slowly because they ally themselves with that morsel of time that is not heading toward decline and decay. That fragment of forever is this moment. Although we're partial to moments that have passed and those yet to come, this moment is the only one we really get. When we recognize and cherish it instead of slighting it or riding roughshod over it on the way to one more noteworthy, we receive its gift.

In this moment, there is plenty of time. In this moment, you are precisely as you should be. In this moment, there is infinite potential. You get to live in this idyllic state when you refrain from worry and regret. Most of us adore worry and regret: they're so dramatic. Lamenting the dreadful thing that might happen or the awful thing that did is as good as watching a soap opera, and the characters are easier to keep track of. But worry and regret are proactive pro-agers. They're like mental free radicals out to rob you of youthfulness and years. When you stay in the now, you're not aging—unless you're staying in the now by lying in the sun smoking cigarettes.

REVITALIZE YOUR LIFE WITH WORDS: *I live in the certainty and safety of the present moment. There is plenty of time.*

JANUARY 10

The Bath as Metaphor

I used to think that if I read one more magazine piece telling me to take a candlelight bubble bath, I'd perish from terminal cliché. That was before I understood that a bath, when you see it right, isn't just a bath. It is rather a metaphor for renewal. Every time you bathe (or shower, for that matter), you start fresh. You make a clean break from all that has gone before. The bath separates you from the argument you had with a coworker and the crowd that crammed you in on the subway. You really can wash that man—or job or deadline or irritation—right out of your hair. The candles and the bubbles simply make a good thing better.

Sometimes you just want a quick shower; it does the job and helps you wake up in the morning. A soak in the tub, on the other hand, melts away the general tensions of the day and can induce the kind of relaxation that nudges back the sands of time. It's no surprise that this should be so pleasurable: when you started life floating in a warm, private sea, you'd never heard of laundry or bills or traffic. Bathing, when no one disturbs you and you've allowed enough time to do it right, takes you back there.

Don't pooh-pooh candlelight and background music the way I used to. If anyone has earned an upper-class bath, it's you. You can get all you need for such a bath inexpensively at the drugstore: a loofah for scrubbing your body, a pumice stone to do away with the rough spots on your feet, an inflatable bath pillow if your tub isn't comfy without one. Collect bath salts and bath oils, and ask for them as gifts. Earmark an unbreakable mug for the cooled lemon water or steamy herbal tea you'll drink as you luxuriate in your bath; and have some oil or lotion nearby for caressing your still-damp self when you emerge from it. You're worth drying off with fluffy, warm towels. If yours have seen better days, those January white sales are going on right now. A soft, roomy terrycloth robe is a luxury that's almost a necessity. Find them at lingerie shops and discount bed and bath stores.

Keep a few candles in your bathroom—mine are lined up on the radiator; they're instantly available and haven't melted yet—and find a safe place (away from the tub and basin) for a little CD player. You won't always light candles or play music, but when you want them, they'll be there. Besides, metaphoric bathing isn't all or nothing. You can light a couple of candles for even a quick shower. At least once a week, though, indulge yourself and go all the way.

REJUVENATE YOURSELF WITH ACTION: *Tonight take a bath that's worth writing home about—or at least writing about in your journal.*

JANUARY 11

The Four-Season Paradigm

You have most likely heard of the three-season paradigm, an old pagan concept that divides a woman's stay on earth into three stages: the maiden, the mother, and the crone. As the first baby-boomers were approaching middle age, this bit of arcana spread like wildfire. Croning parties became popular. When my friend Karen attended her first such fête, she thought it was a joke. Instead of bringing the honoree an earnest poem or something handcrafted in Guatemala as the other guests did, Karen performed a spoof of a Bob Dylan classic. "Everybody Must Get Croned" failed to wow the solemn assembly.

The maiden/mother/crone model was fine when women married at fifteen and few saw fifty. Now that a woman who reaches the half-century mark without heart disease or cancer can, according to statistical projections, expect to live to be over ninety, it's ludicrous to think there are millions of "crones" running around with half their lives left. Three stages aren't enough. We need four.

There is a precedent for this in the three-thousand-year-old health-care system of *Ayurveda*, "the science of long life." Ayurveda arose during India's Golden Age, a period of great wisdom and prosperity that predated the births of Buddha and Christ. The sages then studying human health ascertained that the normal life span was one hundred years, divisible into four sections or seasons of about twenty-five years each. The first was for growth and education, the second for having and raising families. During the third season, people were to contribute their gifts and talents to the larger world, and in the fourth devote themselves to spiritual study and meditative disciplines.

Since living to one hundred is a distinct possibility today, we can adopt this model again. Getting used to the world and learning how things are done here takes you up to age twenty-five. Settling in and going for what you want from life goes to fifty. In the third season, fifty to seventy-five, you can start or continue the work that will constitute your legacy. While we've been told that this is the time for slowing down, it is the age at which people are most likely to lead corporations and nations, and when many artists and writers produce their best work. In the four-season paradigm, middle age is earmarked for branching out and extending your influence as far as it can go.

After seventy-five come the wisdom years, rich in reflection and spirituality. If you're healthy and have your priorities in order, you can relish this time, filling the role of matriarch or wise woman ("crone" if you like, but only if you find the term endearing). This is when you're ideally suited to influence younger people and, while still chalking up delicious experiences on earth, being at ease with what's to come next. Mortality is a dismal subject to broach with the young, but when you talk to people in their eighties and nineties about leaving this body behind, they're usually quite matter-of-fact about it. They're able to see whatever lies beyond this life as simply the next phase, one that's natural and right.

When you entertain the notion that you're entitled to all four seasons, one hundred healthy years or something close to it, you unveil a remarkable new possibility. And you come to regard each season as equal in importance and equally capable of being the backdrop for fulfillment and joy.

REVITALIZE YOUR LIFE WITH WORDS: *All the seasons of the year are beautiful. So are all the seasons of my life.*

JANUARY 12

If There Is a Panacea, Exercise Is It

Exercise counteracts a host of the negative responses to growing older: increased fat and decreased bone, diminished strength, flabby arms and thighs, stiffness, impaired balance, varicose veins, and the slowed metabolism that can make it hard to keep your weight where you like it. And exercise, as you know, lessens your likelihood of having a heart attack or stroke, or developing osteoporosis, diabetes, and even some types of cancer. The term "health club" is well applied.

In addition, active people are happy people. When you're one of them, your moods are more even and you're less likely to succumb to depression. Just getting your muscles in motion releases tension. Beyond that, vigorous activity causes the body to produce a host of helpful hormones—noradrenaline and the eternally cheerful endorphin crew—that shift the way you process the data that comprise your world. In other words, if you saw the proverbial half-empty glass when you were sedentary, you're apt now to say that it was half-full all along.

If you haven't exercised in awhile, get your doctor's okay to start. It seems silly that you can stay on the sofa eating nachos without having medical approval but you're supposed to get it before doing something undeniably beneficial. This is because vigorous activity can exacerbate an undetected heart condition and you could end up dead. So be safe. And if you have arthritis or old injuries, your doctor can refer you to a physical therapist whose help can make the difference between your exercising for life or only until you strain or pull or tear something and give up.

Once you're cleared for action, proceed carefully. This is meant to be forever, like a diamond or a tattoo. We're being told now that for optimum fitness—i.e., getting seriously younger—we need to be doing aerobic activity thirty minutes six times a week (see March 16), weight training three times a week (April 26), and stretching before and after each workout (October 10). Still, if you walk or work in the garden or *simply move*, you're light years better off than someone whose primary exercise is clicking the remote control. This is because the greatest relative gains in fitness, health, and potential longevity come in that first grand leap from a prostrate lifestyle to an upright one.

Start where you are and have realistic expectations. Once you decide what's feasible for you, consider it a sacred commitment. That is, unless you're sick or injured or you have a personal or family emergency, you get to the track or the pool or your yoga class. If you should fall away, start back again as soon as you come to your senses. Don't berate yourself; just get moving again before you lose any more ground.

REVITALIZE YOUR LIFE WITH WORDS: *I love moving my body and feeling supple and strong.*

JANUARY 13

Mastering the Up-Spin

Politicians and PR people spin everything. The movie star who was "resting" may have been resting in rehab; the one who was "spending more time at home" might have been unable to get work. Such people hire professionals to find something positive in their situation and turn it into a press release. Our job is to find the positive in every situation and focus on that. What you focus on becomes more pronounced. When you zero in on the positive, that's what you see and that's where you live.

Practice positivism as life dishes up its specials of the day. For example:

- It's raining again:
  "Terrific—I wasn't in the mood to mow the lawn."

- There's not enough money for a summer trip:
  "Let's take a vacation at home. Then we won't need another one to recover."

- You didn't get the raise/promotion/job/prize/distinction/guy:
  "This one just wasn't mine to have; the next one has my name all over it."

- You did something you interpret as "stupid":
  "Welcome to the human race."

- You discover some sign of aging on your face or body:
  "I'm really something to have come this far."

You get the point. The more you do this, the more instinctive it becomes. At first, you may think that this much positivism is saccharine-sweet and not respectful of the realistic, fact-facing person that you are. So be it. We have the option of living in a world of hard, cold facts, or lush, evolving possibilities. It's no accident that "possibility" and "positive" share a root: the former depends on the latter for its growth and blossoming.

Play with this. People will not treat you less seriously because you refuse to share a worldview with the Grim Reaper. In fact, because negativism is so prevalent, other positive people will sense a kindred spirit and beat a path to your door. Good luck, coveted outcomes, and your share of happily-ever-aftering will come along, too. There is a spiritual law that states: "Like attracts like." Be a magnet for the best that life has to offer.

REVITALIZE YOUR LIFE WITH WORDS: *I live in a world of lush, evolving possibilities.*

A Warm Oil Massage in the Morning

If I were to put a little star by my favorite suggestions in this book, there would be one here. Warm oil self-massage, *abhyanga* in Sanskrit, was lauded in ancient Ayurvedic texts for its youth-promoting properties. Massage gets the life force moving. A head-to-toe massage with warm sesame oil (almond oil can substitute if you find sesame too thick) is also said to enhance immunity, stimulate the circulation of both blood and lymph, and balance the nervous and endocrine systems. I can tell you from experience that doing this with some regularity—at least two mornings a week; four or five is even better—makes me feel calmer, stronger, and better able to take the cold this time of year.

To do *abhyanga* for yourself, buy a bottle of sesame oil at the health food store (plain oil, not roasted) and a small plastic bottle with a lid. Put some of the oil in the plastic bottle and set it in a cup of very hot tap water to warm it. If you can, lie down and do some deep breathing while the oil is warming. When it's ready, pour a tablespoon or so on your head and put some energy into rubbing your head and scalp with the flats of your hands in rapid back-and-forth motions. Then work your way down your body, using more oil as necessary, to massage your temples, ears, face, neck and so on. Use clockwise circular motions around your breasts, abdomen, hips, and joints; and sweeping up-and-down movements on your arms and legs. Pay extra attention to your feet, particularly the soles.

You can spend ten or fifteen minutes at this or do a reasonable job in less than five. It's nice to rest for a little while afterwards (I like to do *abhyanga*, then meditate, then shower), but if time is short and you need to massage in a jiffy and shower right away, you'll still reap surprising benefits. Make this work in your life: even though the head and feet are believed to be the prime areas on which to concentrate, you're welcome to skip your head on days you don't want to wash your hair. Of course, be careful each time you do this since oil is slippery: a bath mat and rubber thongs will come in handy. Every time you perform *abhyanga*, send some gratitude and approval to each body part you massage. They are all good because they are all part of you, and you are part of the Divine.

REJUVENATE YOURSELF WITH ACTION: *Put in your day-planner for one day this week: "Go to health food store and buy sesame oil." Start* abhyanga *the very next morning, and put it in your schedule at least two mornings a week.*

Play Day!

You've been doing a lot for the past two weeks. You've earned a play day. Today, and on the play days that follow on the fifteenth and thirtieth of each month, either take the day off and actually play, or play catch-up by going back to a reading you missed or back over one that you think deserves more attention.

A Rich Inner Life

There is a part of you that is eternal. In fact, *you* are eternal; there are just parts of you that aren't. (Technically, since matter cannot be destroyed, even your parts are eternal. They're just not eternally yours.) If it is difficult for you to entertain the idea that you are not simply a body and brain but the essence that invited your body and brain into being, indulge me here. Allow, just for today, that there might be truth to the notion that you are not an aging body that may have a spirit somewhere, but you are instead an immortal spirit that, for now, occupies a physical body.

This concept helps keep you young because it plugs you in to an endless source of vitality, insight, hope, and promise. Your stress decreases because you understand that what you see is not what you get, at least not nearly all of it. It diminishes discouragement because you come to understand that your work and your being have influence far beyond what you had realized. Besides, you manifest what you identify with. That is, you look and feel the way you think you're supposed to. If you see your true self as the ageless essence that exemplifies and motivates you, you'll age more slowly than someone who takes crow's feet or a crêpey chin at face value.

Women with rich inner lives often retain an uncanny youthfulness, even in advanced age. It's as if they have some delicious secret. They do: they're not old. Iris was one of these women. She never appeared tired, and there was a spark in her eyes that could light up a room. We worked together at semi-volunteer library jobs that only someone under twenty-five (like me) or over seventy-five (like her) would consider. When I complained about a headache or a rude customer or an improperly shelved book, she would smile brightly and say, "The darling physical plane!" In other words: "This is earth, kid. It ain't gonna be perfect."

Iris was a marathon meditator. Other than the day she was in labor with her son, she told me, she hadn't missed a morning in fifty-seven years. She had so immersed herself in great literature that she wasn't just a helpful library aide; she was a fount of wisdom. And she didn't separate her interior pursuits from her external life. She made it her business to spread joy. Iris died young at ninety-six. I don't think she had far to go, since her spiritual life and her daily life were so seamlessly joined.

Your views about spirituality, religion, and the way you see this world and what's beyond it are intensely personal. It's in cultivating an inner life, one that speaks to you and works for you, that you bring some heavenly bliss to this darling physical plane. Then more about life makes sense, and the parts that seem to make no sense are easier to put up with. Your inner life is your anchor, your balance point. You might come to it from the religion of your childhood, from a teaching you discovered later, or from that deep connecting place inside you where there are no names or books or -isms, but where you know you're home. Whatever its configuration, your inner life belongs to you, and it is there to sustain you.

REVITALIZE YOUR LIFE WITH WORDS: *I am an eternal spiritual being living a remarkable physical life.*

The Anatomy of Chic

At their best, clothes tell the world who you are. They show your cleverness in a visual way, even if you can't draw or paint or do any craft yet invented. My mother dressed beautifully when I was a little girl, and Dede, the surrogate grandmother who helped raise me, spoke with near reverence of Chanel and Schiaparelli. Perhaps because one of my first two style mentors was sixty by the time I could do up my own buttons, I never thought that getting older would inhibit my fashionable proclivities. But—one more shocker of this age in the middle—I found myself too old for hip, too young for frumpy, and, for the first time in my life, perplexed about how to dress. I fell into the habit of wearing a lot of black and waiting for inspiration.

That inspiration came when I realized that everyone is too young for frumpy, but that *chic* lies midway between that sorry state and the hipness that belongs to youth. Okay, not quite midway: it's a little closer to hip, but not so close that age affects it one iota. If reaching a certain age didn't cause fashion icons like Jacqueline Onassis and Princess Grace to hide in perpetual mourning or resort to polyester pants and blouses with bad prints, we don't have to either. Just because you're bypassing the skimpy, the see-through, and the skintight doesn't mean that shopping and dressing can't be as much fun as they were when you had your first job and spent more on clothes than rent. It's a matter of making dressing a hobby, a game. Chic is the prize you get for winning.

You win by wearing clothes that fit, flatter you, and are kept in good repair. Clothes like these suit you so well that when you wear them, your personality takes over and the clothes become secondary. Chic is less a matter of the latest thing than taking a touch of what's new—a shirt or a scarf in this season's color, maybe—and incorporating that with the tried and true. Tiny touches can make a big difference: a slit up the side of a long skirt, for instance. Or ripping out the shoulder pads that make an otherwise becoming jacket look like something you borrowed from an NFL lineman. Or getting a hemline to just the right spot: grazing the ankle, or respectably above the knee. If you have great legs, you can carry off something shorter, but probably not so short that the word "mini" comes to mind.

Few clothes in any price range are chic on their own. Chic is more often a combination of the garment and the wearer: its cut and your shape, its color and your coloring, its feel and your lifestyle. Then chic ceases to be the purview of fashion stylists and photo shoots and becomes instead a matter of relationship. You find yourself a more discerning shopper. The process becomes more about mergers and less about acquisitions.

REJUVENATE YOURSELF WITH ACTION: *Take a look at the clothes you own. What do the garments that you really like have in common? Are your favorites in bright colors or subtle tones? Is their character more conservative or flamboyant? Are these clothes cut to show off your figure or offer some camouflage? The commonalities you discover will clue you in on your personal style, the element of chic residing right now in your own closet.*

JANUARY 18

The Best-Laid Plans

One reason midlife disappointment is all too common a syndrome is that we sometimes reach the point of having our plans play out, and we don't like what we see. Someone may have liberally (to her thinking) given her children lifestyle choices A, B, and C, only to find that as adults they've chosen D, "none of the above." Someone else may have done everything right: worked hard on her job and in her marriage, saved regularly for a blissful retirement, and then found herself widowed, or caring for a partner with a debilitating disease.

Such things happen because life on earth is not a sure thing. We can do our best, hedge our bets, put unassailable actions behind well-conceived plans, and still find ourselves the exception to the rule. What do you do in a case like that? First, feel what it feels like—probably rotten. Sit with the feelings. Write about them. Talk about them. But don't reach for them when they start to subside. They're meant to go, and you're meant to go forward.

Going forward means acquiring the kind of flexibility that can make something lovely out of Plan B. It's seeing the big picture, that you're a soul on a path, rather than the little picture of you as a woman alone, or one whose retirement savings half vanished at the whim of the stock market. It's making beauty out of the available ingredients, the way you can make a nourishing soup out of last night's leftovers plus an onion and a few potatoes.

And it's the stalwart commitment to continue making plans and doing the work to fulfill them. If you make them, they *might* not turn out. If you don't, they *will* not. Give yourself the best odds for the best life. Work with what you've got—that onion and those potatoes—and concoct something warm and comforting and delicious.

REVITALIZE YOUR LIFE WITH WORDS: *If one plan is derailed, I have a dozen to take its place.*

JANUARY 19

Move Like a Dancer, Stand Like a Queen

If I told you that you could instantly appear ten pounds thinner, look ten years younger, and make your off-the-rack outfit pass for couture, you'd probably mistake me for an infomercial. It is possible, though, and without three easy payments. The secret is in your carriage, the way you hold your body and move it through the world.

Exquisite posture is so unusual that glimpsing it can be startling—*good* startling, the way spring's first blooming magnolia can catch you off guard. Women who carry vessels of water on their heads have it, but I don't know any of those. Dancers have it (retired dancers, too); soldiers, although they're at the stiff end of straight; and those actors trained to use their bodies as fine instruments.

Slouching compresses internal organs, impedes breathing fully, and compromises the integrity of the spine. Slouchers look like slackers, even if they're nothing of the sort. Conversely, standing straight and moving with grace tell the world you're somebody. You look confident whether you are or not. Even spiritually, the way you hold your body matters. The yogis contend that spiritual energy is meant to travel up your spine, enlivening subtle energy centers along the way. Poor posture may interfere with your enlightenment as well as with your alignment.

You can't force yourself to "stand up straight" or "hold your shoulders back." If that were effective, all the times our mothers told us to do it would have worked. You can, however, notice several times a day the way you're holding your body. Notice it right now, in fact. How are you sitting? Is your stomach distended? Are your shoulders level? Are you closer to straight or closer to sprawled? This isn't a judgment call; it's an awareness call. If you don't like what you discover, you can start to change it. In addition, check your mood. Sometimes poor posture and an indifferent gait are indicative of depression or despair, states not to be ignored.

Throughout the day, give yourself the frequent mental message to stand tall. Then do it by lifting from your solar plexus, the area just above your navel. This not only elevates your overall carriage, it lifts your midriff up from your abdomen and slims your waist. One cause of the thickening there that most of us experience at midlife is that we've lost a little of the cushioning between our vertebrae. As a result the skin around our waist and the fat beneath it compress, resulting in love handles. (Lust handles, unfortunately, they are not.)

Give your kinesthetic memory, the way your muscles have learned to be, time to reprogram itself. Decades of kinesthetic memory won't go away overnight. Keep at it. One of these days, somebody might surprise you and ask, "Are you a dancer?" As far as I'm concerned, you can answer however you like.

REVITALIZE YOUR LIFE WITH WORDS: *I stand tall and move gracefully. I am comfortable with my body and with my place in the world.*

JANUARY 20

Twelve Steps to Happy Skin

Your skin can show your age or deny it. So that it will continue to tell the story you want, keep it happy:

STEP 1: *Cleanse your face gently twice a day.* Cleanse thoroughly at bedtime and lightly in the morning, but even then you need more than a splash of water to do away with last night's product residue and eight hours of sloughed-off cells.

STEP 2. *Feed your skin moisture.* Your skin loves humidity and a cream or lotion that holds moisture in. For a double-whammy of the wet stuff, spritz with water from a spray can and then moisturize.

STEP 3. *Drink lots of water.* This is a way to moisturize from the inside.

STEP 4. *Don't see the light of day without sun-block* (more on May 2).

STEP 5. *Exfoliate once a week.* If your skin is sensitive, using a washcloth with your cleanser may be all the exfoliation you need. Otherwise, choose from a variety of grainy scrubs to ring out the old cells and bring on the new.

STEP 6. *Get plenty of sleep.* Skin positively withers when you're tired. Lack of sleep invites dark circles, blotchy patches, and a pallor that can make you look unwell.

STEP 7. *Do not smoke.* Stopping, if this applies to you, is more to save your life than to save your skin. Still, the sooner you quit, the sooner you'll stop aging your face.

STEP 8. *If you drink, do so in moderation.*

STEP 9. *Use the anti-aging products you need, not every one that comes along.* There are many good products on the market: find a line you have an affinity for and give it a chance to work.

STEP 10. *Eat a balanced diet you're proud of, one with lots of fruits and vegetables.* And do this every day, not just good days.

STEP 11. *Take skin-supporting supplements.* Among the nutrients skin appreciates are the antioxidant vitamins A, C, and E, biotin (a B-complex vitamin), sulphur (in a supplement called MSM), and the mineral silica (which you can find in the herb horsetail rush).

STEP 12. *Do not pull, stretch, tug, or terrify your face.* Your skin is here to protect you, but it isn't armor. Be gentle.

REJUVENATE YOURSELF WITH ACTION: *Choose one of these steps— the one you need most—and practice it until it becomes second nature.*

JANUARY 21

Curiouser and Curiouser

When centenarians are asked their longevity secrets, curiosity invariably comes up. People who are interested in the world, in people, ideas, inventions, trends, and what's around the next corner age more slowly, all other things being equal, than the next person. It makes sense: they need to be here, and in full possession of their faculties, to be in on what's coming up.

If any disinterest tries to sneak into your attitude, eradicate it straightaway. Disinterest can expand, growing from a minor pest to a full-fledged plague. Watch for lines like, "I don't really care," or "I'm not much interested anymore." If you live long enough, you'll have done a lot of things. You either have to find new areas to investigate or experience the old ones over again from a fresh vantage point. It doesn't matter, for example, how many times you've gone skiing in Vermont or watched *The Wizard of Oz*. This is a whole new year. You can do these things in a whole new way.

Guard against a blasé attitude; it may seem sophisticated, but in this case your choice is between aged and sophisticated or youthful and curious. Ask questions: What is this? Where does it come from? How does it work? See if you can draw people out about their life, their childhood, their work, their hobbies. Read historic markers on the highway, the descriptions next to the paintings at the art museum, and every actor's bio in the playbill. Subscribe to publications you're interested in and, when you're at the doctor's office or the library, read publications you didn't know you were interested in. Curiosity is an equal-opportunity character trait; it goes outward in all directions and helps you age in one direction: younger.

REVITALIZE YOUR LIFE WITH WORDS: *I find a million things fascinating, and I'm eager to explore them all.*

JANUARY 22

Starting with the Outside

I believe in changing ourselves from the inside. As the author of a book about losing weight that way called *Fit from Within*, and one about inner beauty called *Lit from Within*, I am heavily invested in this concept. Nevertheless, there are times when it is appropriate to approach the outside first—to change your style, your hair, or your makeup, and allow that to bring your mood up a few notches.

This outside-in kind of transformation is called for when inner change seems too ill-defined or freeform, too "out there" when you're looking for a lift in the rock-solid here and now. At times like these, try bright red polish on your nails or a pair of new shoes (heck, make them red, too). The change you're working for on the heart-and-soul level is in process; in the meantime, you've got the nails and the shoes.

Appearance can be a slippery slope. We don't want to overemphasize it, especially since we live in a culture that overemphasizes it as a matter of course. Doing something lovely for the face or body, however, is a readily available means of elevating the spirit. It's not a sellout: cats groom and birds preen and kindergartners get a kick out of shiny new Mary Janes. There can be serious therapeutic value in a hat or a lipstick or a facial. This isn't "buying happiness," it's just buying a little time.

REJUVENATE YOURSELF WITH ACTION: *Do something nice for your outer self today. You might choose an accessory you seldom wear, style your hair in a different way, or treat yourself to that piece of clothing Santa forgot to bring.*

JANUARY 23

Supplementary Suggestions

Reams of research suggest that certain nutritional supplements can contribute to longevity and delay signs of aging. Most people do not eat optimal diets, and there is growing concern that even those who do are being nutritionally shortchanged. Soil depletion has rendered food less nutritious than it used to be, and the premature harvesting of crops makes the situation worse. A tomato, for example, draws most of its minerals from the soil in the last four hours to thirty minutes of ripening. Few stay on the vine anywhere near that long.

By age fifty, it's more difficult for a body to absorb certain nutrients, so you may need extra after that time just to get enough. It is also believed that many nutrients, when taken in excess of the suggested dietary requirements, have preventive and therapeutic applications. Taking certain vitamins, minerals, amino acids, and other naturally occurring substances appears to eradicate free radicals, the unstable compounds that damage healthy cells, undermine their well-being, and make us old before our time.

The evidence suggests that ingesting antioxidants can intercept enough free radicals to effectively circumvent their destructive rampage. You can get antioxidants in foods, notably anything dark green (broccoli, kale, spinach) or yellow (yams, carrots, pumpkin, citrus fruits, apricots), and you can take them as supplements. If you choose to do the latter, you can randomly swallow dozens of pills a day—I did that for awhile, until my gag reflex let me know I'd strayed from the middle path—or stick with a few well-documented, pro-longevity nutrients in conservative amounts. The literature supports a general recommendation for taking a high-quality multivitamin, plus extra vitamin C, vitamin E, and folic acid, and perhaps additional antioxidants such as coenzyme Q-10 and selenium. Many people might do well to include chromium, vitamin B_{12}, zinc, a calcium-magnesium combination, and/or a supplementary form of essential fatty acids. We'll explore all these individually, starting with a look at multivitamins on February 24.

For now, give supplements some thought, and maybe do a little research. If you're under a doctor's care, let him or her know what you plan to take. Never let supplements, helpful as they are, lull you into thinking that you can get by for long with sloppy food choices. There are nutrients in natural foods that haven't even been isolated yet. Eating well and taking supplements are supposed to work together to help you grow younger and live longer. Do both and glean double the dividends.

REVITALIZE YOUR LIFE WITH WORDS: *I support my health in every possible way. The nutritional supplements I take are helping me grow younger.*

JANUARY 24

Construct a Collage of Your Hopes and Dreams

One secret of eternal youth is this: dreams and decline are opposites; you can choose to grow toward one or the other. Constructing a collage of your hopes and dreams renders them real and solid. The visual image forms the template. All that's left is filling it in.

You're familiar with this process if you've ever done "treasure-mapping," making a collage of what you want to come into your life. The collage I suggest you make is not so much representative of material things you might like to acquire as the life you want to live and the person you want to become. Leaf through magazines for words and images that reflect who you are, what you aspire to, qualities to further develop, ideals that move you, goals you wish to reach, and dreams you long to see take shape. Seemingly impossible dreams are as valid here as the other ones. Cut out pictures and phrases that speak to you in some way. You'll choose some for their literal meaning, others as symbols. Clip everything that catches your eye; it's fine to have more cutouts than you'll use.

Store your clippings in a box, a manila envelope, or a file folder to keep them from getting dog-eared. When you have good-sized stack of them, purchase a glue stick and a blank piece of posterboard, one of the big ones, in white or some other color. Then set aside an afternoon or evening for the time-honored joys of the literal "cut and paste."

You can cover the entire posterboard, or just arrange the images and phrases that appeal to you and leave blank space around them. When they're where you want them, glue them down and admire your work. Then hang your poster somewhere that you'll see it daily and no critical eye will see it ever. Unfulfilled dreams are tender things, like seedlings doing their best to sprout. These dreams deserve to be undisturbed by anyone but the gardener, and uncriticized by anyone at all.

Study your collage for a minute or two every day for at least six months (or until so much of what's there has been fulfilled that it's time to retire this collage and make a new one). When you look at it, mentally caress every quality or aspiration depicted there. Express gratitude for each one already in your life, in full or in part, and for those yet to appear. Do your best to avoid second-guessing: "I may get the trip to Portugal, but I bet I'll never lose the twenty pounds." Instead, trust that every item on this map of your destiny is in the hands of beneficent forces with your genuine best interest at heart.

REJUVENATE YOURSELF WITH ACTION: *Construct a collage of your hopes and dreams. Start today to cut out magazine clippings— words and pictures that can help you build your future. Within two weeks, have your collage finished and hung so you can spend some moments with it every day.*

Your Crowning Glory and How It's Cut

My father held a traditionalist old country viewpoint that girls and women were supposed to have long hair, and when I was living at home I was not allowed to cut mine. I devised all sorts of sneaky ways to have dominion over my hair (and my dad), like cutting it an inch at a time so he wouldn't notice. Having lived through hair oppression, I certainly don't want to tell you what to do with yours. Take what's here as general information, to apply as you wish.

Hair stuck in a decade is pro-aging. I once worked with a woman named Jessie whose hair (and clothes and makeup, for that matter) were twenty years out of date. She didn't use vintage touches; she came to work every day in costume and didn't even realize it. Jessie was the extreme, granted, but if you have the identical haircut now that you had five years ago, it may be time for a change. It doesn't have to be extreme—there is something to be said for having a trademark look—but making even slight variations can keep you in step with the times.

A rule of thumb is that most mature women shouldn't have long hair. It can look unkempt and too casual, and overpower the face, drawing its features downward. For women whose hair is thinner than it once was, the weight of too-long hair calls attention to the loss of volume. But like most rules, this one has a great many exceptions and you may well be one of them. Linda, in her late forties, has the most spectacular long red tresses that look lush and healthy and that match her lifestyle as a clothing designer and fashion stylist. If your long hair defines you, gets you compliments, and sets you apart from the rule-followers, revel in it as Linda does. If it doesn't, lighten your life by shortening your hair.

Think today about your next haircut, whether a mere trim or a major redo. Are you so pleased with the cut you have now that you'll be happy keeping it awhile, or are you considering something new? Are you thrilled with your hair-cutter? So-so is okay for maintaining the status quo; aging in reverse calls for having one who's thrilling (April 5). In the meantime, leaf through some magazines and style books and see if a change is in your future. A well-executed haircut that suits your face can bring out your best features and update your overall look. Wind, humidity, and "sleeping wrong" are no match for a super cut. If you don't have one now, get one as soon as you can.

Your hair should be a pleasure, not a problem. Keep a spirit of play around it. It's a small thing, but all the best stuff starts small.

REVITALIZE YOUR LIFE WITH WORDS: *I always have good hair days.*

JANUARY 26

Bounce Back

Resiliency is a requisite of youth, for rubber balls and human beings. The quicker you can bounce back from a setback, the younger you are, regardless of your chronological age. Whenever you experience a shock, a loss, a disappointment, or an illness, give healing the time it requires, but no more than that. You need to bounce back.

It can be tempting to prolong certain agonies. There is the sympathy vote to start with, and if you haven't felt well or you've been through a difficult period, you certainly can't be expected to work full days or do your own laundry. But bouncing back as soon as you're reasonably able means getting back into the stream of life. This is where the opportunity is. This is where everything is happening. This is where the bulk of answered prayers and fulfilled dreams and realized goals hang out. You have to be there to claim yours.

Bouncing back can seem formidable when you've reached a certain age and you've done as much bouncing as should be expected of anyone. You're tired. You've paid your dues. I know the feeling. Sometimes I think (and sometimes I whine), "Why is this happening? Why do I have to go through this again? Why is what I want taking so long?" If instead of questioning the way things are, I set my sights on bouncing back, the whiny whys fade away. Then I feel the spirit of my dad, a prizefighter in his youth, reminding me that you can either get up and stand in the center of the ring, or be down for the count.

REVITALIZE YOUR LIFE WITH WORDS: *I bounce back as well as if I were made of India rubber.*

Let the Little Things Go

The real trials of life, the ones we can't avoid and have to deal with, can be hard enough on the body, the repository of the aftereffects of mental and emotional turmoil. When we respond to petty annoyances as if they were real trials, our physical selves don't know the difference. A chronic resentment toward a relative or a neighbor or your mobile phone company can be as aging as a chronic illness. We hear of people whose faces are "lined with care," whose bodies are "bent with worry," or who are simply "old before their time." Some of them have had very difficult lives; others have had somewhat difficult lives—in other words, they've had lives—but they've treated every slight, oversight, insult, and irritation as a traumatic experience.

Trauma drama—a lot of folks love it. It keeps life interesting. It also keeps the blood pressure up, the adrenal glands on nonstop sentry duty, and the body in a constant state of anxiety. Anxiety is aging. We may not get a lot of say about our big-time troubles, but the little things, the annoyances and aggravations that crop up every day, we can either make short work of or ignore entirely. This is no small task, but it is necessary. When you feel yourself getting irritated, think "Perspective!" or, as the sign on my friend Tess's desk asks, "How Important Is It?" Value serenity more and winning less. After all, being right is paltry compensation for being miserable. When something comes up today, try to shrug it off or laugh it off. Make it a game, an experiment. See how pleasant it feels to choose peace over chaos.

If your feelings are hurt, talk things over with someone who will listen; then let it go. If someone is doing something stupid that affects your day, work around it as best you can; then let that go. If you got to the interview with a button missing on your jacket, and you uttered two malapropisms, made one grammatical error, and executed a glaring faux pas, leave there and get yourself hugged, listened to, and taken out for dinner. Then let the whole thing go. Your youthfulness is at stake here. Don't risk it to some vexation that will soon be history.

REVITALIZE YOUR LIFE WITH WORDS: *I see the difference between major issues and minor irritations. I automatically let the little things go.*

Hot Water and Lemon

We know about waking up to smell the coffee, but waking up to a shot of hot water and lemon is the stay-young secret of many an ageless beauty. Join them in making your first drink of the day a mug of hot water with the juice of half a lemon (if you enjoy tart flavors), or one-quarter if half makes it too puckery for you. A drizzle of honey or pure maple syrup is allowed, but be sure it's a drizzle, not a dollop. Should you find yourself fresh out of fresh lemons, use a squeeze of the lemon juice you can buy frozen and keep refrigerated. It has no additives and will fill in nicely until you get to the produce market.

An A.M. lemon drink is a gentle wake-up call, since the flavor and scent of lemon revitalize and energize the entire system. Women who swear by this attest that, done long enough, lemon water in the morning keeps things working well in the elimination department without the need to resort to laxatives. Lemon water is also slightly diuretic, to give a cleansing start to the day. Some women report that their skin is less prone to blotches and breakouts when they're consistent about this morning ritual. In addition, the lemon's acidic flavor is an appetite balancer. If you're ravenous when you wake up, that's toned down; if you have no interest in breakfast, you'll get interested.

After your lemon drink, hold off on eating until you've showered, meditated, and dressed. Then you'll be ready to enjoy a simple, nourishing meal, digest it well, and go out and take on the world, or at least that part of it that means the world to you.

REJUVENATE YOURSELF WITH ACTION: *Drink hot water with lemon every morning this week. If it's a habit that sticks, all the better.*

At Peace with the 'Pause

Menopause may be well in your future, or perhaps it happened years ago and you're comfortably on the other side. If it is looming large in your life right now, however, coming to grips with it is essential. Life is a parade of changes unfolding through every day we live. Only one of these, however, earns the moniker *the* change. Whether it happens naturally at midlife or abruptly at some earlier point with a total hysterectomy, we are supposed to understand it and learn what it has to teach us.

Hormonal fluctuations start years before menopause itself, which can be virtually without symptoms, or present you with hot flashes, cold sweats, sleeplessness, forgetfulness, fatigue, vaginal dryness, and as much libido as the average rock. (I wondered why something so natural should be so difficult until I remembered that childbirth was no picnic either.)

Most of us come to menopause having been through quite a bit. We (as a societal whole) took birth control pills, had kids in our thirties and forties, and raised them in our forties and fifties, half the time alone. Accustomed to chronic physical and emotional stress, we've lived on adrenaline (which drops in midlife). Even good stress—trips and promotions and getting the guy—goes through hormones like a teenaged boy goes through groceries. Back when fifty was old, a woman this age could rest when she was tired. Now we're more likely to have to gulp another coffee and go out on another sales call.

Ours is also the first generation to have grown up on processed foods. Our great-grandmothers ate life-giving food, grown in soil rich in minerals and populated with creepy-crawlies that aerated the land while they were living and fed it nutrients after they died. Although Great-grandma might have raised thirteen children in a house with no plumbing, she was not subjected to chlorinated hydrocarbons all her life. Found in plastics, some tampons, and over-whelmingly in the pesticides (and many herbicides) used on our fruits and vegetables, and concentrated at high levels in healthy-sounding foods like milk and chicken breast, chlorinated hydrocarbons are xenoestrogens (i.e., "foreigner" or "stranger" estrogens). Acting like estrogen in the body, they attach to the receptors designed for estrogen, but they're dangerous imposters and potent carcinogens. When natural estrogen production dwindles, those receptors are particularly vulnerable to inviting in a phony.

Knowing all this, it's a wonder anyone has an uncomplicated menopause. For some women, regularly including soy in the diet is enough to ease the transition. Evening primrose oil may help balance hormones at this time, because of its high gamma-linolenic acid (GLA) content. According to clinical nutritionist and registered pharmacist Lisa Everett, my menopause mentor, there also seems to be a basic prescription for menopause:

- Exercise every day.

- Eat vegetables, fruits, soy foods and other legumes, low-fat dairy products, and fish.

- Go easy on refined foods of all sorts, especially sweets.

- Confine oil consumption to moderate amounts of flax, olive, and canola oils.

It's a familiar message in one more guise.

Certainly conventional hormone replacement therapy alleviates symptoms, but studies suggest a link between it and an increased risk of breast cancer, heart disease, and dementia. Curiously, until not long ago, hormone replacement had been shown to protect against these very conditions. I personally feel comfortable with *natural* (or *bio-identical*) hormone replacement therapy. Bio-identical hormones come from plant sources and cannot be patented. A medical doctor prescribes them based on the levels of hormones in a patient's blood; then they're formulated in the prescribed dosage by a compounding pharmacist. There is no evidence at this time that use of bio-identical hormones increases risk of breast cancer or any other malady, but also no scientifically validated evidence that it doesn't.

In the end, you have to educate yourself, consult with professionals you trust, and make your own decisions. These are major decisions and this is a major transition. Getting through menopause is like swimming across the English Channel or climbing Mount Everest or flying solo around the world. You aren't the first woman to have done it, but that makes it no less monumental an achievement.

REVITALIZE YOUR LIFE WITH WORDS: *Every stage of my life is the right one, including the stage I'm in.*

Play Day!

Your Mission, Should You Choose to Accept It . . .

In a patriarchal culture, mature women threaten the status quo. We think for ourselves. We don't believe everything we're told. We realize that consumerism is not the key to happiness and we have the audacity to say so. We like the truth and we're willing to sort through a litany of lies to get to it.

As a woman in this age group (or approaching it), your mission, should you choose to accept it, is to take on the mantle of the valiant, a vocal commitment to fairness and justice, and an unwillingness to back down. This has been the role of older women from time immemorial, even when "older" was thirty-five. It hasn't been easy. You studied in school about the burning times, centuries during which failing to toe the line could get you burned as a witch. The vast majority of "witches" were older women, along with some outspoken younger ones and some gentlemen too gentle for the taste of the times.

These days standing up for your values won't lead to being burned at the stake, although it could get you gossiped about at the country club. Do it anyway. Our planet is in worse shape than our collective arteries. The root reason for a book like this is not so that more of us can stump the age-guesser at the carnival. It is rather to acknowledge that we are alive at a unique time in history. The average woman will live one-third of her life after menopause. Much of that third will be after her children are grown, and quite a bit of it will be after she retires. This is an unprecedented amount of time and womanpower, and it gives us a legitimate opportunity to change the world.

All good people want to leave this place better than they found it, and most do that by raising honorable children or planting healthy trees or leaving a bequest to charity. This is noble and admirable, but we have a chance to do even more, and do it on a global scale. Your mission, should you choose to accept it, entails the following:

- *Take superb care of yourself.* Keep yourself in fighting trim like a soldier or an athlete, because changing a world takes stamina.

- *Formulate a viable spiritual life.* It needn't be religious; in fact, given the penchant some people have for turning religion into mischief, we could use some non-religious spiritual people balancing things out. However your spirituality presents itself, you need it, because you'll have to make decisions based on more than ego and opinion.

- *Take a stand.* Maybe you'll speak for groups even if that scares you silly. Maybe you'll take your case to people in power, or be the voice for those who don't have one.

I can't know your specific path, but I do know it's there for you—should you choose to accept it.

REVITALIZE YOUR LIFE WITH WORDS: *I have a role to play that is bigger than I am. I have a mission, and I choose to accept it.*

February

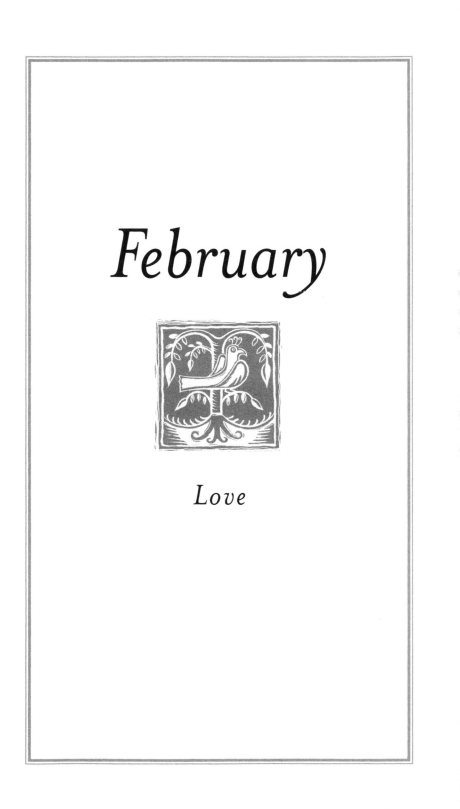

Love

Love Is What You're Made Of

As January ends and February starts, everything is still possible. We're going to shift our keynote this month, however, from *possibility* to *love*. Even though this is the month of Valentine's Day, we needn't confine ourselves to the hearts-and-flowers kind of love, exquisite though it can be. Beyond romance, although at times encompassing it, we find love as a power, healing and renewing. In its grandest expression, love is divine, even a synonym for God. Throughout the ages, mystics, people who have experienced what they describe as "pure being," have also taught that love is what we're made of, and love doesn't get old.

To that end, I suggest that you think from time to time over the next four weeks about how you cannot just *feel* love but *be* love. As you go out into the world each day, toy with the notion that, at the root of everything else you are, you are love in expression. Keeping that in mind, watch how your day goes. Notice how many tiny chances come your way to make another person's life easier. See how creative you can get at expressing love to all sorts of people in all sorts of ways. And enjoy being so filled with love that loving yourself is easier than it's ever been.

REVITALIZE YOUR LIFE WITH WORDS: *I was created by Love, from love, to express love.*

Mixed Company

Your closest friends are likely to be close to you in age, because going through similar experiences around the same time creates a mutuality that strengthens your connection. Even so, life is richer in mixed company, with friends of all ages. Older ones can be advisers and role models, letting you in on their wisdom and showing you how to navigate the path ahead. Younger ones can give you a fresh perspective and help keep you current. When they see you as a peer, you can see yourself that way, too.

The greatest gift of mixed company, I think, is its showing the common bond of humanity that overrides age. We all want love and understanding, good health and good times, and feelings of security and usefulness. The specifics are different for someone thirty and someone eighty, but the basics are the same. When you have friends who span generations, your sense of the world becomes bigger and broader because you're getting a vicarious extension of your own life span. When you get people of different age-groups together, it's like having historians and futurists making engrossing conversation around your table.

To make cross-generational friends, follow up on your cross-generational interests. Take classes and join organizations. Offer your expertise to younger women and your ear to older ones. Appreciate them all. They are to your life like colors to a canvas, brilliant and beautiful. The absence of any one of them would diminish the painting.

REJUVENATE YOURSELF WITH ACTION: *Resolve to end any generational segregation in your life. Make calls today to a friend or relative at least ten years younger and to another at least ten years older. Make plans with one or both of them to get together for a good long talk.*

FEBRUARY 3

Speak Softly and Carry a Big Commitment

All of us hold strong views about something, often many things, and as we mature we may feel less pressure to hide our views. But there is a fine line between being passionate and being a bully. When you believe in something, it should enrich your life so that even people who espouse disparate beliefs admire you for being such a fine example of yours. When you hold a conviction and can express it without shaming or belittling those who hold a different one, or who simply never thought about yours before, you speak volumes for your cause and for yourself. When people have to press you to learn your views, you're a far more convincing proponent of them than one who forces those same views on the disinterested. When you speak softly—not out of shyness or insecurity, but out of confidence and focus—people have to quiet themselves and focus on what you're saying; the ranters they tune out.

The other side of speaking softly is choosing when to speak at all. I love something Bill W., the cofounder of Alcoholics Anonymous, wrote: "Nothing pays off like restraint of tongue and pen." As one who is prone to speak first and regret shortly thereafter, I admire people who by nature weigh their words and wait until a propitious moment to make a comment or elaborate on one. A worthwhile exercise is to hold on to something you intend to say and just keep it yours for awhile. Try this when you're dying to blurt something out. I guarantee you won't die. Or if you're halfway through telling a story or relating a thought and it's interrupted by a zealous waiter or a ringing phone, just let it go when the conversation resumes. Unless someone asks you to finish, check your eagerness to restart the conversation with, "As I was saying. . . ." This is how you can increase your humility *and* your confidence   an unbeatable combination.

Because words can't be recalled like a defective product, don't send them out until you're sure you want them on the market with your name on them. When in doubt, strategic silence is a wise choice.

REJUVENATE YOURSELF WITH ACTION: *Work today with well-placed silence and fully audible but (usually) softly spoken words. See if you find yourself better heard.*

FEBRUARY 4

The Weather Is Permitting

We've all received invitations that included the caveat "weather permitting." Obviously, you can't ski when there's no snow, and if there's a thunderstorm, the garden wedding will take place somewhere other than the garden. For daily life, however, we need to go past thinking in terms of "weather permitting" to "the weather *is* permitting." Certainly exercise good sense when a dangerous weather condition looms. Otherwise, go out. Routinely staying home because of weather is a pro-aging proposition.

It's time to put mind over thermometer. First, make the decision that you're going to get out and live, whether you're comfortable or not. Tell yourself that, short of heatstroke, frostbite, or some other valid threat, discomfort at least lets you know you're alive in a body. Next, find things to do that make braving the elements worth your while. When I lived in Wisconsin, I learned that the people who found delight in winter were those who did delightful things: they skated on frozen lakes and made their way to work on cross-country skis. While others complained, they played.

Finally, dress for the weather. The wicking property of cotton and other natural fabrics draws moisture away from your body to keep you warmer when it's cold outside, and these fibers' ability to breathe can also keep you cooler in summer. If the cold is hard on you, or seems to be getting harder with each passing winter, give serious consideration to the way you dress for going out in it. Never leave home without a hat, and a scarf to protect your neck and throat. Keep your core extra warm and layer, layer, layer. The air between the layers gives you additional insulation, as does the extra clothing itself. When you go in, or you're being active and build up body heat, or, heaven forbid, you have a hot flash, you have only to remove a layer or two.

Beyond this, you may find that regular clothes from regular stores are simply not warm enough for you to be outside in on the coldest days. Should that be the case, get yourself some serious outdoor gear from a camping and hiking store or catalog: long underwear, thick cotton and wool socks and gloves (some even come with little batteries to warm them up), and a coat lined with a modern insulating material (better than down and more humane, this is one concession I make to synthetic fibers).

The forecast calls for either outfitting yourself for the weather or missing out on life. The former helps you grow younger; the latter makes you old.

REJUVENATE YOURSELF WITH ACTION: *How are you holding up this winter? If the weather is keeping you from exercising, seeing friends, or living as fully as you'd like, invest in some chill-fighting clothing to give you more of your life back.*

Forgive Yourself Thoroughly

Guilt ages people from the soul on out, and there's no plastic surgery for a wrinkled soul. Of course be responsible for your actions, but get over guilt by forgiving yourself for every lapse, every fall from grace, and every time you came up short of your own standards or those of someone who mattered to you.

Start your forgiveness process in the here and now. It's easier to forgive yourself for a fresh misstep than for one that has taken on epic proportions from years of mental embellishment. Most of our crimes are verbal—the foot-in-mouth misdemeanor, saying something we shouldn't have, or hurting someone's feelings. Getting into the habit of the quick and sincere apology can take care of most of these.

The old stuff can be harder to make right: a wallet found and kept when you were in high school, a test cheated on in college, an angry word to a child that no mere apology can erase. Everybody has black marks in their history. As humans we respond to action, so take some. Give to charity the amount you found in the wallet, adjusted for inflation. Atone for that test by tutoring a youngster whose chance to go to college could come from your efforts. Be honest with and loving toward that child who is now an adult, and be the best possible grandmother to his children, and the best possible friend and mentor to the other children in your life.

This is not perfect, a flawless tit-for-tat that makes everything okay, but it makes things as okay as they get. You may want to do a ritual to put to rest something you've felt guilty about—writing it out and burning it, maybe (see December 27); or after making amends and talking it through with someone you trust, going for a steam bath and a long, hot shower, metaphorically cleansing the memory from your pores as well as from your conscience.

Having a past won't keep you from growing younger. Beating yourself up with it will. Forgive yourself. You will feel lighter, and you will live with greater effectiveness.

REVITALIZE YOUR LIFE WITH WORDS: *I forgive myself completely, and I allow myself to grow.*

Romancing Your Life

February is the month of romance, which is great if there is romance in your life and not so hot if there isn't. It is essential, for a happy February and a revitalizing year, to grasp the concept that romance is not just about coupling. As much as it adds to sex and relationship, it can exist exquisitely outside sex and relationship.

Candlelight dinners and delivered bouquets barely scratch the surface. Romance needs to wend its way through your days and nights, whether you're newly in love, partnered for decades, or, by choice or circumstance, on your own. Even when you're by yourself or with a platonic friend or your platonic dog, it is romantic to walk in the moonlight, or the streetlight, or the dawnlight (a word I just made up that is really romantic). It is romantic to light a candle for any reason or no reason. A little romantic thrill runs through any gift of flowers, whether they come from Prince Charming, from your niece in Chicago, or from you on the great day when you treat yourself to something that is not practical and will even wilt.

It is romantic to shop for lingerie or perfume, or tie your hair with a black velvet ribbon—or attach hooks and eyes to that selfsame ribbon, pin on Grandmother's cameo, and clasp it around your neck. It is romantic to read the classics or poetry (or nearly anything if you're on a park bench or a fainting couch). The presence of a lover intensifies all this, of course, but even in the absence of one (or in the company of one who just doesn't get the romance piece), the romance is there.

My friend Frankie had been divorced over a year when she bought her charming little house on a cul-de-sac. One bedroom was for sleeping. One was an office. The third was *Lady Penelope's Room*—an ever-changing shrine to Frankie's imaginary alter-ego, a Victorian aristocrat who fancied a chamber outfitted with hatboxes and cut-glass atomizers, photograph albums and hats with plumes, fringed throws on the rocker and velvet pillows on the loveseat. Few of us have a whole room to devote to our romantic proclivities, but let's give them a corner, or at least a thought.

Romance your life, then, this month and this morning. With

your partner, in spite of your partner, or on your own, let a rose or a ribbon, well-chosen music or a crackling fire, weave a bit of romance into the fabric of your February.

REJUVENATE YOURSELF WITH ACTION: *Put some romance in your day—for yourself alone or for yourself and someone you love.*

Meet the Floor

The simple act of sitting on the floor (and getting up again) can increase the strength and flexibility of your legs, hips, and back. Excessive sitting in chairs, on the other hand—unless you're acutely conscious of your posture and the placement of your body in space—encourages relaxed abdominals and rounded shoulders.

Floor-sitting requires some flexibility in your hip joints and the adductor muscles of your inner thighs. It calls for knees that can bend and, when you're not propped against a wall or a back-jack, a back strong enough to hold itself straight without assistance. If all this is hard for you, start by sitting on a low stool or a well-stuffed cushion and, over days and weeks, work your way down. If you're capable of sitting on the floor, do it often.

As a yoga or Pilates student, you'll get down on a mat quite a bit. Should you choose to meditate in the traditional fashion of a yogi or a Buddhist monk, you'll sit cross-legged on the floor or on a cushion designed for meditation, one that supports your hips so you can sit without squirming from here to enlightenment. You can also sit on the floor more often by simply staking claim to your share of carpet when you're watching TV or talking on the phone. The more you do it, the longer you'll be able to.

REJUVENATE YOURSELF WITH ACTION: *Sit on the floor every chance you get.*

Wise Woman Remedies

When you collect natural remedies, you have ways to deal with some of life's discomforts without the side effects of strong medicine. Although there is certainly a time for the doctor and the drugstore, your body has to deal with every drug you take. The less of this detoxing you have to do, the younger you get to stay. Moreover, knowing a bit about herbs and teas and home remedies lets you become a wise woman in the most traditional sense of the term.

Those that I use include:

- *Fennel seeds.* Chew a handful after a meal to aid digestion, or ease indigestion once it sets in. (Fennel seeds, plain or candied, also freshen the breath.)

- *Ginger tea, ginger ale, and candied ginger.* Nothing beats ginger for alleviating nausea or motion sickness. I nibble candied ginger before going to the airport as a defense against taxi drivers' lurch-and-brake driving.

- *Honey.* A tablespoon of honey seems like a lot to gulp, but if you have a cramp in your leg or foot, it can provide nearly instantaneous relief. (Honey is predigested and makes a beeline to the bloodstream.) If you're prone to exercise cramping, pack honey sticks in your gym bag.

- *Licorice tea.* Luscious and sweet without sugar, licorice tea is calming anytime you're upset or nervous. It also takes the edge off an appetite and can dissipate a craving for sweets.

- *Peas and plasters.* Any muscle strain, backache, or athletic injury at our house gets treated with peas—a bag of frozen peas makes a perfect, pliable ice-pack—and a "back plaster" or "medicated plaster." My favorite plasters are Chinese imports, sold in pharmacies and Asian markets; they provide soothing heat and temporary pain relief via ingredients like camphor and cayenne.

- *Sage*. For hot flashes, or just hot summer, sage provides quick relief. The sage plant "sweats" to cool itself, and it can apparently pass the cooling on. Buy liquid sage extract (*Salvia officinalis*) at a health food store and mix a few drops of it in cool water. Alternatively, make a sage elixir by letting a handful of the fresh herb age for twenty-one days in a bottle of sweet white wine. (Strain before drinking. Half a wineglass full should cool you off for some time.)

- *Salt and pepper*. If gargling with warm salt water doesn't do enough for a sore throat, try adding a pinch of powdered cayenne pepper. I use a tiny amount, $1/8$ teaspoon to half a cup of hot salt water, and find it effective.

- *Thyme for a bath*. I buy dried thyme in bulk and keep it in the freezer. If I feel a cold coming on, I make a couple of sizable soaking bags from cheesecloth or old pantyhose fabric and a cup and a half each of thyme. I place these in the tub and run a hot bath, squeezing the bags periodically to impart more of the thyme essence into the water. After a twenty-minute soak, I put on my terry robe and get under the covers for thirty minutes. About half the time, this seems to "sweat out" the cold so I don't have to come down with it.

Start your collection with these and with remedies you already swear by. As time passes, add more that you remember hearing about from your mother and grandmother, and those you pick up from reading and from friends. Consider compiling a looseleaf notebook of them: *Wise Woman Remedies*, by you.

REJUVENATE YOURSELF WITH ACTION: *Jot down the home remedies you can bring to mind. If you like doing this, start a notebook of them.*

Do Work You Love

I hope you're already doing work you love, because the earlier you started, the younger you'll look and feel. If you don't love your work today, can you love what it's doing for you, prospering your life or getting you out and getting your mind off yourself? If you don't love anything about your work, you have a challenge on your hands: either to get a different job or to do some work outside your day job that you really, truly love.

Changing jobs at forty or fifty or sixty can be tricky. There's the benefits piece. The retirement package. The stock options. All you stand to lose if you leave now instead of later. Then there's the matter of getting another job, and the gray ceiling somebody installed when the glass one was lifted. It's a huge decision that only you can make. Some women carry off such a transition masterfully.

Ellen was a high-powered, highly paid executive secretary in New York City who opted for a 180-degree turnaround from stressed-out to fulfilled-no-matter-what. She left the corporate world and started a dog-walking business. Her simpler life gave her a higher level of fitness and health than she'd had in years, along with genuine contentment.

This road less traveled is not for everybody and may not be for you. Still, if you don't love what you do from nine to five as much as Ellen loves Yorkshire terriers and golden retrievers, you need to get that enthusiasm from somewhere. Perhaps a duty that fascinates you could be added to your present job, or maybe there's another job in your department or your company that would suit you ever so much better than the one you're doing now. If this isn't possible, what about staying with the job you've got and volunteering, working for a cause, training for some new kind of work, or starting a business on the side? One of these days, if you haven't already, you'll look back on your life and say, "What have I done?" You want to be able to say, "Plenty!" and believe it with all your heart.

REVITALIZE YOUR LIFE WITH WORDS: *I love the work I do enough to put my heart and soul into it.*

Deodorant Versus Antiperspirant

Deodorant keeps you from smelling bad when you perspire. Antiperspirant attempts to keep you from perspiring at all. And here lie pros and cons, facts and fables, urban legends and Internet myths. Will using antiperspirant lead to toxic buildup in your body? Breast cancer? Alzheimer's? The respective answers: "Sort of," "Nope," and "Possibly."

I'll explain. The skin is a major organ of elimination, and perspiration is one way the body rids itself of toxins—the rationale behind saunas and steam baths. If you wear antiperspirant, its active ingredient, aluminum chlorhydrate, interferes with a process your body feels compelled to engage in. This interference is clearly unnatural, but whether or not it's harmful remains unclear.

As for breast cancer, there is no solid evidence that antiperspirant use has anything to do with it. It's not as easy to give a blanket reprieve on the Alzheimer's issue, to which aluminum has been tied for years. We apparently ingest small amounts when we drink from aluminum cans, cook with aluminum cookware, or eat a foil-wrapped potato, and people who take aluminum-based antacids get quite a bit. Using antiperspirant entails rubbing an aluminum compound onto the skin, and a tiny percentage is absorbed with each application. In theory at least, using antiperspirant over time could cause a buildup of aluminum in the brain, possibly contributing to Alzheimer's disease.

I'm conscious enough of the "could" and the "possibly" that I use antiperspirant only on very hot days, if I'll be under TV lights, or if I'm wearing something that would cost a bundle to have dry-cleaned. (There is speculation that antiperspirant can damage clothes even more than perspiration, so I may have to scrap reason number three.) The rest of the time, I use one of the natural deodorants you can find in health food stores and drugstores; the active ingredient is usually baking soda. Or you can use plain old baking soda, suggests Debra Lynn Dadd, author of *Home Safe Home*, or baking soda mixed with a little cornstarch.

REJUVENATE YOURSELF WITH ACTION: *Experiment with natural deodorant and see how it works for you.*

Nighties

You'll feel better about yourself in the daytime if you dress for bed at night. You're not alone if you frequently fall asleep in front of the TV and awaken in whatever you had on when you became engrossed in the movie. Similarly, you are not in some small minority if your standard slumber attire is an old tank top, sweats, or something once purchased as a nightie that now looks more like a cleaning rag with sleeves.

But since we spend one-third of our lives sleeping, it stands to reason that we require one-third as many nightgowns, sleepshirts, and pairs of pajamas as we have outfits for day. Ideally, we'll have summer and winter nightwear to change when the seasons do, the way we trade T-shirts for sweaters and then trade them back again. We'll have nighties to match moods and situations: sexy (which can show either a lot or a little; only you know which is which); warm and cuddly (flannel gets my vote); formal (the pajamas and matching robe you take visiting); or whimsical (weight-lifting teddy-bears? kittens with angel wings?).

In every case, the garment ought to be one you like. It needs to be comfortable (okay, the sexy negligees don't have to be all that comfortable), and, ideally, it should be made of a natural fabric like cotton or silk. A little polyester probably won't hurt (35 percent or less—the label will tell you), but more than that will interfere with your skin's "breathing" during the night. Sleep delivers a period of repose and fasting that bids your body to detoxify; synthetic-fiber sleepwear can impede the process. And if menopause brings you nocturnal hot flashes and night sweats, synthetic clothing will only intensify them.

You're growing younger because you're taking care of yourself every day. It may as well be a twenty-four-hour proposition.

REJUVENATE YOURSELF WITH ACTION: *Peruse your sleepwear drawer. Is it time to discard some of the contents and treat yourself to a new nightie?*

Keeping Up

Growing younger asks that we become enough a part of the present time that we don't find ourselves caught "back in my day." It's still your day, and it will be all your life.

I personally took the Luddite route as long as I could. In my mind, older was almost always better, especially where technology was concerned. I refused to retire my typewriter and get a computer. Once the lack of repair people and spare parts forced the issue, I held out against opening an e-mail account until threatened with family rebellion and professional blacklisting. My stuck-in-the-old-days stance aged me. While living without a computer can be a laudable testimony to simplicity and self-determination, I wasn't avoiding technology to take a stand: I just didn't want to change. It's that stubbornness—a cover-up for boldfaced fear—that is aging.

So keep up, to the degree you wish or the degree to which you can stretch yourself, with not only the latest ideas and influences, but the gadgets and gizmos, too. Any of these you choose to own, choose also to operate adeptly. Any appliance or electronic contrivance that you see every day and think, "My husband knows how to work this," or "The kids can always figure this out" will age you where it causes the most trouble: in your self-image. Learn to use these contraptions, and know that this learning is an ongoing exercise. There will always be a new model or a new version, something else to master, one more way to stay alert and aware and on top of things.

REJUVENATE YOURSELF WITH ACTION: *Ensconce yourself more comfortably in our back-to-the-future present by increasing your skill with one of the tools of the information age—learning a new computer program maybe, or how to use some of the more esoteric features on your mobile phone.*

R-E-S-P-E-C-T

If you didn't start life with high self-esteem, you've probably worked hard to get it—reading books, taking classes, going to therapy, attending workplace training sessions. However you got here, you're beyond building basic self-esteem. You're all the way to loving and respecting your being. That's more than just knowing you're okay. It's knowing you're amazing.

This love and respect is not to pump up your ego but to acknowledge your essence. The more you're able to do this, the more wondrous your life will become. You'll no longer worry about your own worth, so you can be fully present to others. When you set out to help someone else, you'll be helping that person in earnest—and you'll be respecting that person in earnest, too: you learned how by respecting yourself.

Every kind thing you do for yourself helps build this love and respect. Many of the affirmations you're saying and writing down as you work through this year will expedite the process—even more if you say them into a mirror, looking at your own face, with or without makeup: "I am one of a kind, extraordinary, a woman with a destiny. . . . I am comfortable with my body and my place in the world. . . . I am an eternal spiritual being living a remarkable physical life." When you can say these to your own face, and believe them through and through, you're well on your way to the kind of radical self-acceptance that can revolutionize a life at any point in it. This is how you come to see that it's fine to be proud of what you do, but it's essential to be awed by who you are.

REVITALIZE YOUR LIFE WITH WORDS: *I love and respect my being.*

If It's This Good, It Must Be Chocolate

You don't need me to tell you that fine chocolate tastes fabulous. It also contains a caffeine-like substance called *theobromine* that produces a slight mood enhancement, so you're not just eating something delicious, you're getting a baby buzz from it as well. Some people are so adoring of chocolate that once they start eating it, they can't stop. If you are the proverbial chocoholic and truly can't eat just one, do yourself a favor and don't. Some people find that treats made of carob, although certainly not the real thing, can fill in for chocolate so that giving it up isn't as hard.

For the rest of us, some little chocolate something on Valentine's Day and some other days, too, isn't such a bad thing. You need to make it special, though, and become a connoisseur. Enjoying a beautiful piece of hand-carved chocolate is a very different experience than grabbing a candy bar when you're paying for gas.

If you want to eat chocolate that might actually support your growing-younger efforts, choose the dark stuff. It contains polyphenols that can lower blood pressure and furnish antioxidants that scavenge and do away with harmful free radicals. Milk chocolate doesn't do this, and even drinking milk with your dark chocolate appears to cancel out the effect.

In a nutshell—or perhaps I should say, in a heart-shaped box— a little chocolate won't hurt and a little dark chocolate may even help. If you don't care for dark chocolate, have a little of the kind you fancy and eat lots of broccoli.

REJUVENATE YOURSELF WITH ACTION: *Make this a sweet day, with or without chocolate, and, for that matter, with or without a lover. Just for fun, look up St. Valentine and learn the history of this holiday, which grew out of friendship rather than romance.*

FEBRUARY 15

Play Day!

FEBRUARY 16

Light Up Your Life

If you feel a little droopy in winter or during a spate of gray days, it means you're human. If you feel miserable in the winter or during a spate of gray days, you may have SAD, seasonal affective disorder. This is a real condition. If somebody who's supposed to know better tells you it's all in your head, you're talking to an arrogant fool.

Standard treatment for SAD is a special lamp that provides the missing "happy light" from the sun without harmful rays. You can find these lamps online by doing a search on "seasonal affective disorder." If your doctor agrees that you are genuinely suffering from SAD, insurance sometimes helps pay for the lamps, which are in the $125 to $250 range.

Other ways to help light up your life when the sun is nowhere in sight are these:

- *Wear colors.* Black is elegant. It goes with everything, makes you look thinner, and if you spill coffee on it, nobody has to know. But if you're feeling blue, don't wear black. Or brown. Or gray. Instead, parade your pastels. Triumph in turquoise. Wear winter white (fashion jargon for any white worn between New Year's and Passover). Wow everybody with a red coat, a scarlet hat, a crimson umbrella, or ruby slippers. In China, red is considered good luck. Why not? If it lifts your spirits, you can better see the luck you've already got.

- *Put full-spectrum bulbs in every lamp and ceiling fixture in your house and, if you can, your office.* Designed to mimic natural light, these bulbs supply a pleasing ambience and are great to read or work by. If you surreptitiously change all your bulbs and don't tell anyone, people will comment on how nice your place looks, or how comfortable it feels. Full-spectrum bulbs cost more than the others, but they also last longer than most standard bulbs. (If you have to use fluorescent tubes in a certain room or in your office, these come full-spectrum, too.)

- *Paint your rooms white or a sunny pastel.* A gray sky is bad enough; with a gray sky and gray walls, you may as well commit yourself until Memorial Day. Ditto for brown, khaki, or whatever other color someone tries to convince you is stylishly drab. When light is hard to come by, you need light colors (and light-reflecting colors) around you.

- *Schedule a vacation somewhere warm and bright for February or March.* With all due respect to teachers, your kids will learn as much during a week in the Caribbean as they would in school, and they'll remember it longer.

REJUVENATE YOURSELF WITH ACTION: *Do a little something to light up your life. Purchasing even one full-spectrum bulb and installing it in the room where you spend the most time is a good start.*

FEBRUARY 17

The Gift of Nonattachment

In the yogic tradition, nonattachment is a prized value. It has to do with giving your all to everything you do without getting caught up in the outcome. With attachment set aside, you can go after the impossible and not be devastated when you find out that it really was. It's nonattachment that lets you work for a candidate whose platform inspires you, even if he is the personification of *long shot*. When you're not attached to having to look like you did ten years ago, you're suddenly able to care for yourself in a way that makes you feel like you did twenty years ago.

Working without attachment to a particular outcome involves showing up and doing what's expected, whatever the future holds. In the context of *Younger by the Day*, you read the selections, do the participation exercises, write the affirmations, and adopt the habits of rejuvenation without being attached to wowing people at your high school reunion. It's a lot to ask, I know, because that reunion, or something like it, may be the reason you're reading this book. That's fine: we're all human and we all want things. But if you can keep in mind as you care for your skin and eat better food and get to the gym in the morning that you're doing all this because you deserve to be cared for and not so you can look better at forty-five than the erstwhile prom queen, you'll find yourself growing younger on a whole new level.

Nonattachment keeps you in the present with what you're doing, rather than in the future with an unknown payoff. It prevents disappointment when results take longer than you'd expected, because in your nonattached state you weren't expecting anything. And when the causes you put into motion yield their effects, they'll be the right ones.

REVITALIZE YOUR LIFE WITH WORDS: *I do what I need to do today. The results are none of my business.*

FEBRUARY 18

Food the Way Nature Grew It

Until quite recently in human history, people ate whole foods—i.e., food the way nature grew it. Most processing was done at home, not in a factory. That's all changed now. White flour, for example, lacks 30 percent of the whole wheat; white sugar lacks a whopping 90 percent of the cane or beet from which it came. Eating foods made with these means that we're taking incomplete substances into our bodies. This lack is not lost on the innate intelligence of our trillions of cells. They go looking for what's absent—in more food, junk food, late-night refrigerator forays, or too much caffeine.

Whole foods are unfragmented. They have been minimally tampered with by humans. They include:

- Vegetables that are fresh or freshly frozen

- Fruits that were, until not long ago, growing on a tree or bush or vine

- Dried beans and other legumes (soybeans, mung beans, kidney beans, navy beans, chickpeas, split peas, lentils, etc.)

- Whole grains—brown rice, oatmeal, whole-wheat bread. (The best whole-wheat bread is made from wheat grains that have only been crushed, not ground into flour. The label typically says "flourless whole-wheat bread.")

- Nuts and seeds (unsalted walnuts, almonds, filberts, pumpkin seeds, sunflower seeds, and the like)

- Fish from the ocean or a clean river or lake

- Eggs, milk, and meat from animals who were fed real food and who weren't unnecessarily medicated with antibiotics or growth hormones. (Don't overdo on these, though—see March 26.)

Make eating natural foods an adventure. Be open-minded about brown bread if you're used to white, or about some vegetable you think you dislike but haven't tasted in twenty years; it could be delicious to you now. Explore natural food stores. Read their bulletin boards to see if they're having a lecture of interest. Peruse natural food and vegetarian cookbooks. Frequent farmers' markets for a festival atmosphere and the freshest food you're likely to find. Grow vegetables in the garden or tomatoes in a window box or sprouts on a counter. Get a sense of the wonder of it all.

REJUVENATE YOURSELF WITH ACTION: *Start today to eat more whole grains than refined ones, more fruits than sweets, more beans than meat, and more vegetables than anything.*

Do Something Purely for Yourself

I know you're doing a lot that you're supposed to. You're exercising and making good food choices and keeping your attitude in the right place. Equally important is doing a little something each day just for you, for the unabashed joy of it all. Most days this won't be anything big because time is limited and there are plenty of demands on yours already, but do *something*. Duck into an art gallery on your lunch hour. When they're giving out hand massages at the cosmetics counter, get one. Read the entertainment section of the paper first; it might tell you about your next favorite movie. Put bubbles in your bath. Wear pink underwear. Call the friend who can always get you giggling.

I don't know what makes you happy, but you do. It's important that you visit that happy place inside yourself every single day, no matter what. Linda, my beautiful, elegant literary agent (she's my age, but I still think I want to be like her when I grow up), had done this for years by the time her mother fell ill with the cancer that proved to be fatal. "I told my mother that I did this, and that she needed to do it, too, even now. Especially now." It was a small but ideal gift from one generation to the one before, proving that circumstances are never too dire to preclude some little joy.

Be careful: in your quest to improve yourself, you might say, "I did something for myself: I went to the gym." If you loved going to the gym, if you felt like a kid again, and you never once looked at the clock and wished you were somewhere else, it can count as your happy thing. If the experience was anything less, you owe yourself pink underwear.

REJUVENATE YOURSELF WITH ACTION: *Get into the habit of giving yourself a bit of fun every single day. Write what you do in your journal for the next week or two to cement the practice in your mind.*

A Humidifier Can Help

With age, skin gets drier from the inside. We unwittingly aid the process from without by spending the winter in indoor deserts, our centrally heated homes and offices with parchingly low humidity levels. The healthiest humidity range is 35 to 65 percent. You can find out how your rooms rate with a five-dollar humidity monitor you can buy at any hardware store. If it tells you that you're sleeping in the Sahara, a humidifier can help. This doesn't have to be a major purchase; an inexpensive tabletop model can humidify a bedroom all night long. (Some people prefer small steam humidifiers to the larger, cool-mist kinds, since steam humidifiers are largely self-cleaning.)

If you go from arid air to moist air, even just when you're sleeping, you should notice a difference in your skin in a few days' time. In addition, your immune system will get a shot in the arm and you may find yourself with fewer colds this winter. Even your plants and your paintings will be in better shape.

Watch your little humidity monitor: if the moisture in the air goes over 65 percent, it could encourage the growth of mold and bacteria. Keeping a happy medium is, well, happy—and healthy, too.

REJUVENATE YOURSELF WITH ACTION: *Monitor the humidity level in your bedroom and other places where you spend a lot of time. If it's low, a humidifier can help.*

The Proper Conditions

When a student has a well-lit, well-appointed study area, her grades pick up. When the family dog has a comfortable bed, a regular schedule, and plenty of attention, he is tail-waggingly content. When a plant grows in good soil and gets the right amount of sun and water, it can thrive sufficiently to burst into bloom. There is an atmosphere for rejuvenation, too, and when we have it, ours gets a notable boost.

A rejuvenating milieu consists of:

- *Physical conditions.* Pleasant surroundings, healthy food in your kitchen, well-chosen products on your dressing table.

- *Mental conditions.* Thinking positive thoughts, reading inspiring books, and remembering that you're part of the interconnectedness of life.

- *Spiritual conditions.* Setting aside a place for interior pursuits (prayer, contemplation, journal writing), and having people in your life who see your inner light and their own.

You can help yourself grow younger in ways that seem to have nothing to do with "anti-aging." (This, you might have noticed, is not my favorite term.) A good deed will do it, or getting your windows washed, inside and out. Reading poetry counts, and making amends. Getting away to the country this weekend, or staying home and giving yourself a private vacation. Contentment creates a rejuvenating environment, as do laughter and good company, including your own. Contemplating the mysteries of life will do it, as does letting yourself feel awestruck by ostensibly ordinary things. Providing little treats for yourself and others is a lovely way to construct an environment in which to grow younger. Practice every day.

REVITALIZE YOUR LIFE WITH WORDS: *I surround myself with an atmosphere of rejuvenation.*

FEBRUARY 22

Your Beautiful Nails

The state of your nails gives an astute physician clues about your state of health and tells anybody looking about certain nervous habits, how much time you commune with a computer, and whether or not you have cleaning help. Nails tend more to peeling, breaking, and ridges as time passes. Too much fraternization with water, and cleaning products and other chemicals, adversely affects them. So does going ungloved in the wind and weather, and treating your nails like a Swiss Army knife designed to peel and pry and scrape things.

Nails are living tissue, predominantly a protein called *keratin*. To stay healthy, they need to be fed from the inside with protein, minerals, and essential fatty acids. They also thrive on moisture. While water can dry them out, oil holds moisture in, so cream your nails often, especially the cuticle that protects and nourishes them. (Don't let anybody cut your cuticles either—some manicurists can hardly contain themselves since newly cut cuticles can look ever so neat and nice. Stand firm; you'll have better nails in the long run if you just push back the cuticle but leave it intact.) There are special nail and cuticle creams, too, but your favorite hand cream can easily pinch-hit.

Beautiful nails call for a manicure every seven days, professional or self-service. Non-acetone polish remover won't weaken nails the way acetone does. Nails filed squarish stay stronger than ovals, and short ones are easier to maintain than long ones. A neutral or pale shade of polish shows nicks less, and touch-ups are nearly invisible. Bright or deep reds can be stunning, of course, if you're willing to do the upkeep. A base coat keeps nails from yellowing, especially if you wear colored polish. Choose a therapeutic base and top coat formulated to mitigate whatever peeling, chipping, or breakage to which your nails are prone. (Open a window when you use nail polish; even if the smell doesn't bother you, you're better off not inhaling the stuff undiluted. And choose a nail salon with good ventilation: some of the ones that do a lot of artificial nails smell like they should be shut down by the EPA.)

You may wish to skip polish altogether in favor of the romantic ritual of buffing your nails. There are buffers for eliminating roughness and ridges (these need to be used only every month or two) and smoother ones for bringing the natural oils to the surface and giving nails a glossy shine. Don't do this too energetically—excessive buffing can weaken nails. It's quite freeing, though, to know that there's no polish to peel away and that you can be blissfully self-sufficient in the manicure department.

At the other end of the spectrum, you may have artificial nails and love them. I gave up on them years ago. They wreak havoc on natural nails, and if moisture gets trapped under one of them, you're asking for a fungal infection. A legitimate concession to artificiality is a temporary wrap for a broken nail. Otherwise, my vote is for the nails you grow yourself.

REJUVENATE YOURSELF WITH ACTION: *Book a professional manicure or schedule a trade with your daughter or a friend.*

FEBRUARY 23

Incidental Activity

Incidental activity is exercise that is (usually) free and doesn't call for special attire or an extra shower. If you're active, you will stay younger longer. You'll digest your food better and get to eat more of it. And you'll have energy to spare, like a battery that is constantly being recharged.

I once met a boatman in rural China whose back and chest and arms and shoulders were sculpted as if God and Michelangelo had collaborated to be sure they were perfect. He had the definition bodybuilders yearn for and the strength athletes strive to attain. In this man, however, these had been innocently acquired through living his life, supporting his family by ferrying people along the river in his rowboat. Now, when I see someone at the gym who is obviously taken with his own physique, I remember the boatman and how his muscularity was incidental and therefore all the more enticing.

We can be similarly enticing, and with far less exertion than it takes to row a boat several hours a day. According to the US Department of Health and Human Services, ordinary physical activities like gardening and brisk walking can do much that formal exercise does. Biking, scrubbing a floor, mowing, and raking rank as moderate endurance activities; climbing stairs or hills, shoveling snow, and hiking are "vigorous." In other words, incidental activity isn't wimpy. It deserves respect. And every bit counts: Hang the picture. Feed the cat. Get the clothes out of the dryer. Answer the door, even if you have to walk upstairs to do it because you were getting the clothes out of the dryer. Provided you're phsyically able, do this stuff—even if you have a willing, retired partner and a live-in maid. They can get their own incidental activity.

Housecleaning is a good one because it can be light or intense, and there's always some to do. I like cleaning to music—Strauss waltzes, Sousa marches, or Judy or Liza belting out something sublime. And with housecleaning your actions count for something, like ferrying a visitor across a river. If this doesn't appeal, just stand up. Stand up during phone calls (which, say business gurus, has the added benefit of making you sound more in control). Stand to do other things you used to sit to do—stapling handouts, opening mail, snapping beans. Stand in the bus or on the train, unless you're tired or carrying bags.

Have an "I'll do it" attitude. Be one of those people—one of those trim, energetic people—who sets up the chairs for the meeting and helps the hostess clear the plates. Take active vacations—hikes, tours, spas—and even at home find active ways to have fun. Go skating (rinks are safer than roads and ponds), go biking (wear a helmet and assume that drivers don't see you), or take lessons in ballroom dance or square dance or tango. (That last assumes you're either coordinated, gutsy, or someone who saw *Evita* several times.)

REJUVENATE YOURSELF WITH ACTION: *Observe your activity level today. Are you active on your job? How much do you walk? Who cleans your house and cares for your garden? How many hours each day do you spend in a chair? Do you regularly pursue an energetic hobby? (Formal exercise counts here, as well as anything active you do purely for fun.) If you find yourself short on incidental activity, what can you do to change that?*

FEBRUARY 24

The Right Multivitamin

Health food stores have a staggering array of multivitamins to choose from; so does your neighborhood pharmacy. I like to buy vitamins with the same care I use when buying food, reading the labels and researching the companies that make the products. Although nearly everything I read tells me that "natural" vitamins are no better than the other kind, I feel better taking vitamins from a nutritional supplement company than those from a drug company. It's worth shopping around to find a brand that appeals to you. You also need a form that suits you. That may mean a chewable or a liquid.

Especially if a multivitamin is your only supplement, be sure it contains antioxidant nutrients such as beta-carotene (a precursor to vitamin A); vitamins C and E; the full B-complex (including folic acid); vitamin D (especially if you avoid the sun and don't drink milk—dairy, soy, or rice—fortified with vitamin D); zinc (at least 25 milligrams; zinc is thought to promote immunity and aid in the prevention of Alzheimer's disease and arthritis); and selenium, an immune booster and heart protector (at least 50 micrograms).

Women after menopause and men at any age are less likely to lack iron than they are to have excess iron stores; this can increase free-radical damage to cells and may raise the likelihood of a heart attack. Therefore, once you stop menstruating, unless your doctor tells you that you're anemic, choose a multi that does not contain iron. (The blends designed for older people are iron-free. If the thought of buying something that says "silver" or "senior" makes you cringe, look at it as an exercise in ego reduction.)

Also, understand that although your multi is in no way a substitute for eating right, it may supply an adequate daily dose of vitamins. It cannot do that for minerals. Minerals are larger, in the molecular sense, than vitamins; you can't get much in a single pill. If you believe you need supplementary calcium, for example, you'll have to take that in addition to your multi. Also, if you're under a doctor's care, let her know what supplements you plan to take. There are some cases in which supplementary nutrients can aggravate an existing condition or intensify the effects of a medication.

REJUVENATE YOURSELF WITH ACTION: *Visit a natural food store and spend some time in the vitamin aisle. If you're new to this, look only at multis right now; more than that can be overwhelming. Read the labels. Find the store's vitamin expert and ask him or her questions.*

FEBRUARY 25

Still Sexy, After All These Years

There are fortunate women who feel at home with their sexuality throughout their lives. Some are comfortable with it only when they're young and getting wolf whistles, others when they're older and more sure of themselves, and still others not then, not now, not ever.

The particular challenge in midlife is to keep the focus on yourself as a sexual being and not on the images around you that imply that sexual appeal and expression are the exclusive province of the young and anatomically gifted. Sex itself is less about the body than the mind anyway. There are populations—the South Sea islanders of whom Margaret Mead wrote, for instance—that revere older women as sexual experts and teachers. This is small consolation for those who live here, where the tight young thing is idealized. If a woman has undergone a hysterectomy, mastectomy, or other major surgery, it can be even harder to feel desirable. But we need this. It's not just part of feeling young: it's part of feeling incarnate.

Judith Sachs, coauthor of *Getting the Sex You Want*, told me, "The road to feeling sexy at this time is to take charge and figure out what you want. Sometimes, it's holding hands; other times it's a quickie on the kitchen floor. As the body and mind change, sex needs to change, too. You have to talk with your partner *and* spend enough time alone to experiment with new fantasies and new activities, maybe reading erotic literature or watching some good female erotic films." (For me, *Gone with the Wind* counts as an erotic film. It's all a matter of taste.) Sachs also suggests standing in front of the mirror, appreciating all that's good instead of criticizing the bad, and spending some time naked to start feeling good in your skin.

I think it's also important to be willing to change your sense of how you see yourself sexually. You're way grown up. You know what you like and what you need, and especially after your hormones stop helping, you may need a great deal more spice in your sex life—toys and role-playing and acting out fantasies and staging your own sexual revolution, whether you were around for the previous one or not. If you're holding on to inhibitions—I spent some time in an old-school Catholic school where inhibition was a required course—let go of every one except those you need to stay safe and true to yourself. If there is ever a time to have wild and crazy adventures with a partner you trust, this is it. Despite the barriers to fabulous sex that may exist now, you could be at that luscious time of life when your parents aren't coming home, your kids aren't coming home, and you can't get pregnant. The possibilities are endless.

REVITALIZE YOUR LIFE WITH WORDS: *I always have a great time in bed.*

Find What Thrills You and Stick with It Like a Life Vest

It could be flowers or a sport or a grandchild. Mystery stories or independent films or big shiny magazines with impossibly pretty clothes. It could be singing or running or reading or volunteering, your work in the world or your life of the spirit. Anything or anybody that reliably gives you joy, brings you out of the doldrums, and gets you out of yourself is a treasure. It's all right if you and that special someone or something seem to be joined at the hip; you're already joined at the heart.

Every time you're near someone or something you love like the dickens, you get an influx of revitalizing emotions and brain chemicals. Even thinking about those special people and things does some good. There is great value in having family photos on your desk at work, associating with people who adore the same hobby you do, and reading coffee-table books about the tropical paradise you love to visit but don't get to nearly enough.

Many spiritual teachings insist that love is the most important thing and that learning to love is the main reason we showed up on this planet in the first place. *Love* without something *to* love is a verb without an object. This makes who you love and what you love beings and pastimes of eminent consequence. Never judge them as less than that, and don't let anyone else judge them either.

Of course I'm not talking about "loving" in a harmful way, whether the attraction is to an unwise habit or to a person who is unable to value you as you deserve. But if orchids or Siamese cats or Chopin sonatas just about make your heart stop with the utter grandeur of their existence, they're making you younger, each and every day.

REJUVENATE YOURSELF WITH ACTION: *Regardless of what else the world asks of you today, give someone or something you love a high priority.*

Treat Your Cells Like Somebodies

"It's my body, and if I smoke/eat like a pig/never exercise, it's nobody else's business." Even if you've never thought this, you know people who have. There is a flaw in the reasoning, though. Maybe "my body" isn't really "my body." Maybe it's a loaner. In fact, it has to be a loaner since one day I'll leave it and its atoms will become parts of other objects and other beings. What this means in the here and now is that the way you treat your physical self *is* somebody else's business—quite a few somebodies' business, in fact, if you think of the cells that make up your physical organism not only as parts of yourself that are too small to see, but as entities in their own right.

If you've given birth, you may relate to the experience I had when I was pregnant. I did everything perfectly. My meals could have come from a nutrition textbook and I took every supplement the doctor recommended, even on the mornings I felt nauseous. If my nose was stuffy, I didn't take anything for it except a spoonful of horseradish, which worked more or less and either way didn't matter: it wouldn't hurt the baby. That was all-important. You tap into a similar kind of biological philanthropy when you decide that your cells are somebodies and that your choices affect them.

This rethink changes self-care from a dreary sort of hygiene-class assignment into a rewarding new way of doing things. You might let your coffee cool a bit more before you drink it. It could be easier to spend a little more for the instant soup that's just soup instead of the one laced with chemicals. You might take an unprecedented interest in precisely what is in your face cream and shampoo and toothpaste.

The new physics attests that every speck of matter, if we can think in terms of matter at all, is alive. In the molecular sense, our cells are huge and sophisticated, certainly worthy of being seen as somebodies in their own right. When you see them like this, you'll treat them lovingly, and you yourself will benefit.

FEBRUARY 28

Play Day!

(If there is a February 29 this year, have two play days back-to-back.)

March

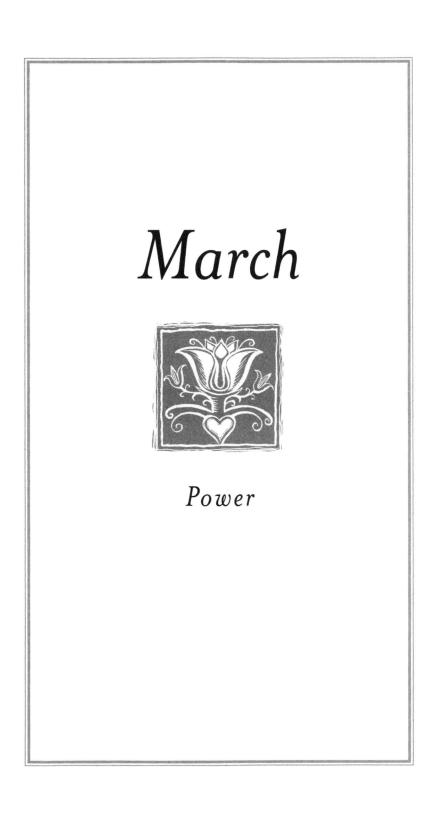

Power

Assume New Power

Every stage of life's journey gives people in that stage a kind of power. Babies, for instance, are helpless but not powerless: their power comes from being round, cute, and cuddly so that any normal person wants to protect and care for them. Teenagers find power in physical vitality and the conviction, however foolhardy, that they know all there is to know. Well into midlife, women (and men) wield the power of their sexual attraction. While we can certainly still be attractive to a partner, often more than ever, and have a most satisfying sex life, the time does come when we're not going to flirt our way into a discount at the sample sale or a better seat at the restaurant. This isn't bad, any more than growing out of "round, cute, and cuddly" is bad. It's simply life, operating on schedule, urging us to look for new and ever greater sources of power.

Power can come from the talents and intelligence we've had all along—and which we may have had to insist upon the world's noticing when it seemed more interested in our breasts or our hair. Other, newer springs of power include the wisdom we've appropriated and the knacks we've developed for devising strategies, reading people, timing moves, and using silence and speech to our best advantage. Like a chess master who has played the game long enough to understand every nuance of a knight's prowess, a bishop's scope, the queen's formidable strength, and the king's imperial vulnerability, we come to know the game of life, the maneuvers that can further our cause, the tactics that can give our dreams solidity.

Throughout this month, consider your power, its sources, its uses, and its limits. Your sexuality may still be a primary reservoir of power in your life. Enjoy it. But recognize other founts of power as well, especially those that will deepen in scope and strength over time. Grow into your power today, and use it for good.

REVITALIZE YOUR LIFE WITH WORDS: *I am a woman of power, a force to be reckoned with.*

First Thing in the Morning

You can set the tone for your day with the thoughts you entertain as soon as you realize you're awake. First, deal with the alarm. You can learn to awaken on time without that noisy reminder by going to bed on the early side of your regular time and giving yourself the mental suggestion, "I wake up every morning at six-thirty [or whatever time you like] without an alarm." Otherwise, invest in a clock that nudges you into the day rather than blasting you into it and taking the memory of your dreams with it. There are clocks that usher you awake with dulcet chimes, or that gradually light up the room, so you awaken the way people in traditional cultures do, with the rising of the (in this case simulated) sun.

Awakening gently, try to recall what you dreamed. If something about a dream seems significant, jot down the gist of it in your journal. The more you do this, the more of your dreams you'll remember. Then, even before your feet touch the floor, envision this day as the best it can be. Keep it reasonable—"I'm here in Bermuda and the butler has just brought my tea" probably isn't—but you can envision doing what you need to do to feel good about yourself and having plenty of time to do it. You can envision commuting in easy traffic and working with people in good moods. Set forth on your morning affirming all good things.

Get up early enough that you don't have to rush. *Decide* that this day will have enough hours and minutes in it to accommodate all that's required of you. If there is chaos around you in the morning—"Have you seen my shoes?" "My jersey is still damp!" "Where's the scraper? There's ice on the windshield and there's no scraper!"—be in the situation without being of it. You can look for the shoes (or not), dry the soccer shirt (or let your son do it), and produce the ice-scraper (or a credit card that can do the job) without getting caught up in the turmoil. This is your day. This is your life. It's worth more than shoes and scrapers.

REJUVENATE YOURSELF WITH ACTION: *Discern what you need to do to get your day off right. Figure out how long it takes and what time you have to get up in order to make it work. If it's unrealistic, pare down. If it just means arising a little earlier, start to do that in fifteen-minute increments that you give twenty-one days to set in before attempting your next quarter-hour shift. I find that if I get up at six, I can do it all: journal and meditate, exercise, self-massage and shower, feed the dog, the cat, and me, straighten up a little, and be at the computer by nine. If I sleep in till seven, one thing or several have to go. Sometimes the lesson comes in being able to let them.*

MARCH 3

Fifty Fabulous Adjectives

In order to remember how wonderful she is, a woman needs fifty fabulous adjectives for herself. Brainstorm in your journal positive adjectives that describe you best and that describe the best of you. Some of these can be about how you look, but let most of them be about who you are. A few will jump out and make you as pleased as punch: *engaging, irrepressible, scrappy.*

Of course you are. And more besides.

If coming up with fifty emphatic descriptors of yourself seems like a lot, think of all the roles you play—lover, mother, worker, friend, student, seeker, and all the rest—and know that each of these parts of you deserves fabulous adjectives all its own. If you get stuck, ask good friends or members of your rejuvenation circle for words they think describe you. Once you have your list, it has a function: to remind you that you're terrific on days you forget. Dog-ear the journal page or put a sticky note on it so you can look at your fifty fabulous adjectives whenever you wish. I suggest Sunday nights, when you're getting things in order for the week ahead, and anytime you'd like some reassurance that you are indeed *talented, tolerant,* and *loyal; friendly, funny,* and *generous; elegant, enthusiastic,* and *articulate.*

You might be thinking, "Nobody's perfect. Shouldn't I recognize some of the bad things about myself, too?" Maybe you should and maybe you shouldn't. Either way, you already do. You and I and nearly all the women we know are acutely aware of our shortcomings. We have noted, examined, and cataloged each one: the disappointing math grade freshman year, an offhand comment made last week, the misbehavior of our hair this very morning. At least even the score with fifty little adjectives, fifty *fabulous* little adjectives that give you your well-deserved due.

REJUVENATE YOURSELF WITH ACTION: *Get out your journal and write the numbers one through fifty. Then, off the top of your head, write fabulous adjectives that describe you: who you are, what you do, and what you've got going for yourself inside and out. Maybe you won't get to fifty right now. That's okay. More will come to you, and people who care about you can fill in the blanks.*

MARCH 4

Invent Yourself Some Holidays

If you read my book *Lit from Within*, you might recall the holiday of March 4th. It was devised by Deborah Shouse, entertaining guru and all 'round wise woman, who cites today as a day that, in English anyway (and with the homonym accounted for), announces its own holiday status as it invites us to *march forth* into the newness of our lives. Celebrate March 4th by marching forth, going forward, forgiving yourself if you feel you haven't been up to snuff, and erasing any regret about New Year's resolutions as yet unresolved. This is a new opportunity, your chance to march forth. Tell everyone you see today about March 4th and give them a chance to march forth, too.

Invent holidays for yourself. Celebrate those from other countries and other religions. Make something grand of a disadvantaged holiday like Arbor Day (the last Friday in April) that everybody has heard of but few do anything about. Make a big deal out of personal achievements, your own and other people's, and the anniversaries of them. Observe saints' days, regardless of your religion, and the birthdays of people whose lives have had an impact on yours. When my daughter was little, we took to having parties for Mozart's birthday, which happens to fall in the holiday-barren final week of January. I got a kick out of hearing her once ask a little friend,

"What did you do for Mozart's birthday?" So celebrate Amadeus on January 27, Beethoven on December 16, and Bach on March 21 with food and music, candles and a toast.

I have a sense that the day comes for most human beings when they regret having earmarked too few days as special. That is a day you can do without. Let the revelry begin.

REJUVENATE YOURSELF WITH ACTION: *Play with the idea of March 4th today. Then every month for the rest of this year, either invent a holiday or find an unusual or little noticed one to celebrate.*

MARCH 5

Come Into Your Own

I was born a New Yorker, just not in New York. Shortly before I moved here from Kansas City at fifty, I had lunch with my friend Carol at a Vietnamese restaurant. Over the spring rolls she said, "You know what I really want? I want to be a biker chick." I heard in her voice the same conviction that was motivating me to leave a lovely home and longtime friends to attach myself to the sliver of island where books are published, and where Dorothy Parker and F. Scott Fitzgerald met their colleagues for lunches around a fabled table at the Algonquin Hotel.

Even so, I was not prepared for biker chick—but this wasn't my dream, it was Carol's. I asked her what it would take to fulfill her vision. She told me that she'd have to go to bars where bikers go, and that it would be hard since she wouldn't know anybody and she didn't have the lady biker look down, and she was basically shy. "Well, if this is what you really want," I said, "get thee to a biker bar. And no matter how out of place you feel or how awkward things seem, keep it up until it happens."

In a way it felt funny to think that I was counseling a friend into a motorcycle gang, but at a deeper level I realized that what I was seeing in Carol that day, and what I was experiencing myself, was the midlife urging to come into our own. Moving thirteen hundred miles or reenacting *Easy Rider* is the exception. More often this coming into our own is subtle, internal, but still profound. Because it is not widely recognized or celebrated, there is a risk of letting the visionary insight of midlife pass you by, writing it off as some mental variation on the hot flash. It is instead an invitation to come into your own in a way you might never before have imagined.

Two years after our lunch, when I was firmly ensconced in New York City, I got a thick letter from Carol telling me how she'd come into her own as a bona fide biker babe. She said she'd used my words like a mantra: "Get thee to a biker bar." For weeks she'd sat alone and felt foolish, but eventually she got to know people and became part of a group of riders. Being who she wanted to be gave her confidence in other ways, too. She bought her first house and deepened her faith in God. "All I do now is trust," she wrote, "and I know I'll be taken care of."

I'm telling you Carol's story because each one of us deserves to come into our own in the exact way we want to do it. If this is a struggle you're facing now, it won't be easy, because for years people have been telling you, in words and intimations, who you are and what is expected of you. Insist now that those voices quiet down so you can listen to your own.

This is your chance. This is the prime of your life. You have the opportunity to move forward with the invaluable guidance of all that has gone before. None of us has forever, but we do have a future, and it's starting now. We can choose to live it in a way that any regrets, if we have them, will predate today.

REVITALIZE YOUR LIFE WITH WORDS: *I come into my own today and every day that I live.*

MARCH 6
***

The Keeper of the Keys

You are the keeper of the keys to your inner world as surely as you hold a set of keys to your house. Just as you invite in those people you choose to and keep others behind the screen door, you can invite in certain ideas and keep others out.

One easy way to start living more positively is by carefully selecting how you get your news and from whom. I prefer reading a good paper to watching a lot of TV news. There is room in a newspaper to cover a wider variety of stories and to do so in more detail, so you get to see the events of the day in a broader context. This is a big world to condense into twenty-two minutes of televised sound bites.

When I do watch the news, I carefully choose my channels for both local and international news. If you do some critical observation, you'll see that many programs are slanted slightly toward an attitude, if not an outright ideology. Choose the ones that you feel come closest to impartial reporting and minimal sensationalism. Favor programs that feature anchors and reporters with whom you resonate, and who can deliver any news, even the kind we all wish weren't happening, with both dispassion and compassion.

In addition, find ways to protect yourself from upsetting images and information. You might imagine a protective white light around you, allowing in data but filtering emotionally negative overtones so you're less likely to feel fear, frustration, anger, or a desire to respond to hatred or cruelty with more of the same. This is a way to be both informed and at peace.

Redecorate your life more to your liking by developing more discernment about which parts of the general world you allow into your specific one. Be well informed about the world around you, but do it on your own terms.

REJUVENATE YOURSELF WITH ACTION: *Consider your relationship to the news of the day. Are you a news junkie? Do issues over which you have absolutely no power affect you in a negative way? Compare different newspapers and television channels. Be sure you're getting your news in the way that suits you best, helps you be an effective citizen, and doesn't interfere with your being an effective human being.*

MARCH 7

Brush and Floss

When I was seven, Dede, the woman who took care of me, got dentures. Her friend Mrs. Ferguson went with her to the oral surgeon's office, and when she came home she had new teeth. They looked just like her old ones, but after that she couldn't eat apples without slicing them, and she took to using a knife and fork for fried chicken. She said that's how the sophisticated people back east did it all the time.

It seemed so natural then. To me she was old (sixty-three), and being old meant having false teeth and wrinkles and maybe a cane. I see it differently now that sixty-three isn't so very far off for me. I want to smile with the teeth I've had since the tooth fairy's last visit, and I'm sure you do, too.

Most of us brush our teeth often enough but not necessarily at the right time or in the right way. To be most effective, brush your teeth two or three times a day *within one hour after a meal.* After that, the pH in your mouth has dropped (become acidic), especially if you've eaten any sweets or refined starches. The bacteria that cause tooth decay and those that precipitate periodontal disease both thrive in an acidic environment. If you remove the irritants (food particles and potential plaque) before the drop occurs, they're gone before they cause trouble. When you awaken, then, you can rinse your mouth and scrape your tongue to do away with morning breath, but hold off on brushing until after breakfast.

Carry a toothbrush with you and forge the habit of reaching for it after eating the way a smoker reaches for a cigarette. (Not giving bacteria a chance to go to work on your teeth and gums is one argument for not eating between meals. This way you can brush virtually every time you eat.)

The brush you reach for should have soft bristles. A hard brush is hard on gums and doesn't clean teeth any better than one labeled "extra soft." If you brush long and carefully, you can do fine with a manual toothbrush, but most dentists recommend a high-quality electric brush. These are programmed with the right technique, gently stimulating your gum tissue as well as cleaning your teeth. The timer lets you know how long to stay with each quadrant of your mouth. For people with carpal tunnel syndrome or arthritis in their hands, an automatic brush is a godsend. Clean the brushheads after use with lots of running water and change them every three months to be sure they're always soft and pliable.

Flossing removes food particles between teeth where gum disease starts. This extra step is imperative if you want to go off into the sunset with your teeth. Once a day is fine, and you can choose the time. The benefits of flossing go beyond protecting against periodontal disease, though. The bacteria that erode gum tissue may precipitate blood clots, which in turn can lead to heart attacks or strokes. As odd as it sounds, for the past several years cardiologists have encouraged patients to floss for their hearts.

REJUVENATE YOURSELF WITH ACTION: *Review your oral hygiene. Are you brushing two or three times a day within an hour of eating? Is your toothbrush soft and not more than three months old? Do you floss every day or just some days? If you're not up to snuff on any of this, turn that around starting now.*

MARCH 8

The Really Big Three

The Harvard Nurses' Health Study, which looked at risk factors for chronic diseases in over one hundred thousand female nurses, revealed that, by and large, having normal weight, normal blood pressure, and low cholesterol means living healthfully to a ripe old age. Surely there are other indicators of health and disease your doctor will want to keep track of, but these are the Big Three, important health markers over which you yourself may have quite a bit of control.

The Big Three work together, in that many of the same lifestyle changes that can help one will also help the other two. For example, an overweight person with hypertension can sometimes get her blood pressure back to normal by losing a little weight. Similarly, someone might change her diet to lower her cholesterol level and find that she's shedding pounds at the same time. It simplifies things to know that the same diet and exercise prescription works for all three.

As for diet, eating real food, lots of fruits and vegetables, and not too much fat (or salt if hypertension is an issue) is the best choice for the long term. You can lose weight quickly with a high-protein/high-fat diet that puts your body in the disease state of ketosis, but that's not a way to live your life. Exercise can assist you in getting a handle on all three of the Big Three, even if it's nothing more than an energetic daily walk.

Sometimes it takes more than self-help to deal with a component of the Big Three. You may need a support group for losing weight, or medication to lower your blood pressure or cholesterol if diet and exercise can't do enough. Take advantage of whatever you need to get the job done. It's one more aspect of doing all that you can for yourself.

REJUVENATE YOURSELF WITH ACTION: *Do you know your blood pressure and your cholesterol level? Those are good numbers to keep track of. Normal weight, in this context, isn't fashion-model thin; it's simply being within the normal range for your height and build. You don't need to be anxious about it, just honest and persistent.*

MARCH 9

The Fountain of Youth

The fountain of youth is a water fountain. If you want every organ inside you to work properly, you need water. If you want your kidneys, which even in healthy people lose function over time, to last throughout your life, you need water. If you want great skin, bright eyes, and the stamina to make it through the class at the gym with all those twenty-somethings who don't think you can do it, you need water.

Every chemical reaction in your body requires a water molecule. Without water your cells go on strike like uncompensated workers. Well-hydrated people have even been shown to handle stress better. In order to get the standard six to eight glasses a day, you need to be drinking a little all day long. You'll need extra if it's hot (that includes hot weather, hot saunas, and hot yoga), or if you exercise, fly in planes, or ingest caffeine, alcohol, or salty foods. If you're thirsty, you're already on the road to dehydration; drink first. Water is best served hot, warm, or cool but not iced. Icy beverages stifle what Ayurveda calls the "digestive fire," and restoring youthfulness calls for good digestion.

Coffee, cola, and even black tea with all its antioxidants can't count in your water quota, because caffeine is a diuretic—i.e., a dehydrator. Ditto canned tomato and mixed vegetable juice, but here the dehydrating factor is sodium, not caffeine. Alcoholic beverages, whether antioxidant-rich red wine or the cold beer that looks so thirst-quenching, will also increase your need for water. Match them glass for glass with pure water—that's in addition to the water you'd have needed if you hadn't had the Coke or the beer.

What does count as water is water, mineral water (still or fizzy), seltzer (preferable to club soda, which has a fairly high sodium content), and caffeine-free herbal teas. Juice counts as water, but fruit juice has enough sugar that you may want to cut it by half with still or sparkling water. One surprising source of pure water you don't even have to drink: you can eat it. Fresh, juicy fruits, as well as salads and crudités, are full of water, with vitamins, minerals, phytochemicals, and great taste to boot. An apple is 66 percent water, raw cauliflower 82 percent, cantaloupe or uncooked spinach 84 percent. People who eat very high quantities of salad and fresh fruit can drink substantially less water than other folks because they're getting so much of it in their diet. Choose pure water or real juice over any drink containing refined sugar or high-fructose corn syrup. Even for those past the age of innocence, this is a case in which purity is called for.

REVITALIZE YOUR LIFE WITH WORDS: *Water tastes good to me, and I drink all I need.*

MARCH 10

See the World

When I was eighteen, I flew to London on Icelandic Airways, now Icelandair. At the time they had cheaper tickets than other carriers—I remember a lot of nuns on that flight, and guys with guitar cases—and for not much more, you could get an extended stopover in Reykjavik. During those three days, I developed a fondness for Iceland, and over thirty years later two of my books made the Icelandic Bestseller List and I got to go back, this time to give a seminar. I will always believe that the bond I forged with Iceland so long ago is one reason people there are so enthusiastic about my books. Setting foot on a place makes it yours, even if just a little, and that can set wondrous forces in motion.

Since nobody knows what the future holds, *now* is a fine time for seeing the world. Why wait? You can always see it again later. And again. And again. See different places and favorite places—it is a wonderful world. If money is an issue, there are flights so cheap you're almost a spendthrift to stay at home. Bed-and-breakfasts don't cost much, and a great many youth hostels cater to "youths" of all ages. Travel keeps you young by giving you a global perspective. It shows you that the role you play is far more about the ripples you set in motion with your actions than how you look or even how long you live.

Whatever your homeland or your hometown, you can be a good-will ambassador somewhere else. That way, you'll help the world get friendlier, and the world will help you get younger by the day.

REJUVENATE YOURSELF WITH ACTION: *Plan a trip, even though logistics like convincing your husband and getting the time off and the money together may be daunting right now. Plan anyway. Maybe you'll go somewhere that holds older women in high regard—China, France, some idyllic island in the South Seas. Plan away. This is so much fun.*

MARCH 11

Look for Something Different in the Magazines

I enjoy reading women's magazines. The clothes are beautiful, the photography innovative, and there are some thoughtful articles to read. There's also a dose of fluff, a dollop of materialism, and the danger of seeing the images on those glossy pages as something specific to strive for: eternal youth and eternal beauty, eternally made up and precisely posed. Real life is imprecise. It gets smudged, creased, and spotted. Some of your best experiences ever—I'm thinking of real goodies like sex and sleeping—you most often do with no makeup and minimal clothing. Those photo spreads are not the ultimate: they're pictures.

Magazines (and newspapers and TV shows) have to find new things to focus on, so they're always looking for the cutting edge: what's new, what's hot, what's next. What's new isn't necessarily better than what isn't, but it's what you'll read about. If it suits you, add it to your repertoire. If not, let it go. If the magazines you're reading aren't giving you your time and money's worth, explore the newsstand and see what else there is to choose from. There are magazines that celebrate women who could never be mistaken for girls, and others that see their readers as complex beings, with spiritual propensities as well as bodies to dress and spritz with perfume.

Whatever publications you choose, look to them for ideas, information, and a little vacation from the seriousness of life. When they're no longer arbiters of the way you're supposed to look and live, reading them becomes pure pleasure. And you get to be okay, just as you are.

REJUVENATE YOURSELF WITH ACTION: *Get to a newsstand one day this week and read a magazine that's new to you.*

MARCH 12

Assert Your Power Over "the Way It's Supposed to Be"

Among the regular patrons at the library where I worked in my early twenties were a young married couple and their son, a tow-headed preschooler with an infectious smile. As I came to know them, I learned that both parents were distressed, perhaps even depressed, because they had not been able to conceive a second child. "We know what our family is supposed to look like," the wife lamented. "We can't be happy until we have that." It seemed to me even then that their primary problem was not their inability to have another child, but rather their inability to see that they had an enviable life already.

This despotism of "the way it's supposed to be" is not exclusively a youthful affliction. Midlife is, in fact, a prime time for it, because this is when cultural messages start to imply that we're no longer in the swing of things, that our lives by definition cannot be the way things are supposed to be. If you look at TV sitcoms as a reflection of modern life, you find that the main characters, with a few exceptions, are young singles or young marrieds with kids at home or on the way. If someone older is on the show, it's usually to play the intrusive mother-in-law or the wacky neighbor, someone not central to the plot. The implication is that youth is life—at least all the life that matters. But in your real life, *you* are the main character, and whether you're thirty-seven or seventy-three, you will be seen again after the commercial.

Do not let the way it's supposedly supposed to be deprive you of the good of what actually is. This is true whether your version of "supposed to be" comes from the media, from family and friends, or from beliefs you took on so long ago they seem like eternal verities instead of acquired notions. But life is not what others expect or even what we expect: it's what happens. Be there for it.

REJUVENATE YOURSELF WITH ACTION: *Write in your journal about the way your life today stacks up against the way you think it's "supposed to be." Be exacting here as you discern which aspects of your life you have a genuine reason to try to improve and which you think you ought to change to fit some preconceived idea. If that idea does not reflect who you are today or what you value now, relegate it to the "supposed to be" scrap heap.*

MARCH 13

Start the Day with a Power Breakfast

One kind of power breakfast is wheeling and dealing over a morning meal. The one we're interested in here is choosing your first foods of the day with an understanding of how your own body operates and what it wants in the morning. Studies repeatedly show that breakfast-eaters live longer and stay healthier than those who plunge into the day on an empty stomach—and they're less likely to overeat or succumb to late-day sugar cravings.

Some people get their power from a light breakfast, perhaps just melon or fruit salad. They do better starting the day without heavy food to assimilate. Others need a meal that contains a little of each macronutrient—i.e., complex carbohydrate, protein, and fat—so the meal digests slowly and keeps them in the pink until lunchtime. If you're old enough to be reading this book, you're well aware of what kind of breakfast gives you your best mornings. Put that knowledge into practice.

I have two primary power breakfasts, one for summer, one for winter. When it's warm outside, I frequently make a smoothie with soy milk and berries, flax oil and wheat germ, and a scoop of nutrient powder that counts as a multivitamin and is also replete with minerals and protein. My cold-weather power breakfast starts with oatmeal—it's filling and has soluble fiber that lowers cholesterol. I top it with flax oil and wheat germ (toasted tastes better than raw and stays fresh longer), a sprinkling of chopped Brazil nuts (for selenium) or walnuts (which, like flax seeds and flax oil, are a good source of omega-3s), and fresh fruit or soaked dried fruit (raisins, prunes, or apricots) that provide fiber, vitamins, and minerals. Both of these breakfasts are quick to put together, and they make me feel as if I've done well by myself.

If you don't yet have a power breakfast (or two or three) that makes you feel on top of the morning, try out mine or come up with your own. Experiment with breakfasts that are enticing enough that you want to eat them and easy enough that even the rush of getting out the door won't keep you from starting your day with a power surge.

REJUVENATE YOURSELF WITH ACTION: *Come up with one or more power breakfasts for yourself. Note them in your journal and have one tomorrow morning.*

MARCH 14

Concrete Confidence

Concrete confidence is the kind that does not depend on externals. With it, you're as confident greeting the delivery guy in your frayed T-shirt and jeans as you are greeting the maître d' when you're dressed to the nines. When you have this kind of composure, people don't think about your age; they're too caught up in your magnetism.

While concrete confidence is unshakable, confidence based only on how you look or what the world thinks of you is easily lost. Our culture doesn't yet value older women. Truth be told, it is afraid of our untapped power and it deals with its fears by marginalizing us.

One day people will be appalled by this wholesale disregard for women at the time they have the most to offer, the way we're dismayed by the disregard for women in general a few generations ago. Right now, we can either side with the culture by shrinking obediently and denying our gifts, or we can confidently go forth with every year we've lived a further credential.

If your confidence is shaky, pretend that it isn't. A prime tenet of successful living is that behavior can precede belief. That is, you can act as if your confidence is as solid as concrete when, in fact, it may be more akin to tissue paper. No matter. Go about your day as if you have concrete confidence in yourself, your abilities, and the impression you make. Pretend that you live in a society in which women are valued more as time goes by, and create a mini-culture around you of people who actually do that. If you cling to the odd sort of selfishness that singles you out as less worthy than someone else, ask yourself, "Who made me so unique as to be *less* worthy?" Assume that you deserve every inch of the space you take and every blessing life bestows on you. Humility is a fine thing; sackcloth and ashes make anybody look bad.

REVITALIZE YOUR LIFE WITH WORDS: *I believe in myself through and through.*

MARCH 15

Play Day!

MARCH 16

The Exercise That Could Save Your Life

We all want to have toned, taut muscles and look great in sleeveless dresses, but the most important muscle to get in shape, our heart, doesn't even show. Heart disease kills more people in the Western world than anything else. Premenopausal women are protected, but that protection ends when menstruation does, putting women in the same statistically precarious position as men. Beating the odds—aside from what your doctor can do—is a three-part proposition of managing stress; eating whole, natural foods low in saturated fat and trans-fats (April 22); and doing regular cardiovascular exercise.

This is the slow-burn activity you get from walking thirty minutes rather than sprinting for two. If you work too hard, you're out of the aerobic range. You won't do your heart any good and you won't burn fat. Exercising at least twenty minutes at a stretch is necessary to directly help your cardiovascular system, but even doing bits throughout the day will help firm your muscles and trim some fat, and carrying less fat is a boon for your heart in its own right. Choose from running, swimming, biking, dancing, skating, cardio classes (they're getting more creative all the time), the treadmill, the stair-climber, the cross-trainer, and even walking around town or through the mall, as long as you walk like you mean it and do it on a regular basis.

Aim for thirty minutes six times a week, the recommendation supported by current research. You could do this with two lunch-hour jazz classes, Latin dancing two nights a week, and a couple of darned good walks. Or you could just ride a stationary bike or do time on the treadmill six mornings a week and be done with it. If you manage even three times a week, the old recommendation, good for you. This will grow on you—those happy chemicals the brain produces in response to vigorous activity are addictive in a safe and legal way—and you'll work up to more. Just keep at it: it will take years off your body and could add years to your life.

REJUVENATE YOURSELF WITH ACTION: *Plot out a reasonable regimen of aerobic exercise that makes sense in your life. If you're over fifty or have any history of heart disease, clear this with your doctor first.*

MARCH 17

Embracing the Tiger

Dede turned fifty-seven the year I was born and she moved in to care for me while my parents worked. She called movies *picture shows*. Buses were *streetcars* and their drivers *motormen*. We didn't *shop* at Joe's Market; we *traded* there. And when she referred to *the War*, she meant the war in which doughboys in foxholes were charged with making the world safe for democracy. Although Dede's antiquated vocabulary embarrassed me as a teenager, I see it now as oral history. When I recently suggested to my seventeen-year-old stepdaughter, Siân, that we meet at the *record* store, I realized that these days I'm the one sounding historical. It wasn't a shock really. I'm aware that I was alive before diet soda and panty-hose and even ZIP codes. Still, it was a reminder: I am bridging eras. Maybe that's why they call this middle age.

I can warm to certain aspects of this venerable status. I like remembering when people had Sunday dinners and took Sunday drives, when they saved a dollar a week in a Christmas club and got their groceries at places like Joe's Market. Having experienced that, and everything in between, the here and now makes more sense. It has roots and reasons. Besides, you have to reach a certain age before you can hope to enjoy the utopian state my baby-boomer age-mates christened as *having it all*. While you can be forty or sixty-five and feel as vibrant as you did years before, it isn't possible to be twenty and have the wisdom that only life experience bestows.

People who are full of vigor and enthusiasm in their seventies didn't get that way by resenting each passing year, being embarrassed about how long they've lived, or focusing on what the years take away and not what they give in return. They refuse to be intimidated by what is out of their control because they are firmly in charge of what is in their control. They take great care of themselves; some may even get a tweak here and there from a cosmetic surgeon. But they're not obsessed with themselves or how they look, and they certainly haven't been surgically pulled, tucked, and lifted into a caricature more reflective of panic and fear than of youth and beauty.

To be more like them, we can borrow the martial arts concept of "embracing the tiger." Instead of recoiling in fear from an opponent, whether the threat is a flesh-and-blood adversary or an invisible one like a particular birthday, *embrace the tiger*, embrace the fear, embrace the moment. When you do this, choices emerge. You're no longer a victim. You find your power.

It takes mettle to embrace the passage of time, something Western society—American society in particular—has turned into an especially vicious "tiger." A mature woman who looks fabulous and lives fully flies in the face of a consumer culture that suggests with almost every advertisement that beauty, desirability, and fun are only for her daughters and her memories. This is absurd. Let the advertisers do what they think they need to do in order to sell their products. You do what you need to do to live sublimely, crafting each day—*this* day—into a little piece of art.

REJUVENATE YOURSELF WITH ACTION: *What is it, in your heart of hearts, that concerns or even frightens you about growing older? Pick just one thing, but promise yourself it will be the thing. Once you know what your "tiger" is, make the decision to embrace it and let it teach you.*

MARCH 18

Luscious Lips

It probably shows my age that I don't understand the fascination with puffy, pouty, surgically enhanced lips. If these appeal to you, or if your lips seem to have thinned since your twenties, you can cheat your natural line a bit with a lip pencil. Also, some cosmetic shops sell topical solutions that can make your lips temporarily fuller. Then when thinner lips come back into fashion, which you know they will, you won't need reverse surgery.

Full lips or not, nobody wants hers flaky and peeling, so keep them moisturized, especially if you're inside with central heating or out in the March winds, and exfoliate once a week. I like using a cream lip exfoliator: you leave it on for ten minutes, and when you gently rub it off with a washcloth, dead skin goes, too. You can also *very lightly* exfoliate using a delicate, back-and-forth motion with a soft toothbrush. Either way, follow with a nourishing lip balm or vitamin E oil from a snipped gelcap.

Unless *au naturel* is your trademark, wear at least a little lip color almost all the time. It is a pick-me-up that means more in your forties and beyond than ever before. When I was eighteen, my roommate's mother invited me to join the two of them for breakfast. I declined, citing lack of makeup. She said, "Just put on a little lipstick and come with us." A little lipstick! Couldn't she see that I needed concealer and base and blush, liner and shadow and mascara? Now that I'm the age she was then, I get it. Lipstick and sun-block can be enough for the gym or the market or Saturday morning with the newspaper at a neighborhood café.

Obvious lip liner can look unnatural and outdated, but it does forestall lipstick's bleeding into the little creases that form around the mouth of a woman who's old enough to be interesting. One way to get liner's benefits without its shortcomings is to color the entire lip surface with the liner and top that with lipstick for a little shine. This also gives your lip color great staying power.

The pros always use a lip brush, and it's well worth developing the skill. The color will last longer and look more natural so applied, and since you're using less lipstick this way, it will be less likely to smudge. Some women like to have lots of lipsticks and team them with the colors they're wearing. I find that life is simpler when the lipstick on my dressing table is the same as the one in my purse: in the brown family October to March, pinker in spring and summer. However you like your lipstick wardrobe, don't get stuck in a shade. Your complexion changes over time and your lip color needs to keep up.

Follow every lipstick application with this trick from a TV makeup artist: put a tissue around your finger, put it in your mouth and pull it out as if it were a lollipop, removing any color from the inside edges of your lips that might otherwise wind up on your gorgeous teeth.

REJUVENATE YOURSELF WITH ACTION: *Buy yourself a new lipstick.*

MARCH 19

Creative Expression and the Only Brain You've Got

Much of the information we have about improving cognitive function comes from studying those who, tragically, have lost much of theirs. The definitive epidemiological study on Alzheimer's disease looked at nuns in several Midwestern convents. Because these women led almost identical lives, they were perfect subjects for studying the subtle differences between those who succumbed to dementia and those who didn't. One startling finding of this long-term investigation had to do with creative thinking and its off-spring, colorful verbal expression.

The researchers found a marked correlation between mental clarity in aged sisters and the level of descriptive expertise shown in mandatory biographical essays they had written around age twenty. Decreased cognitive functioning was widespread among those nuns whose early biographies had been grammatically perfect but stylistically ordinary, something like "I was born on a farm" versus "The blizzard blew fierce as Papa hitched the team to fetch the midwife."

The researchers in the Nun Study, a project beautifully documented in David Snowdon's book, *Aging with Grace*, cannot yet explain the mechanism by which this operates. It appears that creative thinkers are able to etch new neuro-pathways in their brains. Postmortem examinations bore this out: some verbally expressive nuns who had shown no signs of dementia were found, after death, to have in their brain tissue the "loops and tangles" indicative of Alzheimer's. They had apparently outwitted the disease by their ability to think and express themselves in inventive ways.

The Nun Study gave scientific backing to a suspicion others have long entertained, that some people may be able to protect their brainpower by using it creatively. Although there is no guarantee that someone without a predisposition toward colorful verbal expression can learn this, I am convinced as someone who has taught writing that almost anyone who's willing can develop the skill. It's like mental interior design: you start with merely functional and end up with stunning.

Begin with little word games you play silently by yourself. For instance, you take your niece to the park. As you watch her play, how many words can you come up with to describe her? Fresh, alive, innocent, alert, curious, energetic, animated, adorable—you get the idea. And, as you think your everyday thoughts, pick one and turn it from black-and-white language into glorious living color. Instead of just reminiscing, "Gosh, Hawaii was nice," vividly recall the blue ocean in the distance and the white waves lapping at the sand. *See* the ribbons of waterfall, *smell* the guavas in the rain forest, and *feel* the mist on your face and the mud between your toes.

When you tell friends about your trip, whether you're talking or writing, avoid generalities like "It was fun." Tell them instead about the sticky-sweet smell of the guavas and the soft, gooey coolness of that putty-like mud.

As you do this, your life becomes more deeply textured. You get to enjoy the best of it time and again because you can so accurately recreate it in story and memory. And you just might be carving pathways in your brain that will serve you well years and years after your week on Kauai.

REJUVENATE YOURSELF WITH ACTION: *Utilize your journal for practice in creative verbal expression. Since no one else has to read it, you don't need to feel silly about sounding flowery or overblown. Your brain will approve.*

MARCH 20
———————

The Vernal Equinox

In some traditional cultures, the first day of spring is the first day of the year. You can let it be another opportunity to begin again, with all the awakening power of nature on your side. At this change of seasons, and the others you'll meet this year, do something special to recognize a special time. For example:

- *Look for signs of spring.* Even if the weather isn't showing it yet, spectacular things are beginning to happen. Keep an eye peeled for crocuses, pussy willow, every indicator of nature coming to life.

- *Remember spring cleaning?* This is the week for clearing out, airing out, and making things fresh and new.

- *Play at the makeup counter.* New colors are there now for a seasonal change of face.

- *Do away with the winter body blahs.* You have three months until summer—there's plenty of time to tone your triceps.

- *Put some colors of the season into your life.* Pastels are looking right again. Invite some of them into your home and your wardrobe.

- *Treat yourself to flowers.* Even if they're not yet blooming in your garden, they can bloom on your desk and your kitchen table.

REVITALIZE YOUR LIFE WITH WORDS: *I am as filled with promise as the first day of spring.*

MARCH 21

Acknowledge Your Inner Warrior

Every Sunday night, Elizabeth calls her grandmother in California. They chat and say the rosary. "Grandma is ninety-seven and still living in her own house," Elizabeth told me. "Nobody's been able to get her into a nursing home: she's too full of spit and vinegar." Elizabeth's grandmother also exemplifies the personality type some researchers have pegged as longevity-prone: people who have a little grit to them, who stand up for themselves, and set strong, healthy boundaries. These are the folks nobody "walks all over." They are men and women who honor the warrior inside them.

This isn't about becoming a bully, being belligerent or hard to get along with. There are plenty of people who are hard to get along with and still don't know how to get their own needs met. Acknowledging your inner warrior is instead respecting yourself as well as others, knowing that you have as much right as anyone else to be here, do well, and defend that right. For example, should a doctor say to you, "Well, at your age there are just some things you have to put up with," it's your inner warrior that responds with, "Not until I get a darned good second opinion and try every alternative treatment that could help."

If you shy away from the thought of having a warrior within, realize that this is not a quality most of us were raised to honor or even recognize. Although we all have warrior potential, not every woman is born like the goddess Athena, fully armored with a helmet and shield—and those of us who were may have gotten more punishment than praise for it. For now, just think about how it would feel if you did salute the warrior within. Think about women you admire who show their warrior spirit. If you really want to get this piece, enroll in a women's self-defense class. After that experience, you'll know you have a warrior inside you.

There is no better time than this one for tapping into your warrior energy. Astrologically, this is the day the sun enters Aries, the sign that rules the warrior. This is also a time of tremendous power in nature, with the bursting forth of new life. Draw on this power today. Know that it sometimes takes a little fight to manifest a dream or bring forth a vision, although the fight is more often with your own doubts than with another person. Have your warrior poised and ready: she is as skilled at negotiation as she is at battle.

REJUVENATE YOURSELF WITH ACTION: *Think of your inner warrior today. Write about this quality in your journal. And if you've never taken a course in self-defense, look in the Yellow Pages or online for what is offered in your area. For this purpose, a short-term class in self-defense for women, one that actually simulates attack situations, is more efficient than traditional martial arts training.*

MARCH 22

Vitamin E

In *Stop Aging Now!*, an excellent guide to nutrients and rejuvenation, noted health writer Jean Carper calls vitamin E "the vitamin you *must* take to delay aging." Red blood cells require it, as do muscles; and the body is unable to efficiently break down fats without it. Vitamin E is also essential for a healthy heart. It promotes immune function, helps regulate blood glucose levels, can reverse fibrocystic changes in the breasts, and may guard against cataracts. There is some evidence that it may help relieve arthritis symptoms, as the antioxidant properties of vitamins such as E and C appear to protect joint cartilage.

Wheat germ is one of the best food sources of vitamin E, and although it is also found in vegetable oils, nuts, seeds, and whole grains, getting enough from food to help you grow younger is close to impossible. Therefore, a supplement of 100 to 400 IU daily in the form of "mixed tocopherols," either alone or in combination with the more expensive but highly touted "tocotrienols," is recommended.

REJUVENATE YOURSELF WITH ACTION: *If you're not already taking vitamin E, this could be the day to start. As always, if you're under a doctor's care, consult him or her before adding a new supplement to your regimen. Vitamin E is contraindicated for people on blood-thinning medications or those with bleeding problems; and if you'll be having any surgery, including a cosmetic procedure, lay off vitamin E for two weeks beforehand.*

MARCH 23

Every Breath You Take

It's the common thread between the runner and the dancer, the Wyoming rancher who hikes every morning and the Wall Street trader who takes a yoga class before the opening bell. They breathe more deeply and more consciously than most of the rest of us. They treat themselves to extra oxygen, and that leads to bright eyes, clear skin, a fitter body, increased energy, and a better mood.

If you do aerobic exercise, you can't help but take in more oxygen; *pranayama*, the breathing exercises in yoga class, can get you to the graduate program in breathing. Paying attention to the way you breathe in everyday life is important, too, especially if you're not exercising or doing yoga as regularly as you'd like. In her fascinating book *Jumpstart Your Metabolism*, author Pam Grout focuses on how learning to breathe deeply and exhale fully can help people lose weight by correcting a slow metabolism, improving digestion, and altering the attitudes that lead to binge eating and exercise anathema. She states that 90 percent of us engage in some form of "futile breathing" (taking in only a quarter or less of the oxygen our lungs can hold).

Breathing exercises, whether you learn them through yoga, through martial arts, in a stress management class, or by reading a book, can put you on the road to better breathing. A very basic but very helpful exercise is yogic three-part breathing. To do this, sit comfortably with your back straight and understand that you'll be breathing in by expanding your belly. You can put your hand on your abdomen to be sure you manage this. It's hard for some women because we've been sucking our stomachs in for thirty years, but this is a time when expansion is right and necessary. When your abdomen is fully expanded, continue to fill your diaphragm and finally your chest (those are parts two and three of the three-part breath). Then exhale fully. Focus on the exhalation, squeezing your abdomen at the end of the practice (squeezing we're used to, right?) to push out the last bit of stale air.

Do this slowly and gently; you don't want to hyperventilate. Just practice enough until you feel comfortable with slow, deep inhalations and exhalations that go all the way to your belly. This exercise, like most breathing in your daily life, should be done through the nose, the orifice designed for breathing and constructed to purify the air as it passes through the nostrils. Unless you're already involved in a daily discipline that includes deep breathing, Grout suggests taking ten slow, deep, conscious breaths every day. You can do this when you awaken in the morning, at night before bed, outside during your lunch hour, or before your meditation. Practicing even once a day will positively influence your breathing the rest of the time.

REJUVENATE YOURSELF WITH ACTION: *How is your breathing? If you take a standard breath and your lower abdomen stays flat, you aren't breathing deeply enough. Do yogic three-part breathing once a day, ten breaths in and ten fully out, every day this week. You just might want to keep it up.*

MARCH 24

Understand Free Radicals

You're eating lots of veggies and taking vitamin supplements in hopes that their antioxidant properties will do away with the ill effects of free radicals on your body. But what are these cellular rogues with a name that sounds like political extremists who broke out of jail? Chemically, a free radical is an oxygen molecule with a missing electron. In its quest to right itself, it filches an electron from another molecule, rendering that one damaged, too. When this happens enough, it can result in ill effects from wrinkles to cancer. Some theorists believe that free radicals cause *all* the signs of aging.

We cannot keep free radicals from forming, because many of them are the natural byproducts of cells going about their business. I liken them to the clutter generated by a craft project or the mess in the kitchen left after preparing a multi-course meal. Our normal and necessary use of oxygen creates free radicals; consequently, the exercise that is doing so much to make you younger is also increasing your need for antioxidants. Stress, air pollution, chemicals in the food and water, cigarette smoke (even the secondhand kind), and alcohol in excess of one to two drinks a day create additional free radicals in the body.

These are a problem, however, only when they're not cleaned up—like ignoring that disorderly sewing room or dirty kitchen. The antioxidants in fresh fruits and vegetables and in supplements such as vitamin C, vitamin E, and beta-carotene comprise the cleaning crew. It is undisputed that eating large amounts of fresh fruits and vegetables provides antioxidants that do away with free-radical damage. The evidence supporting supplementation is less telling, but the majority of scientists working in this area seem to be recommending both a diet heavy on produce and supplements just in case.

REJUVENATE YOURSELF WITH ACTION: *Consider writing down what you eat for a week, just to be sure you're getting all the fruits and vegetables you think you are. Recommendations range from five to ten servings a day, with the emphasis on vegetables.*

MARCH 25

Accept Your Authority

Who's in charge here? When it comes to your life, your body, and your decisions, *you* are. This implies responsibility, of course, but it's also freeing to realize that no one who gives a lecture or writes a book (including this one), and not even some professional with walls covered in diplomas, is more of an expert on you than you yourself are. This is true to a large extent throughout your life, but now, with the experience you have behind you and your intuition going full tilt, your level of authority on matters pertaining to yourself is at its zenith.

Like a powerful corporation, you engage advisors and consultants. Hopefully, you choose them carefully and they're worth the price of the book or the ticket or the office visit. It would be foolhardy to dismiss out of hand the counsel you receive from knowledgeable people. Still, the ultimate decision is always yours, because the ultimate authority is always you.

This is hard to grasp when you're young and your default setting is to feel less qualified than someone who outshines you in education or reputation. Even so, none of these shining people has earned a Y.O.U. degree. You have—with honors. It's high time to start respecting your own credentials. This will keep you from blindly following the advice of every expert, genuine or spurious, who comes down the pike or over the airwaves. It will help you make wise choices about physicians and therapists, lawyers and financial advisors, because if one of them doesn't feel right for you, he (or she) probably isn't.

Too many women spend too many years in awe of authority figures. That's easier than being an authority yourself. But you are one. Accept your authority today. Exercise it wisely and well.

REVITALIZE YOUR LIFE WITH WORDS: *I receive valid guidance from qualified people, always remembering that I am the ultimate authority on myself and my life.*

MARCH 26

Firsthand Protein

One thing I did right all along was get my protein firsthand—i.e., from eating plants instead of animals. Then, even when menopause hit me like the proverbial tons of bricks, my really important parts—cholesterol, HDLs and LDLs, blood pressure, homocysteine, and body weight—were still okay.

I must admit to some personal bias here since I am a vegetarian for ethical reasons. I decided years ago that if I couldn't kill an animal myself, it wasn't right to expect someone else to do it for me. I liked, as Franz Kafka once said after he stopped eating meat, being able to look a cow in the eye. And if the yogic texts are true in claiming that this kind of diet aids spiritual growth, that's a bonus. Whether I eat the very healthiest diet, I don't know. Maybe being mostly vegetarian and eating a little meat, or at least fish, is ideal. For me, it doesn't matter, since a little meat is a whole animal. You may have other sensibilities. Still, from a health and longevity viewpoint alone, getting most of your protein firsthand makes sense. Here's why:

- Obesity is one of the biggest threats to youthfulness and long life. Vegans are, on average, fifteen pounds lighter than meat-eaters.

- Plant foods are cholesterol-free and, with a few exceptions (like coconut and palm oils), contain no saturated fat. This bodes well for heart health and prevention of atherosclerosis and stroke.

- The fats in meat and dairy products accumulate environmental and industrial chemicals, some of which are known carcinogens. In this case, the fat itself is less a worry than what it has collected.

- Epidemiological studies, those that look at population groups, invariably give vegetarians the edge. Seventh Day Adventists are often study subjects since about half of them are vegetarian and half aren't. Otherwise, they live similar lives—no smoking or drinking, for instance. In these studies, the vegetarians come out ahead on virtually all indicators of health (fat-to-lean body-mass ratio, cholesterol level, blood pressure, etc.).

- Population groups that include meat in the diet but in much less quantity and frequency than is typical in North America or the UK have a markedly lower incidence of degenerative disease. The Mediterranean diet and the traditional Japanese diet are examples of these.

Despite the popularity in some circles of high-animal-protein diets, these foods are hard to digest, especially as we age and produce less hydrochloric acid. Breaking down meat into its usable components is hard work for a body, one reason people who start to eat less of it find they have more stamina than they did before. The average woman needs about fifty-five grams of protein a day, an amount easily obtained from plant foods. A varied diet with an assortment of vegetables, beans, and whole grains ensures a complete amino acid profile.

You already know that lightening up your attitude will help you grow younger. This is a way to lighten up what's going on in your digestive tract. It can help you grow younger, too.

REJUVENATE YOURSELF WITH ACTION: *Many women find themselves feeling leaner, lighter, and more youthful when they commit to eating two vegetarian meals a day and having one vegetarian day a week. Consider this for yourself. If you'd like to know more, I recommend* The Eat to Live Diet *by Joel Fuhrman, MD, and* Being Vegetarian for Dummies *by Suzanne Havala, DrPH, RD.*

MARCH 27

Give Yourself a Trademark or Two

It will add to your mystique and your reputation if you give yourself a trademark or two. It could be a pin on your lapel or a flower in your buttonhole, the fact that you often wear yellow or maintain a flawless French manicure. Perhaps you host a particular party every year or you're so dependable a feature in the 10K run for kids with leukemia that everybody knows you'll be there.

I have a friend named Linda whose clothing is all vintage and another friend named Linda whose entire wardrobe is designer. One Elizabeth in my life is famous for being able to give you the astrological significance of whatever is going on, while another Elizabeth is renowned for writing poetry. One Barbara bicycles enough that it's one of her trademarks; another has made her trademark out of interpreting fairy tales—*Cinderella* in particular—and applying their meaning to our lives.

Your trademarks can be serious or frivolous; they can have a purpose or be just for fun. Either way, they'll remind people of you and give you a timeless quality in their minds. Your trademarks are less for other people, however, than they are for you. They're reliable symbols of who you are, even when circumstances are behaving in unreliable ways. In the year since you last did that 10K, for example, you may have lost a good friend, taken on a stressful job, and moved to a neighborhood where you're still not quite at home, but you know you'll be at that race, no matter what—French manicure and all.

REJUVENATE YOURSELF WITH ACTION: *What are your trademarks, those attributes or activities that symbolize you? If you were to come up with a new one, what would it be?*

MARCH 28

Do It Your Way

It's time. You've earned it. Start doing things your way.

I don't mean always getting your way in insignificant affairs like where the milk goes in the fridge or what TV show to watch this Tuesday night. But when it comes to matters that matter to you— where you live, the work you do, or a health-care decision—your liveliness, even your longevity, may depend on having your say and getting your way.

Human beings require autonomy as well as community. This can be a difficult balance. Peace of mind, not to mention peace on earth, demands that we listen to one another, respect others' opinions, and sometimes put our wishes on hold for the benefit of a family, company, or community. But when we listen so well that we give up talking, when we respect others so unquestioningly that we forget to insist on respect in return, when we forfeit having it our way in all issues more momentous than style of burger, we lose ourselves and we age like crazy. Only serious illness or repetitive grief can make a woman older faster than losing herself in this way.

Suzanne, a wise and wonderful friend of mine, told me when she heard I was writing this book: "Every woman has lost a part of herself. Let her know she can get some of that back." And you can. You get it back every time you stand up for yourself, speak up for yourself, and make your choice, whether it's a popular choice or not.

There are many ways to get a job done. In your own life, your way is often the best.

REVITALIZE YOUR LIFE WITH WORDS: *I am gracious and generous, and when I need to, I get my way.*

Become Politically Aware and Maybe Even Active

Idealism is disproportionately found among those twenty-five and younger and those of retirement age and over. Even in the time-crunched years between, however, we would do well to look at becoming politically aware and perhaps even politically active. This leads to growing younger because it takes us out of ourselves and possibly back to our own younger days of idealistic involvement in some cause or another. Moreover, it can make our lives count for something beyond our personal concerns.

Don't let the word "political" get in the way. It only means "of the people." When you're politically aware, you know about the issues facing the people in your city, your country, and the world, which has shrunk so in our lifetime. To be politically aware, you do not have to stuff yourself on the hash and rehash of the daily news. You just need to be cognizant of the major issues and where you stand in regard to them.

Being politically active scares some people. They worry that "activist" is tantamount to "radical." It's not at all. Author Alice Walker put it beautifully when she wrote: "Activism is my rent for living on this planet." I think many of us could look at our lives today and see that the rent is due. Being politically active can be as simple as choosing one or two issues that either tug at your heart or bore into your intellect. These are *your* issues. With the time available and the resources at hand, what can you do about them?

My current role model for political activism is the fellow diner who approached my friend Hilary and me at a restaurant. She said, "Excuse me. You look like good women. I thought you might be interested in this," and she handed us each cards about some work being done by the United Nations on behalf of women and children. I was grateful to receive the card and learn about some simple ways I could help. Beyond that, though, I admired the woman who made the effort. Hilary and I could have been rude or brushed her off, but she took that chance. She could have been strident or pushy or disrespectful of our time or space, but she wasn't. She inspired me.

The world has probably always been a dangerous place. People of my generation and younger have lived with the nuclear threat all our lives; now there are other threats besides. None of us alone can solve such enormous problems, but each of us working in our own way can do a little something. It feels fantastic to think that maybe, just maybe, your grassroots efforts can be part of some big-picture change.

REJUVENATE YOURSELF WITH ACTION: *Devote a little time today to thinking about some of the issues facing our world or your community. As you go over them in your mind, which ones seem most pressing, or most relevant, or most personal to you? What would you do about them if you had unlimited power? What can you do about them—or even one of them—with the power you've got?*

MARCH 30

Play Day!

MARCH 31

The Need for Natural Cosmetics

The skin is a functioning organ that absorbs much of what you put on it. For this reason, you can't be too careful when choosing makeup and skin-care products. I've read that in the case of lipstick, the average woman can consume four pounds of it in her lifetime. It had better be good enough to eat.

We may not have much control over polluted air, or sometimes even the food we eat, but we have absolute control over what lipstick and foundation we buy, and what cleanser and moisturizer we use. According to the US General Accounting Office, there are 125 potentially carcinogenic ingredients legally found in toiletries. The best way to avoid these, short of becoming cosmetically celibate, is to stick with those companies that have built their reputations on manufacturing natural, high-quality cosmetics. Many of these exist—Origins, Dr. Hauschka, Aubrey Organics, Arbonne, Aveda, and The Body Shop, among others—and their products come in all price ranges except scrape-the-barrel cheap.

Companies like these have a commitment to the environment. Most support humanitarian causes and test their products for safety without using animals. I like being part of that. If you're going to take the high road in your life, why not take the high road in the cosmetics department? Besides, it's hard for me to imagine that a product with cruelty or indifference in its history is going to make me beautiful, at least not the kind of beautiful I'd care to be.

Many women find that when they switch to using natural cosmetics, they start to look forward to putting on makeup and taking it off, in a way they never did before. True, these products are pleasant to use and they smell scrumptious without relying on artificial perfumes. But beyond that, there is a satisfying compatibility between natural products and natural beings—i.e., between what we put on our bodies and our bodies themselves. The more you eat natural foods, the more drawn you'll be to natural cosmetics. Or begin with the cosmetics and see what happens to your taste in food. It doesn't matter so much where you start as that you do.

REJUVENATE YOURSELF WITH ACTION: *Check your makeup case and medicine cabinet for what you're low on—cleanser, moisturizer, mascara, shampoo. Promise yourself that you'll replace it with the purest version you can find. Do this with one item at a time until all your makeup and beauty and grooming products are as natural as can be.*

April

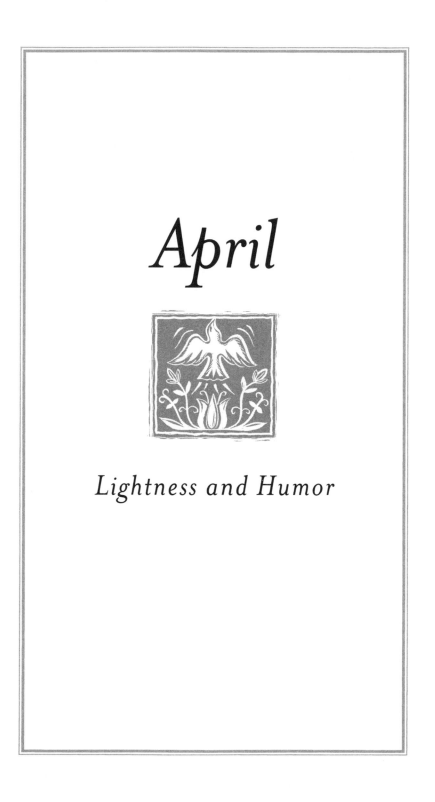

Lightness and Humor

Get the Joke

I don't know if it's true around the world, but in America anyway, this is April Fool's Day. It's not a major holiday—I mean, even the post office stays open—but it is a day devoted to practical jokes and silly fun. If every day were so designated, we'd all feel a whole lot younger, so let's you and I assign to April the dual keynotes of lightness and humor.

Psychologists and physicians are learning that humor can be good medicine. It's known to lower blood pressure, and research has shown time and again that laughing is an immunity-building exercise, measurably increasing the number of on-duty immune cells. There are even official bodies like the American Association for Therapeutic Humor and the International Society for Humor Studies—which sound funny in themselves if you think about it.

Get the joke today and in all the days to come by valuing wit, light-heartedness, and every reason to laugh that comes up. Recognize the humor inherent in just about any circumstance and point it out when your companions are suffering from pathological dourness. Make a point of hanging with upbeat people—not necessarily the class clown grown up, but at least those who can recognize the punchline in a joke or the irony in a situation. Visit the bookstore's humor section or download jokes from the Internet.

Become a connoisseur of the cartoons in magazines and newspapers. I have a friend who covers her fridge with them, and visitors gravitate there for guaranteed chuckles. You can also watch funny movies and TV shows. Choose the style of buffoonery you appreciate: if slapstick annoys you or off-color jokes offend you, avoid those; there's plenty of humor left. Go to comedy clubs. (You can call ahead to find out who's on and the kind of humor he or she is known for.) And if you think you're pretty funny yourself, take a class in stand-up or improv. You'll laugh a lot, often at yourself.

REJUVENATE YOURSELF WITH ACTION: *Get in on the joke today. Somehow, some way, have yourself at least one really good laugh.*

APRIL 2

Shut Off the Worry Machine

Young people tend to live in the future with fantastic daydreams. Older people, unfortunately, too often trade daydreaming for worrying, living in the future in a negative way. This drags them down, sets their face in a frown, and makes them age more than free radicals and abdominal fat do, because it pervades the entire being, body, mind, and spirit.

Worry is not facing facts, dealing with problems, being realistic, or taking charge. It is instead a thumbing of the nose at every natural law except Murphy's, the one that says that anything that can go wrong will. I take exception: things most often go wrong when we expect them to.

Worry is a dreadful waste of energy. Since it is usually about something that either never happens, or over which we have absolutely no control, we invest valuable time and brainpower in a shadow. When we need this energy for real situations, it's used up. Thankfully, worry is a habit, not an incurable disease, even though we can catch it from other worriers, particularly key figures in our early lives. It gets switched on like a machine, and unless we make the effort to turn it off, it just keeps going. Most of us have worry triggers: a woman might, for example, deal valiantly with fire and flood, but throw her the specter of losing a job or losing a man and her worry machine can shift into high gear.

If you're this woman, breathe—slowly, deeply, breathing in the suggestion that you're safe and you're smart and this thing, whatever it is, will not get the better of you. Then talk it out, not with another worrier who can find layers of awfulness you hadn't even thought of, but somebody sane and solid and positive, someone who can see a way out when you see only the way down. Walk or run or swim, to work the worry out of your muscles. Take superb care of yourself: fear and anxiety prefer the company of the minimally nurtured. If some salient action will help defuse this particular worry, take it. Then bring yourself firmly into the present moment, a moment in which something may well need doing, but in which there is nothing to worry about at all.

REJUVENATE YOURSELF WITH ACTION: *If you can't stop worrying right away, at least give up respecting it and excusing it; it won't get you anywhere but older.*

APRIL 3

The Drama Queen Has Left the Building

A drama queen makes a jumbo incident out of one that is really just small, medium, or large. Everything is personal to her, and everything is somebody's fault—somebody who is supposed to make restitution. Favorite drama queen lines include, "This is just not acceptable," "I'm going to report this," "You haven't heard the last from me," and "This absolutely could not be worse," ideally shouted, voiced in a whine, or, for a particular type of DQ, accompanied by tears.

Nobody likes a drama queen, but some people will put up with her as long she's young and cute. Once that's history, DQ behavior is simply humiliating. It's also an immediate pro-ager: a drama queen adds ten years just by opening her mouth—fifteen when she actually says something. A drama queen asks for the spotlight, but it's a glaring, unflattering light that exacerbates every negative feature of maturity and erases the positive ones. If I sound hard on the DQ, it's because I have to fight those tendencies in myself to keep from being a royal pain in the neck. I'm not proud of it, but having had experience with it, I do have a few suggestions for overcoming it. Should you ever find yourself becoming embarrassingly regal, remember:

- *You are one person among millions, not the center of the universe.* This one is hard if you were an only child as I was, but nobody looking at us today sees a child, so it's time to get over it.

- *Whatever has you infuriated was most likely not directed at you.* The dry-cleaning wasn't ready in time for the meeting. The package didn't arrive. The train was late. The only magazine in the doctor's office was *Sports Illustrated.* Any one of these can be irritating, but none is personal.

- *Your fellow humans screw up a lot.* When you stop expecting perfection from the commoners, you'll go easier on them and on yourself.

- *Bad days last twenty-four hours, just like other days.* This is great news since, in DQ mode, a bad day is a life sentence.

- *It's a big world out there.* If you can focus on something outside yourself, somebody else's problem that is huge by any reckoning, whatever seems irritating enough to make this the worst thing that ever happened will shrink quite a bit.

REJUVENATE YOURSELF WITH ACTION: *Be on the lookout for drama queen behavior in yourself and others. When it's yours, nip it in its monarchical bud.*

APRIL 4

A Carb Is Not a Carb Is Not a Carb

One theory of aging suggests that certain carbohydrates keep the body's insulin levels too high, leading to overweight, type II diabetes, and inflammatory conditions such as osteoarthritis and even cancer. Generally speaking, those "certain carbohydrates" are the highly refined staples of the SAD (standard American diet): sugary snacks and desserts, refined flour products (white bread, white crackers, cereal with less nutrition than the box it comes in), along with fattened-up carbs like chips and fries.

Most carbohydrate foods that come from nature, however, are not just exempt from the bad rap carbs have been getting lately;

they promote good health. These include the vast majority of fruits, vegetables, and unrefined (whole) grains. The fiber in fruit slows down the digestion of its natural sugars, and vegetables and whole grains are complex carbohydrates that tend to metabolize more slowly than sweets or refined starches.

There are some exceptions we've learned about from the GI (Glycemic Index), a fairly new classification of carbs based on how speedily they break down and elevate blood glucose levels. White potatoes, for example, have a high GI (meaning they break down into their component sugars more rapidly than other vegetables, including, surprisingly, sweet potatoes). I personally don't do much with the Glycemic Index since meals tend to balance themselves out: I might have a potato, but when that potato is in the company of grilled tempeh and a green salad with oil-and-vinegar dressing, the meal's GI is fine, even though it includes one high-GI component. If you're diabetic or your doctor has told you that you're glucose-intolerant, you may want to look into the Glycemic Index. Otherwise, keep things simple. Choose cereals made from barley, oats, or bran, and substantial breads made with the whole wheat kernel or rye seed before it's been ground into flour. I think of these as medieval peasant foods, chewy and hearty. Enjoy fruits and vegetables (okay, not so many potatoes maybe), give junk food the boot, and dine with gusto and gratitude.

REVITALIZE YOUR LIFE WITH WORDS: *A carb is not a carb is not a carb.*

APRIL 5

One Superior Stylist

In the search for a hair expert, as in the search for a mate, you can't be too careful. I spent two years in New York City, a place presumably overflowing with excellent hair-cutters, before I found Denise Ruidant, a young woman who understands my hair, how I want it to look, and how to bring that about. She translates trends in such a way that I can be current without looking like I think I'm in high school, and although she's young, she doesn't treat me like I should be put out to pasture with a can of hair spray and some curlers.

If you haven't found your Denise, get recommendations from friends or strangers whose haircuts you like. The services of a genius don't often come cheap, but some of the budget chain salons have training programs that rival those of the designer places, so it is conceivable that the cut you fancy came at a reasonable price. Whatever you plan to pay, if you're not adventurous about your hair, book a consultation, not a cut. See if you like this person. Rapport is important. And bring pictures. Even the best hairdresser isn't psychic, and describing something visual can be tough. Although it's unrealistic to think you'll look like the model in the picture—she's a different person and she has different hair—this will at least give your stylist something to go on.

Once you establish rapport, keep it. Be honest. Your hair stylist would rather redo a cut than have you tell all your friends, "I don't know what happened: he used to be so good." This person, like your doctors and your yoga teacher and everybody else on your growing-younger team, wants you to be the best you can be. Help him or her by being clear, courteous, and on time, and by tipping enough to show your appreciation, especially when your stylist goes the extra mile for you. All relationships are worth taking care of, and if you ever want to be seen without a hat, this one is no exception.

REJUVENATE YOURSELF WITH ACTION: *If your hairdresser is fabulous, show your appreciation—flowers or goodies sent to the salon, or a funny card expressing your thanks. If you don't have a fabulous hairdresser at the moment, get recommendations from everyone you see whose hair you like. If more than one person recommends the same stylist, you've hit pay dirt.*

APRIL 6

Introducing Leela

Leela is a Sanskrit term that translates as "God's play." It's seeing the vastness of creation as the Divine's favorite toy, and suggesting that, if there is playfulness indelibly etched into the cosmos, it's probably okay for us to lighten up, too.

When everything seems serious and quite a bit seems ominous, when we feel a lot of fear and carry a lot of tension, we're way out of touch with *leela*, the sense of humor of the universe. You know how it is when things go badly in a way that is almost comedic? *Leela.* When you think, "I may as well laugh because otherwise I'd cry"? *Leela.* When you play with a child or a pet or a half-off coupon at your favorite store and are not one bit concerned about all the "things on your mind," *leela* is operative. It shows up in sentences like "I don't have to worry about this now—let's go out and have fun." *Leela* allows you to chuckle on a rotten day, see beauty in the midst of pain, and find the game inside the dilemma.

Now, if you just miss a bus and it's pouring rain, you can think *leela* and shrug it off instead of ranting about never getting any breaks and catching your death of cold. Should you print a lengthy document and find your numbering is off by a page, you can write it off as *leela*, know your grandkids will get 123 sheets of scribble paper, and print again without going down the spiral of, "I have to do all the grunt work. . . . This isn't why I went to college. . . . This kind of thing only happens to me."

Just knowing *leela* as a word and a concept will help you live with less effort and age with less speed. When you get friendly with *leela*, you'll be lighter of heart and younger in spirit, because you'll be seeing so much of what other people find trying as simply God's play.

REJUVENATE YOURSELF WITH ACTION: *Keep* leela *in mind as you go about your day and your week. When something crops up that looks like a manifestation of* leela, *the playfulness or the irony of life, acknowledge it for what it is. When appropriate, get a little laughter out of it.*

APRIL 7

Change Your Pocketbook

I sometimes think the last unencumbered day of a woman's life is the one before the handbag becomes mandatory. Once you carry a purse, you're responsible for producing on demand a pen or a phone number, a tissue or a breath mint. How can you whirl around a dance floor or breeze through a meadow into the arms of your own true love if you're clutching a clutch, heaving a tote, or bearing a backpack? That's probably why there is more whirling and breezing in movies and commercials than in unscripted, unchoreographed life.

Since we seem destined to shoulder a bag just about every day of our adulthood, the least we can do is make it a lovely bag, housing contents that are well chosen and regularly weeded out. At times in our lives, there is the valid need to carry a book satchel or a diaper bag, but when school is out and the baby has become a child, it's time to downsize.

Now some women love purses—all sizes, all kinds. My friend Leslie is like that. She splurges on purses as if they were shoes. I, on the other hand, have figured out how to get cash, cards, comb, compact, lipstick, toothbrush, pen, and portable phone into the various compartments of a clever little purse that measures just seven inches by four. If you're like Leslie and have lots of pocketbooks, I suggest you display them proudly; stuff them with newspaper when they're shelved so that they keep their shape; and change them often to suit your mood and the occasion. If you're more like me, find a bag you adore (it will be with you for awhile) and clean it out at least once a week. This is important, because carrying around what you don't need weighs on you, both practically and psychically. Snack wrappers, useless receipts, and discarded tissues have no business hanging on your arm. Dispose of them. See yourself whirling and breezing.

Youth is about living lightly, and you can't live lightly if your daily load rivals that of Santa on Christmas Eve. Refrain from hauling anything you don't actually use when you're away from home. Devote part of a drawer at the office and a portion of your car's glove compartment to emergency items you'd otherwise be lugging around like mandatory ID. Decide what you need to have with you at all times. Trust that you will survive, and thrive, without the rest.

REJUVENATE YOURSELF WITH ACTION: *Reassess your relationship with your handbag. Do you love it? Is it in good shape? How heavy is it? Would you be embarrassed if someone you admired looked inside? If you're not happy with what's on your arm, make changes regarding the bag itself or its contents.*

Restful Sleep

It was formerly believed that we require less sleep as we age, but the current thinking is that older people sleep less because of unresolved health issues that interfere with their sleep, not because they actually need less of it. Unless you know that you're in the minority that thrives on six or seven hours' sleep, try for the standard eight. If that's not enough, allow for eight and a half or more. That only sounds excessive: at the turn of the last century, people slept an average of ten hours a night.

It can be harder to get a good night's sleep when you're older and the pineal gland produces less sleep-promoting melatonin; menopausal hot flashes and physical pain or discomfort can be merciless sleep-disturbers as well. If you have serious trouble falling asleep or staying asleep, see your health-care provider; you may need a referral to a sleep specialist. This is too important to overlook.

If you don't have a sleep disorder but you could use a little more of it, homespun wisdom should suffice. Arise and retire on schedule, whether you're actually sleeping the whole time or not. Drink warm milk or calcium-fortified soy milk at bedtime and take your calcium/magnesium supplements then, too. The scent of lavender, the pure essential oil or creams and inhalers made with it, is an olfactory lullaby. Consciously tensing and then relaxing every muscle, toes to scalp, can put the body in the mood for sleep. So can the delicious release of an orgasm.

Soporific herbal teas like chamomile and licorice are also relaxing, especially if you enjoy them as part of a dependable nighttime ritual. Like the bath-and-back-rub, story-and-prayers ritual you devised for your children, a ritual of nighttime grooming, spiritual practice, and reading something scrumptious is dessert at the end of a day. Your ritual will become a wordless hypnotic suggestion to your body and brain that it's time to let sleep take over. You can also affirm a good night's sleep: "I fall asleep easily, sleep through the night, and awaken full of life and energy." Sweet dreams.

REVITALIZE YOUR LIFE WITH WORDS: *I fall asleep easily, sleep through the night, and awaken full of life and energy.*

Fresh Juices

If you eat lots and lots of fresh fruits, salads, and steamed vegetables, your need for fresh juices is far less pronounced than that of someone on a diet of processed foods. I suggest you consider fresh juices anyway. They are an infusion of health: a concentration of vitamins, minerals, phytochemicals, and enzymes you can almost feel your body using to your benefit.

When I say "fresh juices," I don't mean the ones in cans and bottles. By law, all juices, even those whose containers state, "Not from Concentrate," have to be pasteurized—i.e., heated to a high temperature. This decreases the vitamin content, kills the enzymes, and erases the less tangible but still vital sense of "aliveness" in the resulting juice. To get genuinely fresh (and exceedingly delicious) fruit and vegetable juices, you need to either frequent a juice bar or invest in a juicer.

If you're in the market for a juicer, compare prices in health food stores, discount stores, and department stores, as well as online and in catalogs. You can save a lot with a used one. Many people give up on juicing and sell nearly new juicers online, through the classifieds, or by hanging a notice on a health food store bulletin board. Wherever you get your juicer, research the brand and model. My two criteria are power and ease of cleaning. When a juicer isn't powerful enough, it won't extract ample juice, so you'll end up using more veggies and spending more money than you need to. If your machine is a nuisance to clean, you won't juice often enough to realize the benefits. (More people sell juicers because they're sick of cleaning them than for any other reason. Be sure when you get one secondhand that you're not purchasing somebody else's problem.)

Once you're in possession of a well-functioning juicer, start with one glass (eight ounces) of fresh juice daily; if you like it, work up to two or even three glasses. Any more than that and juice may crowd out whole vegetables with their necessary fiber. I do well with one or sometimes two glasses of fresh vegetable juice or a vegetable-fruit blend every day. Sometimes I have fresh juice before breakfast, and a 3:00 P.M. juice break to forestall the energy slump that might otherwise occur then.

It's a good idea to dilute fruit juice half-and-half with spring water to cut its sweetness. Otherwise, use apple, citrus, or carrot juice (although from a vegetable, carrot juice is quite sweet) as the mild base for mixed juice cocktails that include powerful green juices that are important nutritionally but would taste too strong and be too potent by themselves. Sample mixtures are carrot/celery (juice four carrots, one stalk of celery), carrot/apple/parsley (three carrots, one apple, a small handful of parsley), carrot/beet/spinach (five carrots, one beet, one handful of fresh spinach), apple/cucumber/ kale (three apples, two cucumbers, one handful of fresh kale). All measurements are approximate. Experiment. If your drink is bitter or overpowering, you've used too many greens and not enough of the milder fruits or vegetables. If it's very sweet, toss in a few more greens next time.

REJUVENATE YOURSELF WITH ACTION: *If you haven't already, discover fresh juice today. Try different blends at a juice bar, and before long, if you're game, get yourself a juicer. Ideally, you'll enjoy a glass of fresh juice every day this week. (If you are diabetic or on a special diet for another medical condition, check with your physician about whether or not juices are appropriate for you.)*

APRIL 10

The Ten Commandments
of Post-Forty Makeup

1. *Thou shalt not make foundation a mask.* Use it to cover imperfections and discolorations, and use meticulous skin care (and perhaps the services of a dermatologist) to improve them.

2. *Match foundation to your face and neck.* A lot of women judge their facial skin as lighter than it is and choose too light a foundation. Even worse is foundation that's too dark and looks like self-tanner that ended at your chin.

3. *Go easy on blush.* Choose your color carefully and avoid bright pink. Use a good-sized brush (not the little one that comes in the

compact) to apply a bit less blush than you think you need. Clown cheeks add years.

4. *Apply lipstick carefully.* You're better off with clear gloss than a swipe of lipstick that doesn't follow the contours of your mouth and looks like an afterthought.

5. *Play up either your eyes or your lips, not both.* If your eye makeup is dramatic, use a more understated lip color; go light on the eyes if your lips are vamp red.

6. *Leave glitter, metallics, and glaring pastels to the prom and dance club crowds.* A young girl can look dazzling when something she does with her clothes or makeup jumps out and surprises you; a mature woman looks beautiful when she invites you to study her nuances.

7. *Know the ABCs of eye shadow.* A: Cover your entire lid surface with a light, neutral shadow or, ideally, a shadow base. B: Smooth a sheer color, one that doesn't shout, on your eyelid. C: Provide contrast with a deeper shade in the crease of your lid, and highlight with a lighter shade on the brow bone.

8. *Use eyeliner pencil you can purposely smudge.* (If you have 20/20 vision and a very steady hand, ignore this one and carry on with your liquid liner.)

9. *Thou shalt dab thy mascara tip.* Always clean the clump off the tip of the wand with a tissue, lest that clump befall your lashes. A bit of shadow base applied just under your lower lashes will help defray smudges, too.

10. *When in doubt, go easy.* It's not often that you hear someone criticized for wearing too *little* makeup. This is one case in which less is, decidedly, more.

REJUVENATE YOURSELF WITH ACTION: *Choose one of the commandments you haven't been doing and make a habit of it this week. (If you're a no-makeup woman, you've got yourself an extra play day.)*

Eliminate Everything That Weighs You Down

We know longevity is compromised when a body carries too much weight, but what about when a *life* carries too much weight? When a woman's rooms and storage places, her car and her purse, her desk and her calendar are so full there's hardly room for the person in her own picture? She won't feel young and free, that's for sure. And she'll have to work more to pay for this collection of miscellany, not to mention being sure that it's polished or pressed or put away.

There is nothing wrong with having things, as long as you can visualize your rooms and corners and closets and drawers and feel at ease about them. Right now, mentally walk in your front door and look around the first room you come to. How do you feel? Look in the other rooms, the basement and the garage, under the beds and inside the desk and in the glove compartment of your car. At every stop along this imaginary journey, ask yourself how you feel.

If you can breathe freely and feel content, you're not a slave to the various objects you've bought, received, or inherited. If instead your make-believe home tour makes your chest feel tight or your stomach queasy, you may have hardening of the household. In other words, your environment is saturated with clothes and collections, papers and possessions, that clog your life the way saturated fat can clog your arteries. One problem shortens your life; the other just makes it a lot less fun.

So—clean out: drawers, cupboards, cabinets, basement, garage, trunk . . . not all at once, but systematically, and with no iota of judgment about what is left undone. Just moving things around gets an energy going that was stagnant before. Keeping clutter manageable and showing "stuff" who's in charge is inseparable from your growing-younger venture, because youth is about freedom. Maybe you can remember when moving house involved nothing more than loading two suitcases, a portable stereo, a few books and records, and some hand-me-down dishes into a VW Beetle. Few of us would care to return to that level of simplicity, but there is a balance point between *la vie bohème* and being so burdened by possessions we couldn't get away to Woodstock if a time machine offered tickets back to that legendary summer.

You see, everything we own has the option of either serving us or burdening us. Most do both since even serviceable items require cleaning, repairing, insuring, and the like. The ideal situation is that everything you own gives you more in terms of usefulness or happiness than it asks in terms of expense, upkeep, and anxiety.

So clear out a drawer and congratulate yourself. Clear out a cupboard and feel pleased. Clear out the basement and feel darn near reborn. Unless you're naturally organized—some women are (some women are also five foot ten and have to drink milkshakes to keep their weight up)—you'll need to stay with this. Clutter tends to reproduce like the guppies the pet store guy told you were both females. It's okay, though: clutter doesn't have to be annihilated to help you grow younger. It only has to be coming under control.

REVITALIZE YOUR LIFE WITH WORDS: *I let go of every possession and every entanglement that holds me back or weighs me down.*

APRIL 12

Spontaneous Acts

Spontaneity is a youthful trait. Exhibiting it daily will infuse your attitude and reputation with youthfulness. To be spontaneous means to allow yourself a whim, a detour, or a change of plans for no reason other than you felt like changing plans. Like anything else, it is possible to go to the extreme, being so spontaneous that no one can count on you. I doubt you're in danger of that, though. As women, we're well socialized to respect others' feelings and respond to their needs. Those of us who didn't take to these strictures when we were young learned through the rigors of work, partnership, and parenthood to adopt them. I'd venture that you do a dozen dependable things before breakfast; I'm asking for one act of spontaneity in the entire day. You might consider:

- Making a small impulse purchase
- Skipping, running, dancing, or otherwise exhibiting exuberance; you get more points for doing it in public

- Going to the multiplex to see one movie and electing at the last minute to see something else
- Deciding Friday afternoon to get away for the weekend
- Using the good dishes on a Monday when there's no company
- Walking in a rainstorm—all the better if you jump in puddles
- Leaving a great big tip, or giving a homeless person twice as much as you usually would.

Spontaneity is to life what flexibility is to fitness: it keeps you adaptable, supple, and young.

REJUVENATE YOURSELF WITH ACTION: *Try something spontaneous today—something spontaneous and fun.*

APRIL 13

Vitamin B_{12} and the Rest of the Family

The B vitamins are considered the anti-stress family. Tense situations, especially if they're chronic, go through the Bs in short order. Getting extra during times like these could help protect your body from some of the ill-effects. Although each member of the B-complex has qualities of its own, the Bs often occur together in foods. Your diet and your multi are probably providing plenty, with the possible exception of B_{12}, folic acid, and pyridoxine.

VITAMIN B_{12}

Vitamin B_{12} increases energy, protects the heart, is essential for the production of hemoglobin, and boosts mental functioning—even a borderline deficiency can result in memory loss. An oddity as vitamins go, B_{12} is made by microorganisms and therefore not found in the plant kingdom (unless you were to pick vegetables and eat them unwashed, getting B_{12} from less than appetizing "soil contamination"). Otherwise, B_{12} is found in foods of animal origin; thus vegans need to take supplementary B_{12} or regularly eat foods fortified with it (as are many rice and soy beverages and packaged cereals).

Taking supplemental B_{12} may be wise for other people, too, since digestive efficiency decreases with age and supplemental B_{12} is thought to be better absorbed than the B_{12} in food. The suggested supplemental dose is 500 micrograms per day.

FOLIC ACID

Any woman who may become pregnant needs to be taking folic acid (folate) to protect her baby from spina bifida, but the importance of folic acid does not end there. It aids in red blood cell formation; and the Nun Study, that lengthy epidemiological exploration of Alzheimer's disease (March 19), found that high levels of folic acid correlated with strong mental functioning into advanced age. Green leafy vegetables are rich dietary sources of folic acid (its name has the same root as *foliage*); it's also found in beans, avocados, nuts, liver, and wheat germ. A supplemental dose of up to 400 micrograms daily is suggested.

PYRIDOXINE (VITAMIN B_6)

Along with B_{12} and folic acid, pyridoxine plays a role in lowering blood levels of homocysteine, believed to be a factor in both heart disease and loss of memory. Pyridoxine also helps with the manufacture of infection-fighting antibodies. Although it's found in leafy greens, fish, poultry, nuts, and bananas, most diets fall short, so a supplement of up to 100 milligrams—no more than this—could be good insurance.

THE REST OF THE FAMILY

The rest of the B-complex—thiamine, riboflavin, niacin, pantothenic acid, and biotin—are required for metabolism, nerve function, memory, hormone formation, and a host of other tasks. These vitamins are found in many foods, including whole grains, nuts, and legumes. A variety of processed foods are also fortified with several B vitamins, and your multi should get a B+ as well.

REJUVENATE YOURSELF WITH ACTION: *Know the bottom B-line: eat natural foods; supplement pyridoxine, folic acid, and B_{12}; and see a qualified nutritionist if you'd like some help sorting through the complex-ities.*

Grin and Share It

To grow younger, smile whenever indicated—i.e., just about every time you cross paths with another human being. Your smile will put others at ease and give you a good-mood transfusion.

I've heard of women who give up smiling because they're worried it will encourage wrinkles. Please! Let's face it, even with the best care, we're all going to get a few crinkles over time. Let's make them smile lines. As Mark Twain said, "Wrinkles should merely indicate where the smiles have been."

Smiling is healthy. It's relaxing and can pull you out of a somber mood. The very act of pulling up the corners of your mouth sends a message to your brain that things aren't so bad, and the brain responds by releasing the serotonin that promotes a sense of well-being. Before long, you'll be smiling because you mean it, people will smile back, and a little sunshine will get inserted into even the dreariest day.

Smile at people you know and those you don't. Even a chance encounter in a waiting room or on an elevator is a near-miraculous opportunity to come face-to-face with beings who, whether they know it or not, are earthly reflections of the Divine. Smile at young people and old people, objects of beauty and moments of insight, a bit of cleverness here and a wave of happiness there. Smile at yourself in the mirror and your husband when he looks up from the TV. Smile at the server at the diner and the guy at the Department of Motor Vehicles who has to contend with scowls all day. Smile when you're on the phone—it will show in your voice—and when you say your affirmations—it will help them stick. Smile because you're pleased with yourself and because you're thankful to be here.

REJUVENATE YOURSELF WITH ACTION: *Smile more than usual today. Pay attention to the responses you get and the way your day goes.*

Play Day!

(Okay, it's tax day, too. But a lot of people are getting refunds.)

Make a Retreat

I was forty-six when William, now my husband, entered my life. When he asked after our first date if he could see me again, I said, "Not for three weeks. I'm going on retreat." Actually, I was going to get laser surgery for acne scars, information I felt was too personal to tell a man I did hope to see again. He told people later that I'd given him "the old retreat brush-off."

Although I wasn't going on a retreat then, I'd gone before, I've gone since, and I will again. A retreat is time away for inner growth and inner peace. It's a time to gather your thoughts, get to know yourself, and take stock of your life. You can make a retreat at a monastery or an ashram, a cabin in the woods, a hotel room, or right at home (if you have the house to yourself, shut off the phone, and make TV and the Internet off limits). There are group retreats where you grow in community, and private retreats where you spend almost all your time with yourself and the God of your understanding.

A traditional retreat takes a day or a weekend or a week. When you return from a retreat of any length, you're a calmer, more centered human being. "What makes a retreat a restorative healing encounter," writes Jennifer Louden in *The Woman's Retreat Book*, "is not where you go or for how long you do. You don't have to go anywhere. It is all in your intention and commitment."

The makings of a fine retreat might be silence and music, relaxation and walks, prayer and contemplation, writing in your journal and meeting with a retreat buddy, a spiritual director, or someone else whose inner life you admire. The amenities can be minimal—a cot and a shower—or retreat for body *and* soul by including soothing spa elements: a steam bath, whirlpool, and massage. Let nature play a role:

sunrise and sunset, flowers and rain. Since you're retreating from your standard obligations, you have the chance to observe the natural world and the natural you. If it renews and refreshes you, it's working.

REJUVENATE YOURSELF WITH ACTION: *Check your calendar. When can you design a retreat for yourself and treat yourself to it? For ideas on specific kinds of retreats, including mini-retreats you can do over a lunch hour, see* The Woman's Retreat Book, *by Jennifer Louden.*

APRIL 17

The Pheromone Factor

Pheromones comprise a just-below-the-radar scent that attracts others to us. We think of them primarily in terms of sexual attraction, but as I understand it, there are a variety of pheromones ranging from "hot and heavy" to "nice and friendly." Pheromones diminish markedly at menopause, rendering us, if not invisible (January 6), at least less noticeable. You know how a dog or cat can look at an image in a mirror and apparently register nothing? This is because a reflection without scent or depth is meaningless to the animal. Similarly, a full-sized, living, breathing woman without pheromones can elicit no response from the guy behind the counter.

I knew about pheromones from biology class, but I didn't realize their power until I didn't have them, or enough of them, anymore. I can tell you that the last pass a man made at me was the month before my last period when, presumably, my pheromones were still functional. It was at a publishing party. When I told the pass-making person that I was married, he said something lame like, "All the good ones are." Quality repartee is not the point. The point is, I have not been the recipient of a come-on line, either clever or pathetic, since. True, I'm happily married and not looking for that kind of attention from men, but sometimes I really want the attention of a skycap at the airport, an instructor at the gym, or a helpful hardware man who knows more than I do about drill bits.

I'd seen ads about pheromone fragrances, colognes supposedly imbued with the magical secret of attraction, but didn't order any, not wanting to fall under the rubric of "A sucker reaches menopause every minute." Then I watched a TV program about pheromones—an actual network show, not somebody trying to sell something—in which a pheromone-enhanced twin got loads more attention than her identical twin going *a cappella*. All right, I figured I'd order a bottle for the sake of research. I put some of it on my temples and wrists and, in the spirit of experiment, went out into the world. I swear that more doormen said good morning, the guy at the newsstand spoke instead of grunting, and I was called "Miss" twice for every "Ma'am."

Maybe it was the pheromone cologne. Maybe it was that I knew I was wearing it, carried myself differently, and exuded more confidence. Either way, it smells pretty good. If you're curious, go online under "pheromones" and see what you think about what you read. I have no basis for recommending this other than that I seem to be more visible when I wear it. It may be that I am wasting money on over-hyped cologne and the buildings in my neighborhood have just hired friendlier doormen.

REJUVENATE YOURSELF WITH ACTION: *Look into pheromone fragrances and see what you think.*

APRIL 18

Nuts Are Good for You

When I was a pudgy little girl, nuts were a no-no. Today they are, in moderation, a yes-yes, even for those with some weight to leave behind. Raw or dry-roasted and unsalted, nuts contain essential fatty acids, antioxidants, potassium, magnesium, zinc, fiber, and some protein, but the big news is, eating nuts actually helps people stay trim. Although nuts are a concentrated food, meaning they pack a lot of calories into a small space, eating them apparently assists weight loss and maintenance by stabilizing blood sugar levels and keeping cravings for sugar and refined carbohydrates at bay.

All nuts are good, although macadamias and pecans are at the high end fat-and-calorie-wise, and peanuts are technically a legume and not a nut at all. English walnuts are prized for their omega-3 content, but almonds are the golden child of the nut family. Their monosaturated fat content can help decrease LDL cholesterol (the kind to have less of), and they boast a respectable 6 grams of protein in a mere ounce (calorie cost: 160). In Ayurvedic tradition, blanched almonds are said to increase the level of *ojas*, described as the golden fluid of health and radiance, in the system. (Other prime *ojas*-promoters include oranges, mung beans, barley, and raw honey.) Noted psychic Edgar Cayce recommended three almonds a day as a cancer preventive, and current research indicates that eating an ounce of almonds or other nuts four or five times a week instead of some other food of equal caloric value can tame the appetite and make losing weight a more satisfying experience.

REJUVENATE YOURSELF WITH ACTION: *Eat some nuts a few times a week instead of something else. Some people find that soaking raw nuts overnight in pure water makes them easier to digest. To blanch almonds, pour boiling water over them to scald for about two minutes. Drain off the water and, wearing rubber gloves, pop off the skins.*

APRIL 19

Become a Mother of Reinvention

When we reinvent ourselves, we take charge of change. Change is a given, and it often works against us. The scientific principle of entropy states that the nature of matter is to fall apart, wither, and decay. Still, every atom that makes up the known world has been here as long as the world has. When an atom that was part of something (or someone) old becomes part of something (or someone) new, it acts like a brand new atom. It's reinvented itself. So can we.

My mother is active and attractive at eighty-five. Since she retired from her job managing beauty salons twenty years ago, she has had a career in real estate; cared for an ailing in-law; perfected her golf game; learned rug-hooking, ceramics, and stained glass; volunteered at a hospital, a nursing home, and a library; gotten involved in online bridge; joined a new church (and is teaching bridge there)—and I'm sure there's something more recent, but I haven't talked to her in a week. My mom has the ability to pass through circumstances without their branding her for life. She is devoted to every job or activity for its time. When its time is up, she goes on to the next one, and her next role, without looking back.

Like her, you're open to reinvention or you wouldn't be reading this book. Given that, here are some exercises to try:

- *Rewrite (or simply rethink) your life story.* Ponder how different you might be if you had your same mother but another father, or vice versa. Or if you'd been born in a different country or a different era. Or if one key event were erased from your life, or one key person never existed. This exercise shows that what we think is so solidly *us* may not be so solid after all.

- *Spend a week watching no TV except shows you've never seen before.*

- *Try something for fun you're not sure you'd enjoy.* Hear choral music, country music, opera, jazz. Try birdwatching, croquet, poker. Sample the cuisines of India, Korea, Vietnam.

- *Listen to someone whose views diverge dramatically from yours.* Stay neutral. Arguing defeats the purpose. The point isn't to change how *you* think either; rather, it's to understand why someone else might think differently.

- *Try on clothes you think you would never wear.* Experiment with a sexy, low-cut dress; a corporate, tailored suit; or something inspired by old hippies or New Agers that flows all over the place. If the idea of having such an outfit on makes you nervous, you can really use this. Alternatively, experiment with hats, wigs, jewelry, or makeup well off your beaten path.

Every time you reinvent yourself, even a little, you keep attitudinal adhesions from forming. You convince your body and brain that they belong to someone younger than they thought they did. At the same time, you're telling other people that you are a multifaceted and fascinating woman. They may never know what to expect from you, but they'll always expect *something*. Even years and years from now, they won't think of you as old, because thinking of you as interesting has become such an ingrained habit.

REVITALIZE YOUR LIFE WITH WORDS: *It is safe for me to explore new things and great fun to reinvent myself at will.*

APRIL 20

Size Is Just a Number on a Tag

Too many women in every age-group are hyper-critical of the shape they are and the size they wear. Women going through menopause can become despondent when they realize that their proportions aren't what they were six months ago, that some clothes don't fit right anymore, and others don't hang the way they used to. Take heart: if you're eating right and exercising, you're doing all anyone could, short of liposuction. Whatever your physical dimensions at this point in time, you are fully deserving of owning beautiful clothes and looking beautiful in them.

Women of all sizes can dress becomingly. The first step is to stop criticizing your body the way it is now. If you think it's too fat, too flabby, or too old, redouble your efforts on those parts of the younger-by-the-day program that deal with your self-esteem. If you are indeed too fat, you won't eat less or eat better until you believe you're worth the change. If you are too flabby, you won't make exercise a regular habit until you believe you're worth the effort. If you're feeling old, you won't feel younger until you accept the age you are—the youngest you'll ever be. One way to jumpstart any of these improved attitudes is to start having fun with clothes—right now, at your current age, weight, and state of fitness.

The clothing industry (if not the "fashion" industry—there is a difference) has awakened recently to the fact that most real women do indeed have curves, and these are not grounds for reducing one's wardrobe to sweats, elasticized pants, and oversized tops. Microfiber, soft knits, and other fabrics that drape the body and move with it are becoming on women of a variety of shapes. Experiment with them.

The best training for looking fabulous in what you wear is the fitting room tutorial: shopping for clothes season after season with an eye to the colors, cuts, and fabrics that truly become you. In time you'll know when it's still on the hanger whether a dress or a shirt will bring out your best or do the opposite. It's a matter of optics—clothes that take the eye away from your less-than-perfect parts and draw it toward what you like most about your figure and your coloring. The more clothes you try on and see yourself in, the easier it will be to pick out those that downplay the negative and accentuate the best you've got going.

Image consultant Mari Lyn Henry works with women in New York and Los Angeles, places renowned for furthering the mystique of the immature and underfed. Even in these cities, she tells her clients of every age and shape: "When you give yourself permission to be beautiful and real, you have found who you are." I think that should go on a sign in every fitting room in the land, right next to "We Prosecute Shoplifters."

REJUVENATE YOURSELF WITH ACTION: *Go shopping with the conviction that you're setting out to (1) learn more about what looks great on you, and (2) become willing to see how great you look.*

APRIL 21

Trading PMS for PMZ

We all know about PMS: feeling puffy and cranky and able to cry at the heartbreaking poignancy of just about anything. PMZ comes later. It's *postmenopausal zing.* You get it from surrendering to maturity and daring it to give you at least two gifts for every one limitation. If you are currently dealing with hot flashes or other unlovely side effects of menopause, the zing may seem hyperbolic at best. Hang in: it's coming, sooner or later—sooner if you help it along, later if you don't.

When I was forty, I attended a tea with nearly a hundred women, all ten to fifty years my senior. I was struck by the strange phenomenon that the *older* older women, the ones in their seventies and eighties, almost all looked lovely, while many of the youngest ones did not. They seemed to be trying so hard it hurt. These younger elders were dressed to impress at any cost. The women my mother's age, on the other hand, were relaxed, smiling, and obviously comfortable with themselves.

I promised myself that afternoon that I would never go through the desperate quest to hang on to youth that I saw in those women. Then I spent another ten years on the planet and I was embarrassed that I'd judged anybody else. Now that I was walking in their shoes (albeit with shorter heels), I understood them completely. I recalled the quotation from Cher: "I've been rich and I've been poor, and rich is better. And I've been forty and I've been fifty, and forty is better." Was it ever!

This was a watershed moment: I could desperately attempt to hang on to youth, or be true to the promise I'd made when I was still young enough to blithely vow such a thing, that I would allow my life to ripen on schedule. I didn't want to get any riper than I already was, but the choice was obvious: I had to both accept the facts *and* make the most of them. Fifty was a fact; making the most of it would come from diving into the day and soaking it up like a French pop-up sponge.

Take this idea of accepting what is *and* making the most of it for yourself. Apply it to the particulars of your life. For example, if you're not ready to go gray (I'm not), you might consider lightening or highlighting the color you have. Or it could be that you're willing to wear a little less makeup instead of a lot more. Or perhaps you'll choose to be open about the age you are, whether you look it or whether you don't. Such consideration and willingness and choice-making are the raw materials of postmenopausal zing.

As I said, you will come to it eventually. If you live long enough, stay in good health, and gain from your spiritual life a sense of optimism to carry like an emergency fifty-dollar bill, you will have PMZ. But there's no reason to wait twenty years for it. You can have it now—call it perimenopausal zing if that's the phase you're in. Gradually, patiently, but persistently modify those parts of yourself or your life you wish to change, unless it's something etched into your genetic material or otherwise unalterable. Enjoy being infinitely pleased with both the changes you make and the facts you make do with.

REVITALIZE YOUR LIFE WITH WORDS: *I do maturity exceedingly well.*

Get Your Fats Straight

Fats are the most confusing aspect of nutrition for lay people, and registered dietitians have told me that the complexities of fats perplex even them. They have to understand the biochemistry, though; we only have to know how to eat for growing younger. This chart details the basics:

THE FATS	THE PROS	THE CONS
Fat One of the three basic macronutrients; the others are protein and carbohydrate	Concentrated energy source, necessary for warmth, production of certain hormones, soft skin, and lustrous hair; source of essential fatty acids	Just over twice the calories of the other macronutrients; some types of fats have been shown to contribute to heart disease, cancer, and increased inflammation
Saturated fat Found in animal products (i.e., meat, whole milk, cheese, butter) and some tropical oils (notably palm oil and mature coconut oil)	Because butter and coconut oil are stable at high temperatures, some experts suggest using them in moderate amounts for frying	Can raise cholesterol levels and contribute to clogged arteries, heart disease, and stroke; possible link to Alzheimer's disease
Polyunsaturated fats The fats in most plant foods; also the liquid vegetable oil extracted from them, such as corn, soy, sunflower, and safflower oil	When eaten as part of whole foods—i.e., nuts or soybeans—these are health-promoting; in food or extracted, they do not contribute to elevated cholesterol as saturated fats do, and at least one study suggests they offer protection against Alzheimer's disease	When used as extracted oils, these are artificial (since oils out of context do not occur in nature); they are also highly unstable compounds prone to rancidity, and they cause free-radical proliferation
Trans-fats Made by hydrogenating vegetable oils—i.e., artificially saturating unsaturated fat molecules with hydrogen; recognize them by the words "hydrogenated" or "partially hydrogenated" on a label	Cheap, so manufacturers use them widely; can also turn liquid oils into spreadable margarine	Mimic saturated fat and share its hazards, along with the instability of polyunsaturates; implicated as causative for both heart disease and cancer; can block conversion of essential fatty acids to their active end product

THE FATS	THE PROS	THE CONS
Monounsaturates The kind of fat that predominates in olive and canola oils, oils that are liquid at room temperature and thicken if chilled	Oils the body seems best able to handle; staples of the healthy Mediterranean diet, monounsaturates have a higher smoking point than polyunsaturates, for greater safety and versatility	Too much, as with any fat, can make you fat; canola oil is often genetically engineered, so choosing organic is especially wise in this case
Essential fatty acids The nutrients found in fats that are required for life and health	Supply the fundamental building materials for the body's cells; essential to all tissues and organs	Most of us get too much of the omega-6 fatty acids and not enough omega-3 (see August 8 for details)

Translating this to the grocery cart can be fairly straightforward:

- Keep your overall fat intake modest by avoiding anything greasy or deep-fried, too many rich sauces, and even a heavy hand with salad dressing.

- Cut your saturated fat intake by eating less meat and more vegetarian entrees and fish. Put olive oil and fresh black pepper on the table as a classy alternative to butter.

- Improve your balance of omega-3 to omega-6 fatty acids by eating whole foods, having fatty fish like salmon or mackerel twice a week, including flax and walnuts in your diet daily, and/or taking an EFA supplement.

- Toss most bottled oils with the exception of cold-pressed, extra-virgin olive oil for salad dressings and cooking; and organic, expeller-pressed canola oil to use when you want a lighter oil for desserts or baking.

- Eliminate all trans-fats by purging your kitchen of everything that says "hydrogenated" or partially so. Shortening, margarine, conventional peanut butter (as opposed to natural peanut butter containing only roasted peanuts with or without salt), and conventional baked goods are the primary culprits.

- Learn some low-fat (they're also low-calorie) ways to prepare your favorite foods: steaming instead of sautéing, or sautéing in water, tomato juice, or wine instead of oil; enjoying all-fruit jam on toast or roasted garlic on bread; using seasoned rice vinegar on its own to dress a salad.

With all this fat trimmed from your diet, you can enjoy a few more of the rich foods you may have been denying yourself—avocados, almonds, walnuts, Brazil nuts, sunflower and pumpkin seeds—with their healthy oils the way nature packaged them.

REJUVENATE YOURSELF WITH ACTION: *Do a fridge-and-cabinet cleanup, eliminating the trans-fats and polyunsaturated vegetable oils.*

Look for Little Graces

The most agreeable things can happen in a day. The odd fellow from upstairs who's known for being grouchy might front you the quarter you're short for laundry. Your son might come in from college on a weekend you weren't expecting him. You could take the car to the repair shop expecting the worst, only to find that ten minutes and twenty bucks solve the problem. These are little graces, small gifts from life that make your life flow more smoothly. We don't have to earn them and we may not even deserve all of them, but they come anyway.

When bad things enter our lives, either really bad or nominally annoying, we instantly lament, "This isn't supposed to be happening," or we ask, "Why me?" We need to respond just as automatically to the good stuff, the little graces. They like being noticed. When they are, they show up more often. When the first one presents itself to you today, say a silent thank you, or tell a friend about what just happened. Write about it in your journal, or take the experience into yourself as wherewithal for passing the good along to someone else.

The psychologist Abraham Maslow said that as a person approaches self-actualization, he or she goes from one peak experience to another. Little graces are peak experiences in miniature. Look for them today and enjoy each one.

REVITALIZE YOUR LIFE WITH WORDS: *I am a magnet for little graces.*

APRIL 24

All the Gloomy People, Where Do They All Come From?

Moods are as contagious as last winter's flu. When you're around positive, happy people, you tend to be positive and happy.

Certainly come to the aid of anyone in difficult straits, but avoid entering into the dramas of those whose difficult straits are continually of their own making. Sometimes we feel guilty about feeling good when someone else isn't. The urge to commiserate is strong. When a friend presents you with her laundry list of woes, you may be tempted to say, "Things aren't so great at my job either," or "I know what you mean: I've been feeling tired lately, too." Resist the temptation to mirror misery. Don't even bring up your analogous difficulties unless it's to segue toward something optimistic and helpful: "I was having some trouble at work, but I set up a meeting with my boss and it's made a big difference," or "I used to be tired all the time, but since I've been swimming in the mornings, I've got more energy than I've had in years." There is a fine line here: you want to relate to people, but if you get down to their level, you're like a doctor who succumbs to the disease he's supposed to be treating.

If you want to feel younger, live the life of your dreams, and look back on brilliant memories, you can't let anybody rain on your parade. And if you yourself are playing the role of thundercloud, cease and desist. There is always something going wrong in life. That's the nature of the physical world. Still, we are fully within our rights to say, "Everything is great," when things are just okay. Even when they're terrible, we can say, "They're getting better," because chances are good they are.

Certainly there are times for opening up, telling it like it is, and getting another person's advice and counsel, but such discussions should be planned and focused, not random and repeated. Take the middle path: recognize, when something is wrong, whether it can be changed or must be lived with. Talk about it as much as you need to when talking will help, but know that negativity is a habit. When you see yourself indulging in it, change the station in your mind as surely as you'd click the remote if it were on TV. When others continually try to bring you into their distress, be so annoyingly optimistic that they'll take their distresses elsewhere.

REJUVENATE YOURSELF WITH ACTION: *Think about the people you're around most: family, friends, co-workers. Who is positive and who is negative? You needn't be judgmental, just aware. Can you find ways this week to spend more time with the positive people and less with the negative ones? When you must be in the company of someone mortally glum, be extra-positive and see how far you get.*

APRIL 25

Discern the Important from the Urgent

If you look up "important" and "urgent" in a dictionary of synonyms, they'll come up as interchangeable, but they're not. The *important* is what matters for the long term. The *urgent* is what supposedly needs to be done right away. Some things are one, some the other. A few are both, and most are neither.

We live in an age of inflated emphasis on the magnitude and timeliness of just about everything. Sometimes a voice-mail system will let you flag a message as urgent. Think: When was the last time you left a truly urgent voice-mail message? Maybe you were calling from the emergency room, or you were stranded by the side of the road at midnight next to your burning vehicle. These things happen. They just don't happen often (thank goodness), and most of those "urgent" messages aren't.

The problem with urgencies, and plain old stuff that likes to buoy its own reputation by pretending to be urgent, is that they get in the way of what's important. When a project deadline at work is urgent, it can interfere with spending time with a child—a task that's important. When rushing to an appointment is urgent, it can impede driving safely—which is important. When making an impression seems urgent, it can thwart being yourself—the most important person to be.

Today, and as you proceed through life, be on the lookout for what is truly urgent and what is genuinely important. Don't be led astray by someone else's assignation of either label. Ask yourself, "Is answering this e-mail really urgent? Does it have to be done right this second, within an hour, within a day?" "Will getting involved with this task someone else believes is urgent or this activity someone else says is important keep me true to myself, or would it detour my destiny?" When you have lucid answers to these questions, you'll conserve your life force and steer the energy you've got in all the right directions.

REVITALIZE YOUR LIFE WITH WORDS: *I see the difference between the urgent and the important, and I always spot imposters that are neither one.*

APRIL 26
―――――――――

The "Iron Pill"

Weight-training or resistance exercise is working against an opposing force. The health reformers of the early twentieth century called lifting weights "the iron pill," seeing its value as akin to a miracle drug. Proper use of free weights or weight machines will give you toned muscles and more lean tissue so you burn extra calories, even when you're sitting at your desk or sleeping in your bed. Resistance exercise is more beneficial after forty than before, and remarkable gains in strength and muscular endurance can be made even in advanced age. Strong muscles prevent injuries, and weight-training lessens the risk of osteoporosis, gives the quick reactions and stability necessary to prevent falls, and may reduce blood pressure and minimize the belly fat that makes a person more susceptible to both heart disease and adult-onset diabetes.

Don't worry that strong muscles will translate as bulging muscles. Without taking steroids or becoming a full-time bodybuilder, women simply can't bulk up that much. Besides, since we start losing muscle in our thirties and that loss becomes relentless after menopause, getting to worry about being "too muscular" would be a luxury problem.

Plan to do weight-training three days a week, two days minimum. Taking a day off between workouts both gives your joints a chance to rest and gives your muscles a chance to grow stronger. Weight-training works by pushing your muscles close to their full capacity and tearing tiny fibers. When these microscopic tears heal—that takes a rest day—you've got yourself a stronger muscle.

You can certainly get an instruction book, invest in some dumbbells or a resistance band (a thick rubber-band–like contraption that provides the same resistance you would get from weights), and exercise at home. Doing this consistently takes more discipline than most of us come equipped with, but if you're motivated, it can work. Still, the easiest way for most people to have a realistic weight-training program is to join a gym. This way, you can get some guidance as to how to proceed safely and effectively, and for efficiency's sake you can piggyback weight-training onto aerobics (half an hour with the weight machines, half an hour on the bike or the treadmill). Most health clubs also offer classes that use weights. These have hopeful names like "Body Sculpting" and are particularly popular with people who like people, contagious energy, upbeat music, and the structure of knowing there's a reason to show up at 7:15 A.M.

Of all types of exercise, weight-training is first to reveal its positive results in a visual way. As early as two weeks after you start, you'll see some muscle definition. Before long you'll be giving yourself approving glances in shop windows, the way teenagers do. And that's just the part you can see. Strength also endows you with a sense of personal power. This is thrilling anytime, but in middle age and later, when the culture wants to grant women less power than ever, it is particularly exhilarating to know that you have a demonstrable reserve of it in your own body, a reserve you can tap without anyone else's assistance, approval, or permission. You couldn't buy that with fifty IRAs, but it's yours if you want it.

REJUVENATE YOURSELF WITH ACTION: *Determine a realistic way to fit regular resistance exercise into your weekly routine. Write this in your journal; then follow up.*

Allow for Some Discrepancy Between How You Feel and How You're Perceived

"I feel like I always have." "It surprises me that I look older because I still feel young." "People don't respond to me the way they used to, but I don't feel any different." You hear this quite a bit. Maybe you've heard it from yourself. In fact, these are positive statements: I mean, it's good to feel young. Where it gets troublesome is when the way you feel contradicts the way you're perceived. Other people, younger ones in particular (and there are getting to be more of them all the time), see your physical shell and make some rapid assessment: "She's my mom's age; we couldn't possibly have anything in common." "She's somebody's grandmother; this must be the wimpy aerobics class."

Younger people are going to think this way because it's the way they routinely think. If you're about my age, you remember the admonition, "Don't trust anybody over thirty." Don't think that advice hasn't trickled down. Still, with the exception of a daughter just entering her teens, the younger people who really know you won't think this, and the opinion of strangers is meaningless. It's not just total strangers who are prone to writing off a mature woman and her concerns, though. Doctors are notorious for it. So are repairmen. It's all perception. If you visit a home for the aged, you'll be on the other side of the perception. The residents will say, "When I was young like you . . ." and "Enjoy life while you're still young." Wherever you are and whomever you're with, hold firm to your truth, *your* perception of who you are and where you fit in the world. "You're as young as you feel," the saying goes. If you feel it, you are it, regardless of anyone else's perception.

REVITALIZE YOUR LIFE WITH WORDS: *I feel young today, and I'm looking younger all the time.*

Dressing Table Essentials

We think of makeup in terms of software—the foundation, the blush, the lipstick—while the hardware, the tools of application, are equally important and often overlooked. It's a pity, too, since this equipment is easy to locate, easy to use, and easy on the wallet. The tools I find indispensable for putting my best face forward are:

- *A headband.* Skin is skin and hair is hair and the twain aren't supposed to conflict when you're washing your face or putting on makeup. A simple stretch headband sees to it that they don't.

- *A lighted mirror.* If you live in a new house or you've had your bathroom updated, the lighting around your mirror could be providing the clear, even light that's ideal for makeup application. Most of us aren't that *au courant.* If you're not, price a stand-alone, lighted makeup mirror at a bed and bath store. Some of these let you change the settings for daylight, evening, and office ("office" means fluorescents, the least flattering light of all). Most of these mirrors have a magnifying side, too— helpful if things blur when you take off your glasses.

- *An eyelash curler.* When wand mascara made its debut in the late 1950s and promised to "lengthen, curl, and separate," the eyelash curler headed out of fashion. It's back. We finally realized that curl takes more than a swipe of mascara. When your lashes have the benefit of an upturn, they're easier to see, even when you're not wearing makeup.

- *Wonderful brushes.* Get yourself a really big brush for loose powder, a fairly big one for blush, an eyebrow brush (to make brows look thicker, brush them straight up and then smooth down the tops to give a natural line), and a lipstick brush (your lipstick will look more natural and it will last longer if applied with a brush).

For eye shadow, you have the choice of brushes (wide for the base, narrower for lids and crease) or sponge-tip applicators, which I find easier to use. Take your pick. When choosing brushes, go a little high end. Otherwise, they're liable to shed and you'll end up with hairs sticking to your face that aren't even yours.

- *Makeup sponges.* Wedge-shaped sponges are easiest to work with. Dampen slightly if you'll be applying liquid foundation—it will give a youthful, moist glow—or use dry with a cream foundation. Sponges give you more control than fingers do over the amount of coverage you're getting and the evenness of your blending.

- *Cotton swabs.* Mistakes happen. Erase a mascara smudge, lipstick that's outside your lip line, or shadow that extends out a bit too far with a cotton swab. Use a dry swab to deal with most goofs, or add a bit of makeup remover for the more stubborn ones.

Remember the old rhyme about Monday being washday? Well, make Monday (or some day of the week) washday for your beauty tools. Launder sponges with very hot water and a little soap or shampoo. For makeup brushes use warm water; ditto for hairbrushes and combs.

REJUVENATE YOURSELF WITH ACTION: *Inventory your beauty hardware. Are you adequately supplied? Are your tools clean and functional?*

APRIL 29

Don't Miss Anything

Within reason of course, and without running yourself ragged, don't miss anything. At least don't miss anything you have a nagging suspicion you might later regret having bypassed. This is a two-part proposition: not missing events and not missing incidentals. An event could be a wedding, even if it means leaving town; a play, even when it means juggling your budget; or a chance to see the president, even if he didn't get your vote. An incidental is, in this context, one of those details of life that gives it its sensory richness. Just as you don't want to miss an event like a touring production of *The Iceman Cometh,* you don't want to miss an incidental like the indomitable daisy that's pushing its way up through the sidewalk.

You ready yourself for not missing events by paying attention to what's going on with the people in your life and your community. Keep track of friends' birthdays. Read the entertainment section of the paper and keep your calendar up to date. Get tickets for the concert or the baseball game as soon as you hear about it, not days later when the good seats are gone.

You won't miss incidentals if you train yourself to be observant. With spring here, there are all sorts of natural events you can be part of as you remind yourself that this year, you're not going to miss anything that's budding or blooming or awakening because you're busy at work or preoccupied with a problem. You may be busy, and problems are part of life, but from now on you aren't missing anything lovely because of them.

REVITALIZE YOUR LIFE WITH WORDS: *I don't miss a thing.*

APRIL 30
_____

Play Day!

May

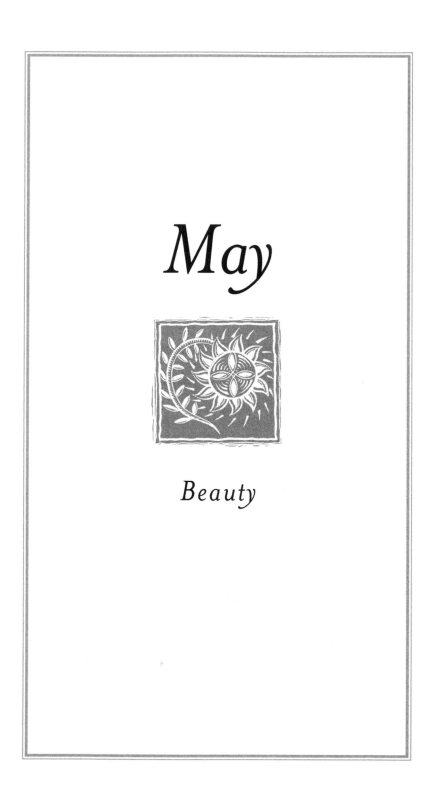

Beauty

MAY 1

Beauty as a State of Being

"Beauty is before me and beauty behind me," says a Native American prayer. "Above and below me hovers the beautiful: I am surrounded by it, I am immersed in it."

In this eminently attractive month, I suggest that you stay close to the idea of beauty as a state of being and a positive force in your life. Pay attention to beauty where you would expect to find it and where it comes as a surprise. Look for beauty as it comes to all your senses—sounds and textures as well as sights. Look for beauty in people, in their hearts as well as their faces.

Realize your own beauty as well, not by comparing it to arbitrary standards but by accepting it as a given. Part of your beauty can be those ways in which you look younger than your years, but another part can be the evidence of those years, their grace and their depth. Barbara Barrington, LCH, LCPH, a homeopathic physician who embodies the doctor's role as teacher, puts it this way: "I realize now that my vehicle may indeed show some wear and tear, but the quality of the maintenance on every level—physical, spiritual, and everything in between—is what counts."

An enjoyable exercise in "beauty appreciation" is to give yourself an hour with a book of photographic portraits, preferably black and white, by some skilled photographer. Study the faces and look into their eyes. Open yourself to the stories they tell. Most people who do this are more entranced by the old faces than the young ones. There's more to see in an older face; its stories are more intriguing, more inspiring. Use this activity in the library or bookstore as your springboard for a keen observation of beauty all month long. The more of it you see, the more you can take into yourself and reflect back to the world.

REJUVENATE YOURSELF WITH ACTION: *Treat yourself to some time with a book of photographs of all kinds of people—anything by Annie Liebovitz works for me. Allow yourself to see the beauty in all these faces. Let it fill you and make you richer.*

Sun-block Savvy

When I was growing up in the 1950s and '60s, a tan was a sign of both beauty and health. To burn first and then tan was "normal" for some people, and a blistering burn at least once each summer was as inconsequential a part of childhood as a skinned knee. Now we know that getting a sunburn is like signing up for wrinkles and even skin cancer, that simply tanning without a burn is a response to cellular damage, and that we chalk up our most harmful sun exposure before our eighteenth birthday. We can't redo birth to eighteen, but we can stop adding to the sun damage we've accumulated thus far:

- *Wear sun-block with a minimum SPF ("sun protection factor") of 15 and UVA and UVB protection.* Apply it over your moisturizer and under your foundation (if you wear foundation), whether these contain sunscreen or not. A barrier (reflective mineral) block like zinc oxide or titanium dioxide is unlikely to cause an allergic reaction, and it goes to work right away; chemical blocks can take up to half an hour to be effective. There are also safety questions regarding certain chemicals typically used in sunscreens. Swiss research suggests that several common ones may mimic estrogen and, in a laboratory at least, were shown to encourage the growth of cancer cells.

- *Review the numbers.* An SPF of 15 means you can stay in the sun fifteen times longer without burning than you could without the block. Most experts agree that 15 SPF is adequate, since no sun-block lasts all day and you'll be reapplying, although people with very pale skin might benefit from a product with a higher SPF.

- *Store sun-block within easy reach and reapply often.* Keep a tube in your desk drawer and another in the glove compartment. Touch up every two hours if you'll be outdoors. And use enough. You need a silver-dollar-sized dollop for your face and neck, a full ounce for a swimsuit-clad body.

- *Choose face powder with SPF.* Nothing is easier than touching up your powder and reprotecting.

- *Remember your forgotten parts*—ears, back of the neck, arms (especially the left one if you go sleeveless and drive), the tops of sandal-clad feet, and your décolleté, the area between your neck and your breasts that, when neglected, can become an ugly patch of dry, discolored skin in sharp contrast to a face that's been pampered and those parts that have been covered up. Apply sun-block (or a hand lotion containing it) to the backs of your hands every time you wash them.

- *Understand that clouds and windows do not a sun-block make.* You'll need to be more vigilant when you cruise to the Bahamas than on a rainy day in Oregon, but sun exposure is cumulative. Protect yourself every day. When you're indoors but sitting by a sunny window, pretend you're outdoors. Aging UVA rays in particular have no problem passing through glass. Outside, even a lightweight T-shirt can let harmful rays through. This isn't cause for alarm if you're just shopping in the city, but if you're walking ten miles to raise funds for something, be aware.

REJUVENATE YOURSELF WITH ACTION: *Get into the sun-block habit. Have it where you can see it and practice putting some on before you go out, after you wash your hands, and when you notice how good it feels to have the sun warm you through the window.*

Solution-27

Sometimes an energy shortage is due less to the years you've lived than the space in which you're doing it. Clutter is the number-one environmental energy-zapper. For starters, it's depressing. It's possible to wake up feeling refreshed, then open your eyes to piles of paper and clothes and mountainous miscellany, and immediately feel as tired as if you'd never slept. Since clutter isn't going anywhere you don't take it, but it's got you too tired to deal with it, you're in a catch-22. This catch-22 calls for solution-27: picking up twenty-seven items in your house or even in a single room.

In *feng shui*, the Chinese art of placement, twenty-seven is a magical number, signifying completion, putting a problem to rest. The teaching is that you can change your life by moving twenty-seven objects in your home. *Feng shui* practitioners mean furniture and paintings and the like, but I've found it works beautifully when applied to clutter, the leftovers of daily living. When you pick up twenty-seven items and put them in their rightful place, you will make a visible dent in the clutter level of any room. I've made solution-27 a regular part of my morning routine. Right after I meditate, shower, and dress, I pick up twenty-seven things that either are out of place or otherwise require attention. For example: 1. The teacup on the end table. 2. The dog's bowl. 3. The cat's dish. 4. The bed: make it. 5. The towel on the bathroom floor: hang it. 6. The paperwork I was doing on the couch. 7. The basket of laundry to put away (sometimes that gets extra counts: sheets and towels are number 7, socks and underwear 8, everything else 9). And on to 27.

I promise that if clutter is a problem for you, solution-27, regularly practiced, will bring you a rush of energy and the thrill of accomplishment. You can use solution-27 on a desk, a closet, or any other space. The great thing about it is that once you've tended to the twenty-seven items, you can be finished for the day. If there's more, and there may well be, just come back tomorrow.

REJUVENATE YOURSELF WITH ACTION: *Give solution-27 a try in some clutter-prone part of your environment. (If you have no clutter, take the day off.)*

Boning Up: Calcium, Magnesium, Vitamin D

In the United States alone an estimated ten million people, mostly women, are believed to have osteoporosis. Another eighteen million are likely to have a low enough bone density to put them at a heightened risk for fractures, especially the dreaded broken hip, responsible for one-fourth of all nursing home admissions. One factor in strengthening bones is a complement of nutrients with which you're already familiar: calcium, magnesium, and vitamin D.

By way of review, calcium is essential for healthy bones, and taking extra may help reduce the risk of osteoporosis, although calcium intake early in life appears to be more beneficial than trying to make up for a shortfall later. This mineral is also needed for strong teeth, and it helps muscles and nerves do their jobs. In addition, it may mitigate anxiety, insomnia, depression, and high blood pressure.

Calcium is abundant in a variety of natural foods, and many packaged foods are now fortified with it. Even if you don't use dairy products, you can get your day's worth of calcium from leafy greens (notably collards, kale, mustard greens), almonds, sesame seeds and tahini (sesame butter), dried beans and peas, shellfish, and whole grains. Calcium-fortified products include orange juice, soy milk, rice milk, and many cereals.

The World Health Organization currently recommends a calcium intake of 1000 milligrams for women nineteen to menopause. For postmenopausal women, for whom bone loss is an issue, as well as for females ten to eighteen who are building the bone meant to last a lifetime, the recommendation is 1300 milligrams. If you're uncertain about how much you're getting, keep a food diary for a couple of weeks and have it checked out by a nutritionist or dietician. You want enough, certainly, but don't go overboard: there are indications that an excess of calcium in body tissues may contribute to heart disease, dementia, or arthritis.

Vitamin D is essential if you intend to absorb the calcium you get; it may also offer some protection against breast cancer. If you have dark skin, live in a northern climate, or use sun-block resolutely enough to substantially slow the aging of your skin, you may be short on this vitamin. Even if you get some sun (see September 14), age makes it more difficult to manufacture vitamin D. Some foods are fortified with it (milk, soy milk), and there is some in liver and fish oils; in addition, you'll find vitamin D in your multivitamin, a modest but safe amount since fat-soluble D can be toxic in high doses.

Magnesium works with calcium and vitamin D to keep bones strong. You need half as much magnesium as you do calcium, but most people don't get this much, especially now that so many of us are loading up on calcium and don't give magnesium a second thought. This is a pity, since magnesium's prowess extends beyond bones to scavenging free radicals, normalizing blood pressure, and protecting against heart disease. Get it in whole grains and wheat bran, nuts, soy foods, and leafy greens, particularly when eaten raw. Around 200 milligrams daily in supplemental form could be advisable, but anyone with heart or kidney disease should check with a doctor before taking more supplementary magnesium than is included in a multivitamin.

REJUVENATE YOURSELF WITH ACTION: *Assess your intake of calcium, magnesium, and vitamin D, either on your own or with the help of a nutritionist. Make changes as indicated.*

MAY 5

Boning Up: The Rest of the Story

Keeping strong bones for life is more than a matter of calcium and its nutritional henchmen. Risk factors for osteoporosis include:

- Being female (women's bones are smaller than men's and we lose more bone as we age.)

- Having a slight build

- Being Caucasian or Asian

- Reaching menopause before age forty-five

- Family history of osteoporosis

Whatever your risk category, it's a good idea to get a bone-density test from your doctor when you're in your forties and again after menopause. If there's appreciable loss, there are medications that can help. You'll also improve your odds if you:

- *Stop smoking if you smoke, drink moderately if you drink, go easy on the salt, and keep your caffeine intake down to two cups of coffee or four cups of tea per day.*

- *Eat plenty of fruits and vegetables.* These are the source of the little touted nutrient vitamin K, once believed to aid in blood coagulation and not much more, but now thought to protect against brittle bones just like its more celebrated colleagues, calcium and vitamin D. Collards, spinach, Brussels sprouts, romaine, and broccoli (in that order) are where K resides. One serving a day of any of these (half a cup of cooked greens, a cup and a half of romaine) will get you the daily requirement of 90 micrograms with some to spare.

- *Give a thumbs-down to soft drinks that contain bone-eroding phosphoric acid.* Colas are in this group, regular and diet. If you don't want to cut out soda, read labels to find those that do not contain phosphoric acid, or choose natural brands that are refreshing combinations of juice and carbonated water.

- *Keep your protein intake adequate but not excessive.* Much research attests that excess protein—animal protein in particular—causes the body to excrete more calcium in the urine than it would otherwise. Other studies indicate that older folks on low-protein diets have weaker bones than those who get more protein. The answer seems to be to stay close to the RDA of .4 grams of protein per pound of body weight—i.e., 56 grams for the average (140-pound) woman.

- *Discover the joy of soy.* The isoflavones in soybeans and soy products like tofu and tempeh may help sustain bone density.

- *Get weight-bearing exercise six days a week.* This means weight-training and/or any aerobic exercise except swimming (which, of course, has other attributes to recommend it).

REVITALIZE YOUR LIFE WITH WORDS: *I am aware of what I need to do to protect my bones, and I do it every day.*

MAY 6

Flowers and Plants

Giving flowers is a disarming way to remember another person, but flowers were first a gift from nature to all of us. They look beautiful, they smell beautiful, and they make us feel beautiful. Kevin Kelly, master flower-arranger and author of *Letting the Lotus Bloom*, says, "If we're looking at flowers, which are naturally beautiful and vital, we take that image into ourselves. It helps us identify our own beauty."

Flowers are an energetic life form. As long as they're fresh and colorful, they put energy as well as beauty into a room. Give yourself this energy. When flowers start to go, you can get an extra day or two by trimming away the spent petals and tossing wilted stems, but don't hang on too long. Droopy flowers are worse than no flowers. Besides, part of the enchantment of a bouquet is that it is temporary. It forces us to look now, enjoy now, and appreciate now; if we wait until we get around to it, it could be too late.

Potted plants have more staying power than cut flowers and they assist rejuvenation not just by being attractive and alive, but by cleaning the indoor air. Plants produce oxygen and absorb harmful chemicals such as formaldehyde and benzene. Among the best air-purifying choices are chrysanthemum, peace lily, ficus, and English ivy. Plants require some attention, but caring for growing things, whether houseplants or a garden, is a rejuvenating activity. It is life-affirming and gives us more life.

REJUVENATE YOURSELF WITH ACTION: *Have cut flowers within eyeshot this week, even if it's just a bunch of daisies. If you're interested in the air-cleaning properties of houseplants, take a look at* How to Grow Fresh Air: 50 Houseplants That Purify Your Home or Office, *by B. C. Wolverton.*

Every Little Thing You Do

The way you sign your name. The way you fold the laundry. The straightness of the stamp on the envelope. The tone of your voice when you answer the phone. Making your bed, even though no one will be home to see it. These details and hundreds like them are little things that give you a little edge. They can be the difference between being pleased with your life or discouraged by it.

Of course you don't want to be bound by an absurd perfectionism—"Good grief! The stamp is crooked!"—just aware of the little things and willing to give each one enough time and care to do it in a way that pleases you. If you have so many little things to tend to that you can scarcely give any this kind of attention, can you limit their number? Can you delegate certain jobs and let others go? Can you give yourself totally to each task and honor it with your focused attention? When you do, days get longer, life gets richer, and more beauty fills your world.

REJUVENATE YOURSELF WITH ACTION: *Pay particular attention today to the little things and tend with finesse to each one.*

Make a Beauty Smoothie

A smoothie can be a yummy serving of health and beauty. Use smoothies as an easy way to get a variety of fruits and some supplementary power foods (green concentrates, supplemental protein, wheat germ, flax oil, B-complex-rich nutritional yeast) into your body in an easy, tasty fashion. These creamy shakes virtually always turn out, and they never have to be the same twice. The basic recipe that follows can be modified by substituting nonfat milk, soy milk, almond milk (blend ¼ cup blanched almonds with a cup of water), or yogurt for the apple juice; by using an unfrozen banana instead of a frozen one for a thinner, not-so-cold smoothie; or, if serving for breakfast instead of dessert, by adding nutrient powder, wheat germ, flax oil, or other supplements. When the recipe is used unmodified, each serving yields 116 calories, 1 gram protein, 27 grams carbohydrate, and no fat at all.

Strawberry Smoothie

FROM *THE PEACEFUL PALATE*, BY JENNIFER RAYMOND

1 large frozen banana, cut into 1-inch pieces
1 cup frozen strawberries
½ to 1 cup unsweetened apple juice

Place the banana chunks and strawberries into the blender with about ½ cup of apple juice. Hold the lid on tightly and blend at high speed until thick and smooth. Stop the blender occasionally and move the unblended fruit to the center with a spatula. Add a bit more juice if needed to completely blend the fruit. Makes two dessert portions. Serve immediately. (Note: Freeze bananas unpeeled, broken into inch-long pieces, and placed loosely in an airtight container; they'll keep about a month. Frozen strawberries stay good for six months.)

REJUVENATE YOURSELF WITH ACTION: *Fix a smoothie for breakfast this morning or tomorrow.*

MAY 9

Always Have a Future Project

There is a story that Irving Berlin's standard "Always" was wanted for a film—wanted so much that ten million dollars was offered him for the rights—but the composer refused. When asked why, Berlin answered that he had that song in mind for a future project. He was ninety-nine years old.

To stick around, and be glad you're here, you always need a future project, something to look forward to that excites you. Sometimes you can get involved in such an energy-intensive and time-consuming project—getting a degree, renovating a house, writing your memoir—that finishing it catches you up short because there is nothing to do next. There needs to be. The healthiest response to completing something huge is a vacation, either at home or away, a time to rest up, regroup, and plan the next exploit. If you can, consider your next project in a different vein or a different genre. If you've been working alone, perhaps your next project could be in company. If you've been doing brain work, maybe you can do something physical. If your major projects always involve your work, can you make the next one charitable or recreational instead? Above all, just be sure there is a future project waiting in the wings, ideally one you think is worth at least ten million dollars.

REVITALIZE YOUR LIFE WITH WORDS: *I always have a project and a future project.*

MAY 10

Ramp Up Your Passion Potential

Passion is vigor for life. The more you have, the more you get. None of us can afford to let life get boring. That starts a downward spiral of passionless living: no interest, no energy, no youthfulness. The most obvious example of passion is the romantic kind. People newly smitten with true love (or what seems like true love at the time) are different creatures, whether they're seventeen or seventy when Cupid comes calling. Life takes on a new finish: glossy instead of matte. Having passion for life or anything in it gives us a similar glow.

Think about the things you're passionate about, or used to be before you got so busy that just keeping up with it all crowded some of the passion out. Put your passions on paper, both those that are personal—pursuits you find fulfilling, fun, and exhilarating—and those that extend your reach beyond yourself and your family, those that make you part of effecting change in the larger world. In the first category you might have genealogy, painting, and traveling; in the second, you could have working for peace or helping AIDS orphans in Africa. These are just examples. Your passions are your passions, and you can have as many as you want.

Once you have a sense of what your passions are, promise yourself that you'll visit at least one of them every day. Some days you'll have five minutes, other days an entire afternoon. Start today with the time available today. Watch your life become more joyous, more meaningful, and more significant.

REJUVENATE YOURSELF WITH ACTION: *List your passions in your journal. Involve yourself with one of them this very day.*

MAY 11
_____

Defy Gravity

Certain time-honored teachings contend that by inverting yourself, either with yoga postures like the headstand and shoulderstand, or by relaxing on a slantboard a few minutes every day, you can reverse the effects of time. There are also legions of anecdotes from women who believe that defying gravity in this way has resulted in thicker hair and sometimes even the restoration of color to hair that was formerly gray. These could be suburban legends, but I do know some extremely attractive women who swear by "slanting." They find the time to do it by meditating on a slantboard, or watching their favorite TV shows in this unusual but potentially beautifying position. The idea is that blood nourishes the hair and skin, and since our precocious ancestors decided to walk on two limbs instead of four, our faces and hair get less blood than they're entitled to. Lying on a slantboard or performing inverted postures rectifies that.

If you're a yoga student and have access to personal instruction in the headstand and shoulderstand, doing these is an option, and the shoulderstand offers the additional benefit of stimulating the thyroid gland. I don't recommend your trying these postures unassisted, however, because there are a slew of contraindications. Anyone with a neck problem is advised to avoid them, as well as pregnant or menstruating women and anyone with high blood pressure, a heart condition, recent surgery, or weak eye capillaries. Even if none of these applies to you, it's best to get in-person training from a flesh-and-blood teacher.

Otherwise, look into purchasing a slantboard. Internet retailers offer these, as do some large natural food stores. They're usually fold-up foam contraptions. Alternatively, you can rig up your own slantboard by placing one end of an ironing board on a heavy chair or sofa. Then spend a few or several minutes every day with your head lower than your feet and your heart. When you get up, you'll have the rosy glow synonymous with youth. Arise slowly so you won't get lightheaded. And don't do slanting right after a meal when your digestion needs to take precedence over your hair.

REJUVENATE YOURSELF WITH ACTION: *Rig up a makeshift—but safe, of course—slantboard and spend a few minutes today defying gravity. If you like the sensation and agree with explanations of its alleged benefits, go online and order a real one.*

MAY 12

Favor People Who See Your Beauty and Acknowledge Your Value

One advantage of adulthood is being able to choose many of the people who populate your immediate world. This means that you can favor people who see your beauty and acknowledge your value.

I understand that the woman in the next office may dislike you for some mysterious reason, or that the man your sister married hasn't been congenial in your presence for sixteen years. There are such unpleasant people and we have to interact with some of them. Even so, there are plenty of others who are sensational. Cultivate these people. Encourage these friendships.

The men and women who see your beauty and acknowledge your value aren't just people-pleasers who prop up their own self-esteem by telling you what you want to hear. They really do see your beauty; and because they do, they help you see it as well. They really do acknowledge your value; and because they do, so can you. If I asked you to tell me the people who could help you grow younger, you might say a dermatologist, a personal trainer, a terrific hair stylist, and so on, but deserving a slot high on the list are those folks who know without question that you're beautiful and valuable. And their services don't cost a penny.

REJUVENATE YOURSELF WITH ACTION: *Write the names of the people in your world who see your beauty and acknowledge your value. Put yourself in the physical presence of at least one of them in the next twenty-four hours.*

MAY 13

Walk the Path of Mindfulness

To be mindful is to pay life such thorough attention that you glimpse the heartwarming beauty of all that is. With mindfulness, you don't just *do* what you're doing: you *become* what you're doing. And when one task or conversation is finished, you move on to the next with the same attentiveness, the same conviction.

A mindful person is a blessing to everybody else, because he or she is fully present. So often the person we're talking with on the phone is also writing an e-mail or scrambling an egg. This doubling up is how we get things done. But when you focus on someone to the exclusion of everything else, you give something rare and eloquent.

Do your best to be mindful at least once every day. That's all. Once a day, give another person your undivided attention. Once a day, look at a flower and see its petals and leaves, its strength and delicacy. Once a day, focus on the heat from the sidewalk, the breeze from the fan, the wetness of a glass of water or a shower or a swim. When you do this, you learn to be *in* life instead of just passing through. This slows it down and fleshes it out. It makes you a blessing, yes, but it also makes you blessed.

REVITALIZE YOUR LIFE WITH WORDS: *I practice mindfulness each and every day.*

A Bra That Fits

Few women over thirty have, without benefit of surgery, breasts that stand at attention like a boot-camp roll call. The sagging that doesn't come from time, gravity, weight fluctuations, pregnancy, and nursing will come later when hormone levels fall and breast elevation follows suit. This is nature's course, and some women are happy going braless or wearing the lightest, most comfortable brassiere possible, uplift be damned. I personally feel better every time I put on a bra that takes years off my chest. To each her well-deserved own.

For any bra to do right by you, it has to fit. When it does, the support comes from the cups. The back isn't riding up (back up means front forward, defeating the purpose), the straps aren't digging into your shoulders, the cups don't wrinkle, and no skin bulges from around the bra. You can bend over without falling out of the cups and get the support you're looking for without discomfort.

Getting a fit like this can take more than knowing you're a 38-B. Bra sizes are not perfectly calibrated. They differ a bit from brand to brand, and racer backs tend to run smaller than back-closure bras. Besides, your bra size may well be different than it was five years ago, even if you weigh the same. A bra-fitter—their services come gratis at lingerie shops and department stores—can help you determine your proper size and find the styles that fit you best.

For all a good bra can do for your shape, it is part of prudence to take it off sometimes. Breasts are organs; they shouldn't be caged and compressed 24/7. Sleep braless, and if you wear an underwire or other push-up bra most days, consider something softer for evenings at home and leisurely weekends.

Extend the life span of all your bras by hand-washing them with a little shampoo. Yep, shampoo. Lingerie aficionados wouldn't use anything else. With even the best care, brassieres eventually stretch out, lose their shape, and need to be replaced. Unless you have a special situation—i.e., you're particularly hard to fit or you need a custom-made, postmastectomy bra—you're better off buying lower-priced bras more often than a budget-straining one you feel compelled to wear after it's past its prime.

REJUVENATE YOURSELF WITH ACTION: *The next time you shop for a bra, have it professionally fitted.*

MAY 15

Play Day!

MAY 16

Art for the Soul

One day last year my nineteen-year-old daughter came home from school with more sparkle in her eyes than usual. "Guess what?" she asked, about to burst with her news. "Laura's parents gave her tickets to the Met for tonight and I get to go!" She knew she was in for a soul feast. If a blizzard had been due to hit, or if the city were under siege, I think I would have still said, "Go ahead: enjoy the opera."

Too many of us force our souls into anorexia. There isn't enough time to feed them, or it costs money, or other responsibilities take precedence. But when our souls are taken care of, we put the time and money we have to better use and often end up with more of both. When we prioritize our souls ahead of some more obvious obligations, we tend to meet the obligations with more energy and efficiency. A full meal for the soul—a concert, film, art installation, hike in the woods, whatever does it for you—is also the world's most overlooked beauty treatment. If you treat your inner self only every now and then, you may not notice much, but catering to your soul on a regular basis takes years away and leaves richness in their place.

Look at your calendar for the next seven days. If there isn't at least one soulful indulgence there, schedule one. And every day give your soul little nibbles, like the samples they pass out in the supermarket. Have the radio at home and in your car tuned to a station that plays music you love. When you come in the door, put on a CD that thrills you or calms you or entices you to sing along. Walk and drive through areas that are beautiful or that at least give you a change of scenery. Let your decor and artwork and personal touches give your soul something to enjoy, both at work and at home. Read poetry and essays and novels that inspire you to laugh or cry or support a cause or hug your children, even if they're old enough that they wish you wouldn't.

REJUVENATE YOURSELF WITH ACTION: *Schedule some outing for your soul this week that will let it soak up beauty, power, inspiration, or all of these from art or nature.*

MAY 17

Fab Abs

There is beauty in efficiency, and working your abs is one efficient use of time and muscle. Of course crunches and their kin help flatten you front and center, but a strong midsection also provides a natural girdle of support and protection for your lower back. While tight, toned abs make you look younger, a healthy back means you'll live better. Back pain can be debilitating and its medical toll, according to a Duke University study, is $26 billion a year.

Crunches (curls) and sit-ups target the upper abs. Side-bends and cross-overs reach the oblique muscles that make for a waistline. Reverse crunches (reverse curls) and front leg lifts zero in on the lower abdominals, responsible for tightening the dreaded "pooch." To do away with the fat that tends to settle in the middle reaches, you'll need aerobic exercise (March 16) or aerobics combined with a caloric deficit. ("Spot reducing" was, sadly, debunked before *The Lucy Show* went off the air.) Even so, strong muscles make any abdomen look better, and if you're willing to get down on the floor for sit-ups, getting out the door for a power walk is an easy afterthought.

Here are instructions for a complete abdominal workout you can do in mere minutes. They come from exercise motivator Joan Price in *The Anytime, Anywhere Exercise Book:*

Crunch. Lie on your back, knees bent. Cross your arms over your chest or place your hands behind your neck, elbows out to the side. Do not pull on your head. Take a deep breath. As you exhale, pull your abdominal muscles in and let that muscle contraction lift your chest, then shoulders, then—if you're strong enough—shoulder blades. Hold at the top for 2 seconds before slowly releasing down for 4 seconds. Keep your head and neck relaxed through the whole sequence. Repeat 8 to 12 times.

Twisting crunch. Put the right heel on the left knee. Place your right hand on your right thigh. Start as if you were doing the regular crunch, but when you get halfway up, twist at the waist to the right and continue curling up toward your right knee. Slowly release down. Repeat 8 to 12 times before changing sides.

Reverse crunch, advanced. Lie on your back, legs in the air, arms by your sides, palms down. As you exhale, gently rock your legs toward you and contract your abdominals so that your rear lifts slightly off the ground. Return to starting and repeat 8 to 12 times. Use abdominal power—don't cheat by pushing hard with your hands or swinging your legs to get the movement started.

Now that you know what to do, here's how to actually do it: Roll out a yoga mat at night before you go to bed. When it's right there in the middle of the floor, you will stop on your way back from the bathroom in the morning and do some yoga stretches and this quick, efficient fab-abs workout. And you'll hit the shower feeling that you've accomplished something already.

REJUVENATE YOURSELF WITH ACTION: *Approach your midsection kindly. First, make friends with it. It's tired of hearing, "I hate my stomach!" Give this area some credit for being functional, accommodating, able to expand and contract. Then set yourself up on a regular program of abdominal exercise—the home workout given here (for more, see www.joanprice.com) or classes that emphasize abs. Shoot for four days a week, although this is one muscle group that you can, if you're up for it, work every single day.*

Take Some Small Action on Your Own Behalf

Friend to friend now, this is important: don't let yourself get overwhelmed. That can happen when you're reading a book like this and trying to keep up with everything. In a perfect world, you'd do all this perfectly. So would I. In the world we've got, we never will.

What is vital, though, is to simply take some action on your own behalf. You may be familiar with the theory of the holographic universe. It suggests that any action that affects any part of the picture affects the whole. Your growing younger is like that. Even if you're not doing everything you've read about so far, you can change your whole life by just doing something. Exercise is a great example: it can elevate your energy, your immunity, and your self-esteem; it can help clear your head and your skin, tighten your muscles and strengthen your bones, and give you a better-looking body and a better-functioning heart. That's one action. One. The same is true for eating better, opening up to your spiritual side, drinking more water, taking more chances, and making peace with the age you are because it gives you this day, the best thing going.

If you can't do everything, relax. Just take one simple action on your own behalf. You'll never be the same.

REVITALIZE YOUR LIFE WITH WORDS: *I do something for my well-being every single day. Some days, just doing something is doing enough.*

Phytochemicals

If you think of heart disease, cancer, diabetes, and hypertension as Goliath—big and mean and scary—phytochemicals are David, small but mighty. Phytochemicals are compounds found in plants that offer protection against several degenerative diseases and many types of cancer. They congregate in vegetables, fruits, whole grains, beans, nuts and seeds, tea, and herbs such as basil, ginger, licorice root, mint, and oregano.

There are supplements that provide phytochemicals, but since there are nearly a thousand of them discovered to date, a mere smattering is the best you could hope for in a pill. The way to get a wide array of phytochemicals is to eat from the various plant families every day. Environmental toxicologist J. Robert Hatherill, PhD, gives the easiest-to-follow grouping I've found of these in his book *Eat to Beat Cancer*. He calls them the "Super Eight Food Groups." Including these foods in your daily diet offers protection against a host of degenerative diseases.

Dr. Hatherill's Super Eight Food Groups
FROM *EAT TO BEAT CANCER*

- *Onion group:* onions, garlic, leeks, chives, asparagus

- *Cruciferous group:* cabbage, cauliflower, broccoli, Brussels sprouts, kale

- *Nuts and seeds:* pumpkin seeds, sesame seeds, walnuts, etc.

- *Grasses group:* wheat, rye, corn, oats, rice

- *Legume group:* soybeans (tofu), green and wax beans, peas

- *Fruit:* citrus fruits, berries

- *Solanaceous group:* peppers, tomatoes, white potatoes

- *Umbelliferous group:* carrots, celery, parsnips, parsley

Vary what you're eating according to season and availability, but do your best to get something from each group every day. It's easier than you might think—for example:

- *Breakfast:* Oatmeal (grasses group) with blueberries (fruit) and chopped walnuts (nuts and seeds), and half a grapefruit (fruit)

- *Lunch:* Carrot-ginger soup (umbelliferous group—plus ginger, a phytochemical-rich herb), whole-rye crackers (grasses group), raw cauliflower and broccoli (cruciferous group) with bean dip (legume group)

- *Dinner:* Green salad, whole-wheat pasta (grasses group) with marinara sauce (solanaceous group) and soy "meat" balls (legume group), baked garlic (onion group), and red wine or grape juice (fruit)

To your health!

REJUVENATE YOURSELF WITH ACTION: *Keep track for a few days of how close you come to eating from all these groups. If you would like to read more, see* Eat to Beat Cancer, *by J. Robert Hatherill, PhD.*

MAY 20

The Beauty of Bravery

It may be unfair, but there is a season of life when you get to be beautiful just because of the state of your hair and skin and figure, and another when being beautiful requires actually having to *do* something. To be beautiful when you're no longer young, you have to be brave. That means doing what needs to be done even if you're scared. You have to rise to occasions, come through in the hard times, and be there when a lesser person would have bailed out. It was easier when all it took was the right dress.

You build your bravery by tending to the little things that you'd rather put off: making a dental appointment, getting all your paperwork in order, cleaning the garage this weekend instead of waiting another six months. You become braver every time you open the intimidating legal-looking envelope first and the one you know is a birthday card with a check in it afterwards. You're brave as can be when you deal with the mouse in the kitchen, the noise in the hallway, or the meeting with your boss in as self-possessed a manner as possible, especially if you see yourself as an essentially brave person, except in cases of rodents, noises, and authority figures.

Perform small acts of boldness and daring; then, when you need to do it, you'll know how. Courage isn't just an attractive quality to have—that's the least of it. It is indispensable as you go forward in life. When you have to deal with illness—your own or that of someone close to you—it's going to take all the courage and endurance and determination you can come up with. When someone you care about dies, you have the choice of falling apart or coming together. Courage is the glue. You get it from practice and from observing others who exhibit it. You build it by helping out when someone else has to have great bravery and you need only a little. You add to it when you do what you have to, frightened or not. You guarantee your supply when you have faith in something bigger, in a process or a plan that makes sense of what you can't.

REJUVENATE YOURSELF WITH ACTION: *In the next twenty-four hours, you will have an opportunity to be brave. Take it.*

MAY 21

Meditation and Rejuvenation

One study reported that people who had meditated daily for five years or more tested twelve years younger physiologically than the non-meditating control group. Twelve years! Physiological aging includes such indicators as short-term memory, acuity of vision and hearing, blood pressure and cholesterol levels, and joint flexibility. The idea that simply sitting quietly can affect these is exciting, because it leaves no one out. If you have trouble changing your diet, or if getting to the gym requires herculean resolve, you can sit still and grow younger.

Meditation is simply a state of consciousness, like thinking, dreaming, or deep sleep. You don't have to change your religion (or even have a religion) in order to meditate. It's easy to learn and, unless you opt to pay for instructions, without charge. It is a champion stress-reducer, and recent research indicates that it may help relieve depression by lowering levels of mood-dampening cortisol. The downside of this uplifting practice is that it takes a little time and a little more discipline, but turning the clock back *twelve years* is a strong inducement.

The primary purpose of meditation, of course, is not to lower your blood pressure. It is to connect your ego self, the everyday person you see yourself to be, with your eternal self. When you make this connection and revisit it daily, you gain calmness and courage. The irritations of life don't get to you like they used to, and they don't show on your face the way they used to either.

Meditation itself can be as simple as sitting comfortably with your back reasonably straight (in bed, in a chair, or cross-legged on the floor), resting your hands in your lap or on your knees, and observing your breathing. This is not a *breathing* exercise: it's a *watching* exercise. This simple watching is meditation, what the Buddhists speak of as "mixing the mind with virtue." If you wish to add a cognitive component—in other words, if the thought of just sitting bores you silly—choose a word or phrase that appeals to you and silently recite it with each breath. There is the classic Sanskrit *Om*, believed to be the primordial sound from which all creation emanated. *Love* or *Peace* (*Shanti* in Sanskrit) works fine, too, or a phrase like "All is well" (inhaling on "All," exhaling on "is well") or "God is love" or "I am peace."

To grow younger, I suggest devoting at least ten minutes a day to meditation. The majority of scientific studies have looked at practitioners of Transcendental Meditation (TM) who meditate twenty minutes in the morning and another twenty in the late afternoon. This is a worthy goal, but there is absolutely nothing wrong in starting with the time you've got. In the spiritual realm, time gets hazy anyway. "To meditate," wrote J. Krishnamurti, "is to be innocent of time."

If you've tried meditation and didn't stay with it, I recommend you try again. Some time has passed. In the interim, you may have developed the discipline of mind or the patience you were short on before. Let these qualities aid your practice. If you give it your best shot and it just doesn't suit you, there are alternatives: writing in a journal at the same time every day; reading lofty literature and thinking about the thoughts it provokes; praying, talking to God or Jesus or your guru like your best friend in the universe; or simply setting your mind loose as you swim or stroll and allow yourself to be carried to the state meditators call *restful alertness*. Some will tell you that only standard, sitting meditation will take you there, but you and I are old enough to know there's never just one way to get where you're going.

REJUVENATE YOURSELF WITH ACTION: *Set aside at least ten minutes, preferably in the morning, for meditation. Use a technique with which you're already familiar or one given in this reading. If you prefer not to meditate, you can pray or write in your journal. Just plan to do it every day at about the same time.*

Vitamin C

Your morning glass of o.j., although certainly a good thing, won't give you nearly the vitamin C you need for getting younger. This calls for eating vitamin C–rich foods with all your meals, and probably taking a vitamin C supplement besides. In addition to citrus fruits, foods bursting with this multi-purpose rejuvenator include cantaloupe, sweet peppers, berries, tomatoes, kiwi, and leafy greens like broccoli and kale.

Vitamin C lowers LDL (a.k.a., "bad") cholesterol, raises HDL (the good guy), and helps clean fatty debris from the walls of your arteries. It aids immune function and the white blood cell activity that routinely slows with age. Vitamin C also increases energy, helps produce the brain chemicals necessary for lucid thinking, works to keep gums healthy, protects against cancer and lung disease, and is indispensable in the construction of collagen, a protein required for healthy, young-looking skin.

Because vitamin C is water-soluble, your body can't store it the way it does fat-soluble vitamins like A and E. Therefore, you need to be conscientious about getting plenty every day, and if you take a supplement, dividing it into two doses. The research suggests that a daily supplement of 250 milligrams of vitamin C is good; 1500 milligrams may be better, but there is no reason to go over 1500 milligrams in supplement form unless instructed by your health-care provider.

If pure vitamin C (ascorbic acid) bothers your stomach, buffered versions are available. If you don't like swallowing pills, try chewables until you find one you like. I tend to go for natural everything, but there is no strong evidence that natural forms of vitamin C are more effective than the synthetic kinds. You may want to shop for a bargain supplement and save your money for organic strawberries.

REJUVENATE YOURSELF WITH ACTION: *Eat something rich in vitamin C at every meal today, and tomorrow, and the next day. As you do, tell yourself that you're making this a habit.*

The Opportunity Age

Plastic surgeons and doctors who specialize in extending youthfulness into the later years refer to our forties and fifties as "the youth corridor," the prime time for making changes that will keep us younger later. The ancient healing tradition of Ayurveda similarly contends that youth ends at sixty and getting one's health in order prior to that time is the closest thing to real "health insurance" for the years that follow. This *opportunity age* is that betwixt and between time when we're showing some signs of aging but they're not advanced. Some can be turned around—these are the ways in which we really can grow younger—and others can be halted for a time, or at least slowed down.

A change in diet at this time could, for example, prevent type II diabetes, while waiting could present the more formidable task of attempting to reverse it. Or if a woman gets a facelift in her fifties rather than in her seventies, it will obviously be a less dramatic procedure. All in all, this is a hopeful concept, the idea that just at the time we start getting those "over the hill" birthday cards, we're actually entering the opportunity age. It also makes the years leading up to and following menopause a time to invest in our future.

This is not to say that if you're in your sixties or seventies or eighties you can't grow younger: you can. The body and mind are amazingly resilient. I read not long ago about a study that put people in their nineties on a weight-training program and tracked the subjects' astonishing ability to build muscle. This implies that elements of the opportunity age go on indefinitely for anyone willing to take advantage of them. I believe it is also possible to use the mind to extend the opportunity age for yourself, and today's affirmation is designed to do that. In strictly physical terms, the closer to the actual opportunity age you are, the more mileage you'll get from smaller efforts. If you're at that stage now, take advantage of it. If you have friends who are there—but who may not see its advantages—let them know about the opportunity at their disposal.

REVITALIZE YOUR LIFE WITH WORDS: *I am at the opportunity age, and I take full advantage of it.*

Hang a Childhood Photo

If you have children, their pictures are probably prominently displayed in your home and office. If you have grandchildren, you may have whole rooms that look like photo galleries. Where, in the midst of all this family lore and all these adorable children, are *you* at three or seven or fourteen? At least one picture of you as a girl needs to be displayed where you can see it. It is a reminder of who you are, the eternal you that was once a child and is now a woman with years of experience and insight at her disposal. Find your favorite photo, frame it, and hang it or set it on your desk or your dresser.

Seeing an image of the child you were acknowledges her and the part of her that yet lives in you. Seeing this image daily helps you remember your youthful side; it reminds you that you are not only a woman of sixty but a child of six with wisdom added.

REJUVENATE YOURSELF WITH ACTION: *This weekend or one evening this week, go through old photos and choose at least one of yourself as a child to frame and hang where you can see it.*

Music Therapy

Music can relax you or give you energy, lift your spirits and change your mood. I learned this twenty years ago when I worked as an assistant at Quest Books and helped in the editing of *The Healing Energies of Music,* by Hal A. Lingerman. I used his musical suggestions when I was pregnant, and I played them to my daughter when she was a baby. Then life intervened, I got busy, and music once again became something playing in the background. I've since rediscovered it as a heavenly way to feel less encumbered by age and life's assorted irritations.

I'm most moved when music has lyrics, and I love musical theater. Seeing *Phantom of the Opera* for the first time was a bona fide transformational experience for me. I could feel my consciousness changing, song by song. When I left the theater that Wednesday afternoon, I knew, even though I hadn't been thinking about any of these things, that the man I was seeing would not be my permanent partner, that I would eventually live in New York City, and that the story of my life hadn't begun to be written. I was with my boyfriend another two years and didn't move to New York for six, but the wheels were set in motion, I believe, by hearing music that awakened something dormant inside me.

Although live music is the most powerful, listening on CD to "Can You Hear the People Sing?" from *Les Misérables*, "Only You" from *Starlight Express*, or "Some People" from *Gypsy* invariably makes me believe that anything is possible and there's nothing I can't do. Lingerman would call these "lively songs" that leave people feeling recharged and physically renewed. To follow are some of his specific suggestions. I think any of these can make a person feel lighter and freer and younger. Help yourself:

- *For more energy:* Schubert's *Marche Militaire*, Copland's *Fanfare for the Common Man*, and the overture to Mendelssohn's *A Midsummer Night's Dream*

- *For clearer thinking:* Bach's Brandenburg Concertos, Handel's *Water Music*, and Baroque string music (Telemann, Vivaldi, Albinoni, Torelli, etc.)

- *To relieve fear, depression, or grief:* Haydn's flute quartets, Sousa's marches, Debussy's *La Mer (The Sea)*, and Saint-Saëns's Symphony no. 3 for organ, with its uplifting power finale

- *To make you feel like dancing:* Dvorák's *Slavonic Dances*, dances from *Swan Lake* and *Sleeping Beauty* by Tchaikovsky, and Chopin waltzes

And if you feel like dancing, by all means dance.

REJUVENATE YOURSELF WITH ACTION: *Pay attention to how the music you hear affects you, body and soul. Listen to something today that gets inside you and changes for the better the way your world looks. You might even make a compilation CD of songs that move you—your very own "Greatest Hits."*

Extra! Extra! Most Women Look Like Us

Marilyn was a friend of a friend who thought we'd be friends, too. We scheduled our first meeting at Quintessence, a raw food restaurant in Manhattan. Marilyn said, "That's across the street from the Russian Baths. Do you want to do some bathing first?" So we did. "The Russian and Turkish Baths" in the East Village has been around since the 1800s, and although the establishment's glory is somewhat faded, we had an invigorating morning that included unique steam rooms, an intrepid dip in an icy pool, and an energizing massage.

An unexpected side benefit, however, was being in the presence of self-confident women, the majority of them in the absolute buff. Because we're routinely covered up and the only women most of us see naked are the occasional model and the leading lady's body-double, we imagine that almost everybody else is perfect beneath her clothes. Had you joined Marilyn and me at the Russian Baths, you'd have been quickly disavowed of that notion, as I was. Still, the women there were so comfortable with their bodies, walking around in the altogether like goddesses who had a day off. You can't be around that many women feeling good about themselves and not start feeling good about yourself, too.

If you have any body image problems, believe me: real women look like real women. They look like us. We're not comparing our husbands' bodies to Hollywood hunks' and we don't need to compare ours to starlets'. If you doubt me on this, meet me one ladies' day at the Russian Baths.

REVITALIZE YOUR LIFE WITH WORDS: *I am one hot mama.*

Your Skin Deserves the Services of an Astute Dermatologist

If you haven't seen a dermatologist since the one who didn't cure your acne sophomore year, things have changed. A dermatologist can do skin cancer screening, help with troubles like rosacea and eczema, and do wonders for your face. MDs with this specialty have traditionally treated diseases of the skin; cosmetic dermatologists comprise a subspecialty of doctors who devote their careers to helping people look better.

This sounded to me like the purview of the terminally vain until I attended a lecture by Marsha Lynn Gordon, MD, vice-chairman of the Department of Dermatology, Mt. Sinai School of Medicine. Intelligent, down-to-earth, and with perfect skin to back her up, Dr. Gordon proposed that, while other branches of medicine are helping extend our lives, cosmetic dermatology can provide ways to look more attractive during the extension. It can address dryness, lines, red patches, adult acne, or anything else that's making your skin less than flawless. If you have substantial sagging—i.e., you look ten years younger if you lift the skin beneath your jaw with your fingers—you've entered an area of either acceptance or plastic surgery. Otherwise, a dermatologist can help.

To start with, there are retinoids and other peeling agents that clear clogged pores, exfoliate the top layer of the skin, minimize the appearance of lines, and increase micro-circulation at the surface of the skin, possibly curtailing future line formation. Your doctor can choose the right one for your skin. Applied as instructed, this alone can result in a brighter, younger-looking face. (It does make your skin somewhat more sensitive to the sun, making a good UVA/UVB block all the more important.)

If you wish to go further, there is Botox®, of course, the brand name of the botulinum neurotoxin used most often in the United States to weaken or paralyze, for a few months at a time, the muscle that's causing a crease in your skin. Although I'm still wary (blame it on my sixth grade teacher, who showed us a ballooning can of sauerkraut and gave an overly effective lecture on botulism), Botox has been used in non-cosmetic medical procedures for years, and its track record is excellent. Cosmetically, it's used most often for lines between the eyebrows, but it can also help other movement-related lines, such as crow's feet and frown lines. In some people, a bit of properly injected Botox can lift the aforementioned sagging jaw enough to put off a facelift for those so inclined.

Also in your dermatologist's medicine bag are a variety of injectable substances that fill in lines, creases, and certain scars, and plump sunken cheeks. These include collagen (human or bovine), hyaluronic acid (Restalyn®), or your own fat; your doctor can explain the pluses and minuses of the various options. In addition, discolorations (dark spots, reddish blotches, broken blood vessels) can be erased with bleaches, lasers, and even newer technology. The field is changing so quickly that there is always something promising in the trial stages or pending approval.

Most of these treatments can be performed in the office in a single visit. There is often little or no downtime involved, and those commonly used to date are, in the hands of a skilled physician, very safe, although there is always the slight possibility of an allergic reaction or other untoward effect. These procedures are seldom covered by health insurance, however, and many of them require maintenance—i.e., repeat treatments in three to twelve months, depending on what is being done and the body chemistry of the patient.

Dermatological services can be the bridge between home skin care and cosmetic surgery. Photographer Henri Cartier-Bresson once said, "At a certain point, one gets the face one deserves." A good dermatologist can offer a bit of absolution.

REJUVENATE YOURSELF WITH ACTION: *You have an internist and a gynecologist; you deserve to have a dermatologist on your team. If you don't have one already, get some recommendations or check the list from your HMO or PPO.*

MAY 28
———————

Customized Exercise

To make exercise as attractive as it promises to make you, find those types that will engage you—you, not somebody else. When the activity means something beyond thoughtless motion—that is, if you run for the joy of it, dance for the beauty of it, lift for the power of it, or do yoga for your soul as well as your body—it becomes less a chore and more an enticement. Consider ballroom dancing with your best guy or belly dancing with your best friend. There's tennis if you like combining sweat with strategy, or biking if you love nature and the outdoors. In winter you could try snow-skiing or snowboarding or snowshoeing. If you're adventurous, check out rock-climbing, unicycling, or trapeze school. Health clubs are creating more and more interesting programs to keep minds engaged and bodies coming back to class. If even "stripteasaerobics" or "bring your dog to yoga" classes don't entice you, maybe the key for you is as simple as getting a portable CD player and listening to music or audiobooks while you're on the stationary bike. Experiment until you find what it takes.

Sometimes customizing is necessary because of an injury or the inability to do, for a short or long period, the kind of exercise you formerly did. When you're used to customizing for fun, doing it under duress won't seem like such an imposition. Either way, experiment until you find activities that make you happy as well as healthy. Choose your exercise using the same criteria you'd apply to choosing a date—that is, attractive to you and able to hold your interest for an hour.

REJUVENATE YOURSELF WITH ACTION: *Take a look at your exercise program. Do you like it? Do you look forward to it? Can you see yourself sticking with it far into the future? If not, expand your horizons. Try something new. Try lots of things that are new. Collect enough choices that exercise becomes more a buffet and less a mono-diet.*

MAY 29

Avoid Dowdy, Even at Home

These are the synonyms my thesaurus gives for *dowdy:* bedraggled, drab, dumpy, frowzy, frumpy, slovenly, stodgy, tacky, and unkempt. Seeing them all lined up makes it obvious why dowdy is dangerous. It's a way for someone twenty to look old and for someone forty to look decrepit. Every time you allow yourself to sink to that state, you feel, consciously or not, drab, frowzy, frumpy, and the rest. This is the way someone feels who is too old or feeble or unwell to care, and our plan is to go spunkily into the triple digits without getting that old.

Few of us show our dowdy selves to the larger world—not on purpose anyway—but many of us revert there when we are on our own turf. We confuse dowdy with relaxed, casual, and taking it easy, those states of mind and body for which home is best known and most treasured. We all need to go home, get out of constricting attire, shed constrictive attitudes, and be fully ourselves. We just don't want to start thinking of our true selves as "tacky, bedraggled, and slovenly," believing that we can clean up pretty well for public view but are, in essence, "unkempt, dumpy, and stodgy." No. You want to see your core self as relaxed and comfortable, easygoing and informal, spontaneous and at ease with herself, but not dowdy or anything like it.

Some ways to avoid the frowzy-frumpy-dumpy trap are:

- *Determine your casual style.* How can you feel comfortable and unencumbered but still pleased with yourself when you walk by a mirror?

- *Turn anything threadbare, impossibly stained, or irreparably ripped into cleaning rags, quilt squares, or a contribution to the Dumpster.*

- *Buy a few clothes earmarked for wear at home, so your domestic wardrobe won't be confined to garments retired from active duty.*

- *Appreciate the beauty of your face without makeup and experiment with ways you can wear just a hint of it to feel both unpretentious and pretty.* For one woman that's a little lip gloss, for another a bit of tinted moisturizer and a touch of mascara, for someone else a pat of powder on her nose.

- *Assess your relationship with the elastic waist and the drawstring.* Some women love their comfort; others feel sloppy with that much room for expansion.

REJUVENATE YOURSELF WITH ACTION: *Go through the clothes you wear only at home. Discard anything that has gone beyond the pale.*

MAY 30
———————————

Play Day!

Become Classier Every Day

When you're young, the be-all and end-all of life is to be cool. But once your twenties are behind you, unless you're gainfully employed as a rock musician, *cool* needs to give way to *classy*. Although it has observable characteristics, class isn't a matter of sham and show; it's about what you've got going on the inside. Contrary to widespread belief, this has nothing to do with class in the socioeconomic sense. Affluence can make it easier to have class, and easier to embarrass yourself by the lack of it. Tennessee Williams said, "High station in life is earned by the gallantry with which appalling experiences are survived with grace." At least, that's the way it ought to be earned. I love Williams's words "gallantry" and "grace." The more of both we're able to exhibit in our lives, the classier we'll be.

You have class when you let someone else blabber away because you don't always have to tell everything you know; or when you help someone out and don't let other people in on it because you aren't doing it to earn points with third parties. You show your class when you're wrong and admit it, or when you're right and don't demand that your rightness be acknowledged and praised. You're one classy lady when you're blind to another's position in life and see only this person's humanity, or when you set aside your own priorities for someone else's greater need. And when you start your day asking God or the universe how you can be of service instead of asking for what you can get, you're a class act all the way.

I have a feeling you're pretty classy already. Still, I encourage you to commit yourself to becoming classier every day. Every person you meet, even brief encounters on the street or on the phone, will give you an opportunity to do this. Your best teachers will be the annoying ones.

REVITALIZE YOUR LIFE WITH WORDS: *I am a class act all the way.*

June

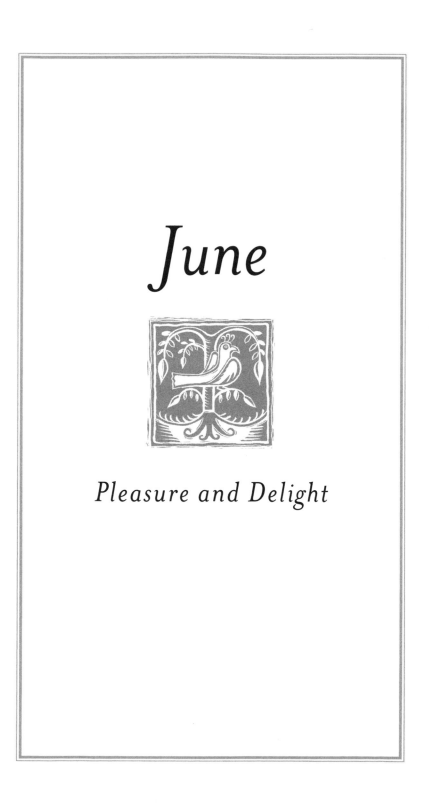

Pleasure and Delight

JUNE 1

Pleasure and Delight Ought to Get More Credit

School's out and that's a kick, even if you haven't been in school in thirty years. The fact that you were once in school programmed you with the idea that June is a happy time, dedicated to having fun and having adventures. This month, let your mind expand on its proclivity for appreciating pleasure, joy, and delight. Oscar Wilde said, "An inordinate passion for pleasure is the secret of remaining young." But too many of us still hold, subconsciously at least, to the puritanical notion that pleasure can't possibly be good for a person. Hard work? Yes. A restful afternoon? Of course not. Running a mile? Certainly. Getting a massage? Are you kidding?

This is a fallacy. Just as the body requires both activity and rest, the body-mind-spirit that you are requires work and play, scheduled time and free time, well-placed effort and well-earned pleasure. Your job this month is to elevate your opinion of pleasure. Find ways in which pleasure improves your health and enriches your life. Give it a higher priority. When appropriate, give yourself over to it. Let your mind be with your body when it's immersed in a hot tub, a soothing back rub, or making love.

Pleasure doesn't just feel good: it *is* good. When balanced with work and service, to which you're committed already, it can play a vital role in keeping you young all the days of your life.

REVITALIZE YOUR LIFE WITH WORDS: *I let myself enjoy life's pleasures. I leave no delight undetected.*

Host a Slumber Party

You can't grow old while you're busy being young. Every kind of pleasure and play you can indulge in counts here. One of the most playful occurrences you can plan for yourself is a slumber party. Ridiculous? Not at all. Create the slumber party experience the next time a friend from out of town comes to stay, or when you visit her. In fact, if you're with your sister or a sister-like buddy, the slumber party ambience will show up with no additional coaxing. The girl in all of us comes out when we're with a tried-and-true girlfriend.

You can also throw a slumber party on purpose. Plan one for the next time you have the house to yourself. Invite over two or three willing pals and commit an evening, a night, and a morning to pure fun. You can talk and talk and talk, or rent funny movies; play CDs and dance, or do a clothing swap; give one another manis and pedis and back rubs and facials, or assemble magazines and posterboard so everybody can make a hopes-and-dreams collage (January 24).

The rationale behind a grown-up slumber party is not to recreate the past but to bring the carefree nature of times long gone to bear on the often too serious here and now. Giddiness produces chemicals in your body that are conducive to rejuvenation, and acting like a kid, at the right times and for the right reasons, tells your cells and your psyche that there is still a kid in you they need to accommodate.

REJUVENATE YOURSELF WITH ACTION: *Do some slumber party research. Call a few friends and ask, should you indeed have a slumber party, if they'd come. Once you have your guest list, you're more likely to have the party. If you're part of a younger-by-the-day support circle, a slumber party would be a most appropriate group activity.*

Historic Preservation

Punctuating your immediate surroundings with a bit of history can help you feel at home in the present, even when it's moving so fast it feels like the future. Have multigenerational family photographs out where you can see them. Outfit your desk with a fountain pen and lovely paper on which to write notes, tangible and touchable, that will get stamps and postmarks. Blend the present and the past with a few pieces of vintage clothing, an antique here and there, and handcrafted items that, even if they were made last week, carry the timelessness of the materials that comprise them and the artisan's skill.

We benefit from including in our space mementos of the times we have known, in the way that people who live abroad include in their adopted location reminders of home. I've seen quaint English village scenes far from England. They were in India. During British rule, expatriates sought to recreate a bit of their homeland, perhaps making it more perfect than it actually was. We can do something similar for ourselves with heirlooms and memorabilia, as long as we understand that these are imports from another time, just as those Victorians had to remember that they were living twenty miles from Bangalore, not Bristol.

REJUVENATE YOURSELF WITH ACTION: *Within the next couple of weeks, treat yourself to a little something old (or reminiscent of something old): a candle, a fountain pen, or the heirloom photographs your mother has been promising to give you.*

Indulge Your Earthy Aspects

Once when my daughter Adair was going through a trying time, I said, "Life can be really tough, but you came to this earth for a reason." "Yes," she said without skipping a beat; "it was for the food."

Food is pretty amazing stuff. So is sex. And walking barefoot along the beach, planting tiny seeds in soft soil, sleeping and waking and stretching and showering, being out in the weather and in by the fire. When you've lived quite a while and done quite a bit, it's easy to take a "yeah, whatever" stance as to these bits of earthly ecstasy. We can't afford to: that's an attitude of rapid aging.

In very old age, physical drives diminish. Sense of taste is less keen, sex drive is low or nonexistent, and bodily aches and pains may take precedence over the joys of the flesh. The exceptional people who stay robust in their eighties and nineties, however, still find gratification not only in intellectual and spiritual pursuits, but in decidedly earthy ones as well. An interest in living thoroughly bodes well for extending one's stay here, perhaps the way taking an interest in the hostess makes one a preferred guest.

We increase our odds for being youthful and long-lived when, in addition to exploring and honoring our inner mysteries, we never fail to be tempted by the season's first strawberries, tingled by an evening kiss, taken with a timeless pleasure. The heart of extended youthfulness is not just staying on the planet: it's being at the party.

REVITALIZE YOUR LIFE WITH WORDS: *I live today in a sensual paradise, indulging in sensory pleasure.*

JUNE 5

Fresh Fruit for Dessert

Like most people, I have a sweet tooth, and if it isn't satisfied with fruit as nature intends, the clearest alternatives are either sugary treats or those made with artificial sweeteners. (I remember in my dieting days putting phony sugar and vanilla extract on cottage cheese and pretending it was pudding. There is just something pitiful about that picture.) Fresh fruit will take care of a yearning for sweetness, once you've been off the super-sweet stuff for twenty-one days. Give yourself three weeks to withdraw from conventional desserts and coffee break accompaniments. Have fresh fruit instead. Get the best fruit you can: ripe, attractive, organic, and in season. If you've been a big sweet-eater, it may not even taste sweet at first.

Stay with it. In less than a month, your mouth will water for sliced mango, orange wedges, Bing cherries, or a bounty of berries.

This doesn't mean you'll never have a fancier dessert. Special occasions are for doing things you don't routinely do and eating things you don't routinely eat. Even for these times (when you're in charge of the menu anyway), you may wish to stick with a fruit-based dessert that gets its extra sweetness from dried fruit or maple syrup or something else that's indisputably sweet but less processed than refined sugar. I'm thinking naturally sweetened versions of baked apples, poached pears, blueberry cobbler, chocolate-dipped strawberries, or a fruit salad so idyllic it gets to be called *ambrosia*, food of the gods.

REJUVENATE YOURSELF WITH ACTION: *Take the twenty-one-day challenge and have fresh fruit for dessert for the next three weeks. This is the ideal season for initiating this healthful habit.*

|UNE 6

Oases All Around You

You know how important it is to drink plenty of water. Most of us don't do it because we forget, or other beverages are more readily available and more tempting. The key is to make drinking water easier than skipping it or drinking something else. You do this by putting oases all around you:

- *A pitcher on the counter, in the fridge, on your desk.* We go for what's effortless. If there's a six-pack of soda all chilled and ready, we're apt to drink soda; if there's a pitcher of water, with or without lemon, in an easily accessible place, we'll drink water.

- *One for the road.* Become one of those attractive people who's always accompanied by a bottle of water. You can buy a fresh one every time or save money and landfill space by refilling a bottle from your pure water source at home. Take it to work, when you go on errands or for a walk, and definitely when you go to the gym. (One study found that 50 percent of exercisers were dehydrated before they even started their workouts.)

- *A bottle on the table*. When you're out for a meal, order a bottle of still or sparkling mineral water for the table. Your tablemates will drink good water when it's there; I've never been stuck having to down a liter of San Pellegrino on my own.

- *A coffee and a water*. If you drink coffee or black tea (or if you're still working your way out of a cola habit), start the practice of ordering your caffeine *plus* a bottle of water. Get used to the fact that you'll never again have a cup of joe or any other caffeine-containing beverage without a water on the side.

- *You get what you ask for*. When you're offered a drink, ask for water. If it's not offered, ask for it anyway. Make mineral water or seltzer with lime your party drink of choice, at least for your second drink. (As with caffeinated drinks, every alcoholic beverage needs an H_2O chaser.)

Let these ideas spark ideas of your own. You'll get younger not from what you read but from what you apply in your life. Customize these suggestions to the person you are and the life you live.

REJUVENATE YOURSELF WITH ACTION: *Start to create oases all around you by making a list of real-life ways you can drink more water—e.g., taking a bottle to the gym, keeping a plug-in water boiler on your desk at work, ordering sparkling water for the table every time you go out for a meal.*

JUNE 7

Massage, or What an Hour in Paradise Can Do for a Body

A full-body massage by a trained therapist can reduce stress, enhance immunity, ease aches, and assist your body's ongoing detoxification efforts. It does this by promoting circulation, thus oxygenating all the tissues of your body, and encouraging both physical and mental relaxation. In this state, your body is best equipped for healing itself on whatever level necessary.

Massage also makes you the recipient of healing touch. If you feel at all inhibited about the condition of your body—perhaps it's not as toned or as taut as it once was—you may be denying it touch on a variety of levels. When you go for massage, you're telling your physical self that it is worthy of attention. It deserves relaxation and nurture and healing. The massage itself reinforces these messages in the language your body understands best, the language of sensation. Every time you take your body to this place of calmness and healing, you imprint upon it how calmness and healing feel. With this information, your body itself can take better care of you by letting you know when you've strayed too far from this state of balance. "Massage is a great tool for taking stock of your physical, emotional, and mental state," says massage therapist (and one of my mentors) Necia Gamby. "The minute you break out of the pigeonhole of 'When I touch, it's physical; when I talk, it's mental,' massage becomes a medium for self-discovery."

You're doing self-massage (January 14), and this is great. Professional massage therapy takes you to the next level. If you can get it twice a month, or alternate massage with reflexology (November 29), you'll be on a program that will result in tangible improvements in your health and well-being. With just one massage every twenty-one days, you'll be gifted with enhanced immunity, and even once a month will tell your body and your budget that *you* have become a priority.

REJUVENATE YOURSELF WITH ACTION: *Book a professional massage if you can. To get one at a substantial discount, see if there is a massage school in your area. I've had some heavenly treatments from massage therapists-to-be.*

JUNE 8

The Gene Pool

There is no doubt that our genes play a significant role in how we age and how we show it. It's a bell curve: some people age more rapidly than average, others less rapidly, while most of us fall somewhere in the middle. Penny Drue Baird, a decorator and mother of four, is a friend of mine. She's my age but she doesn't look a day over thirty-five. Penny is genetically gifted. Her skin is flawless and appears to defy gravity. She had a baby at forty-six without working to get pregnant, and she shows no signs of incipient menopause. If she were obese, however, or a smoker, or had baked herself like a pan of muffins every summer of her life, we might not see her genetic good fortune and she might not even realize she had it. Moral of the story: we can't do better than our genes dictate, but we can do a whole lot worse.

You can get some idea of the kind of genes you've got by looking at your mother, your grandmothers, and your aunts. If your relatives aged well, chances are you will, too. If they didn't, don't despair: their aging may have had more to do with lifestyle than genetic makeup. My mother and her sister Exie have both aged beautifully; their other five siblings did not, and all passed away some time ago. My mom and Aunt Exie were the family rebels who gave up down-home, deep-fried cooking, and who stopped smoking as soon as the dangers of cigarettes came to light. They drew from the same gene pool as their brothers and sisters; they just gave the genes they got a better chance.

If you think you have great genes, you can either slack off a little and still not show your age, or take great care of yourself and be a Penny-like phenomenon for the rest of your life. If, however, you have genes that are less than phenomenal, it's even more necessary that you treat yourself to a youth-extending lifestyle. Although we live in a competitive world, rejuvenation is not a competition. Each of us has to work with what we've got. For one woman, that might be age-resistant genes; for another, it could be gene-defying determination.

REVITALIZE YOUR LIFE WITH WORDS: *I have terrific genes and I live in a way that they can reach their full potential.*

JUNE 9

A Nightly Check-In

I learned about the nightly check-in through the writings of Charles Fillmore, cofounder of the Unity movement. Fillmore suggested that when we lie down for the night, we would do well to scan the day just past from evening to morning, noting any places where we may have fallen short, asking God for forgiveness, forgiving ourselves, and, if we owe anyone an apology, noting that as our first task for the morning. Of course we can—and should—also recall those times during the day when we lived up to our standards with flying colors. Even if nobody else noticed, we can, and give ourselves a mental pat on the back.

This small exercise, easily done in a minute or two, can pave the way for restful sleep since it tends to the completed day and, literally, puts it to bed. It helps us to know ourselves, grow as individuals, eliminate repeat patterns we're not proud of, and give ourselves credit where it's due. It keeps life cleaned up, so we don't find ourselves in over our heads, trying to deal with more missteps and misunderstandings than we can keep up with. When the nightly check-in becomes a nightly routine, nothing goes more than twenty-four hours before it's taken care of.

Guilt, regret, denial, and avoidance promote aging. Awareness, amends, clarity, and compassion do the opposite. Check in tonight; it only takes a minute.

REJUVENATE YOURSELF WITH ACTION: *Starting tonight, put into place the practice of mentally scanning your day when you lie down and turn out the light. This is a time to be liberal with approval, generous with forgiveness, and honest about any need to make something right tomorrow. The day may not have been perfect, but you don't have to take it to bed.*

JUNE 10

The Wonder of Walking

Walking can make a surprising difference in your fitness level, your energy level, and how much "spread" middle age brings on. Some people were shocked by a study that found that Americans were getting fatter everywhere except in New York City, despite its having one of the highest restaurant-to-resident ratios in the world. Those of us who live here weren't shocked at all. We know that we walk miles a day as a matter of course. It's cheaper than a cab, often faster than a crosstown bus, and if we do take the subway, we have to walk to and from the station.

If you don't live in a place where people routinely walk, it is your responsibility, presuming you are physically able to do it, to start walking and hope to start a trend. If no trend transpires, keep walking anyway. Where can you walk to from home, from work, from your mom's house or your kids' apartment or your best friend's place? Can you do your errands—pharmacy, cleaners, post office, hardware store, whatever your routine is—on foot or partially so? Can you adopt a dog or borrow a dog or walk the one you've got? Can you walk for fun with a buddy or two and get some socializing in the bargain? Or join a group that goes hiking or trekking or walking in the mall? And when you take the car, park as far away as if you owned a brand-new Jaguar and you didn't want any other cars near it.

As you walk, remind yourself how fortunate you are to be able to do it. Really feel the sensation of the muscles pumping in your legs. Pick up the pace. Breathe deeply. Notice what's going on around you as well as within you. There is much to be said for changing out of your heels and into your sneakers.

REJUVENATE YOURSELF WITH ACTION: *Do something today that will make walking easy. Buy some shoes that are truly comfortable and supportive. Figure out what places you do (or could) frequent that are within reasonable walking distance of your home or office; plan to get there on foot from now on. Choose some great CDs to accompany you, or burn a mixed CD of your favorite songs that have a good walking beat. Get a walking buddy or put together a walking group. Purchase a clip-on pedometer at a sporting goods store (they're less than twenty dollars) and see how far you go. Five miles a day, or ten thousand paces, is the number to strive for (fewer if you also ride a bike, dance, or swim).*

JUNE 11

Put Yourself in Places Where You Feel Terrific

Where are you going on vacation this year? And where do you go when you're not on vacation but you want to feel as if you are for an hour or a day? We all have places that make us feel terrific. Some are faraway, once-a-year or even once-a-lifetime destinations. Others are around the corner. Spending time in either is a valid rejuvenation strategy.

Give some thought, then, in this traveling season, to the kind of travel that would refresh and renew you. What does it for you? The beach maybe, or the mountains. A luxurious spa, or a no-frills hiking or biking or rafting trip. A country with lots of history, or a city with lots of shopping. Or maybe, because you have many facets, it's two or three of these or more.

If you're like most women, you have taken many altruistic vacations. The kids wanted to go to a theme park. The in-laws expected a visit. Your husband's convention was wherever it was and it made sense to tack your holiday onto that. There is nothing wrong with altruism, but if you tossed coins into the Fountain of Trevi when you were nineteen and you've waited to get back to Rome ever since, it could be time for a little altruism turned in your own direction. Do some writing in your journal about places you truly want to go—places you've never been and those to which you're aching to return. Then make a plan for how you can get there.

In the meantime, those around-the-corner places you like a lot can be godsends. Choosing one supermarket or bookstore over another, one coffee shop or hair salon over the one across the street, the bank or the Laundromat that's farther away instead of the one that's closer, may seem utterly insignificant. It is not. You're spending your *life* in these places. Spend as much of it as you possibly can in the ones where you feel terrific.

REVITALIZE YOUR LIFE WITH WORDS: *I spend my discretionary time in places where I feel terrific.*

JUNE 12

Wanted: One Sex Drive

Who would think that sex drive, an appetite you've had since before you could vote, could disappear like a sock in the dryer? Maybe yours hasn't, and maybe it never will, but for a great many women, especially around and after menopause (natural or surgical), the incredible, shrinking sex drive is a fact of life. An abbreviated list of reasons for this includes:

- *Vanishing hormones.* The hormones that made you sexual in the first place—estrogen, progesterone, and testosterone (yep, we've got that, too, or at least we did)—are taking a nosedive.

- *The betrayal of the body.* When your breasts point down like a dousing rod at the seashore and you're dealing with stress incontinence, vaginal dryness, and an arthritic knee, it can take some serious mental gymnastics to feel sexy.

- *Lifestyle changes.* Becoming an empty-nester or a grandparent, getting divorced or being widowed, even something as seemingly inconsequential as having to wear supportive shoes can change the way you see yourself sexually.

- *Lack of reproductive potential.* Instead of feeling liberated from concerns about pregnancy, some menopausal women come to the subconscious conclusion that since sex has to do with babies, it no longer has anything to do with them.

- *The partner problem.* Maybe you don't have a partner (and nobody is holding Friday night mixers to help you meet people). Or your partner has lost interest in sex and you're not about to "beg for it."

Now, what to do. There is no single, simplistic answer, but these ideas will help:

- *Staying healthy is staying sexy, and seeing your doctor is a fine idea.* She has tools other than conventional hormone replacement that can help you feel more sexually alive. Sometimes all it takes is a good vaginal lubricant or instructions in vagina-tightening Kegel exercises to remind you that you *have* a vagina. These exercises can intensify pleasure for you and your partner, and perhaps help with stress incontinence, a problem that is extremely common after menopause and can make a woman feel horribly unsexy. Let your doctor help: she can.

- *Get turned on by life.* Excitement about a cause or an event or your own creativity is akin to sexual excitement; let one lead to the other.

- *Make a date with yourself.* Turn off the phone, put on some jazz, and enjoy the fine art of masturbation, with or without motorized assistance. While you're at it, rediscover your body. Touch your nipples, the backs of your knees, the small of your back, the outline of your ear.

- *Fantasize.* It can bring on desire like nothing else. Don't edit yourself because you're such a good girl. You may be good, but you're not a girl. You're at the age when, if it won't bring on a broken heart, an STD, or cardiac arrest, anything goes.

- *Celebrate celibacy.* Abstinence, whether short- or long-term, can be an adventure in its own right. The yogis say that sexual energy can be sublimated, turned into energy for spiritual growth. You can use this energy however you want: for working in the world, encouraging your artistic potential, or exploring the depths of life and meaning, heaven and earth, and the unparalleled enticement of unfathomable mysteries.

REJUVENATE YOURSELF WITH ACTION: *Curl up with a good sex book. My favorite is* Getting the Sex You Want: A Woman's Guide to Feeling Proud, Passionate, and Pleased in Bed, *by Judith Sachs (who helped with this section) and Sandra Leiblum, MD.*

Boost Your Enthusiasm

The word *enthusiasm* comes from the Greek *entheos*, "God within." It's no wonder, then, that when you're enthusiastic, it feels divine. This is also a youthful trait and a youthful state. Think about how children respond to every little happiness: "The ice-cream man— hurray!" "A card from Grandma! Let me open it." "We learned the coolest thing ever in school today." You get it. Maybe you even remember it. The point is to reenact it, to feel this power well up inside you and burst forth in a torrent of glee. You want to light up a room? This is where the light comes from.

I know you're grown up and you've probably been told to curb your enthusiasm. Do nothing of the sort. Curbing enthusiasm is spitting in God's eye. Instead, enthusiastically enter this healing state for body and soul whenever life is generous enough to put something worth enthusing about into your experience. It doesn't have to be winning a sweepstakes. It could be a call from a friend or seeing this year's roses bloom or learning some facinating fact that makes life just a bit sweeter.

Ebullience is allowed. Enthusiasm is required.

REVITALIZE YOUR LIFE WITH WORDS: *I have a remarkable talent for curbing any* lack *of enthusiasm.*

Your Sense of Smell

You know the way a certain smell can take you back to your second-grade classroom, your grandmother's boudoir, or some romantic evening years and years ago? This is because our sense of smell is closely related to our emotional selves, and a rich olfactory life can be part of a rich life as a whole.

Treat yourself to delightful smells today and every day. Notice what things smell like and which aromas particularly appeal to you.

Make the connections to times past that scents engender. Smell the stew in the pot, the spice in the jar, and the grass in the morning. Light scented candles. Bury your face in a stack of towels fresh from the dryer and enjoy the subtle scent of clean. Sniff natural fragrances and synthetic ones to train your nose to tell the difference. If you get a headache from chemical smells, you should be able to enjoy more natural ones with no ill effects. All our senses are meant to bring us pleasure. Get your fair share.

REJUVENATE YOURSELF WITH ACTION: *Pay attention to scents today. When you come upon one that's sublime, give yourself the time to enjoy it.*

JUNE 15
_____

Play Day!

JUNE 16
_____

Bio Brio

The closest thing to getting to rehearse the parts of your life you haven't lived yet is to read or watch and listen to stories of how other people have done it. Biographies can provide guidelines, warnings, inspiration, and delicious food for thought. Make part of your revitalization plan reading them, renting them, or checking the TV listings to see whose is on tonight. Enter into the life stories of people who are similar to you and those who couldn't be more different, men and women of the past and present, those from your own country and from faraway places, the famous, the infamous, and the unknown.

Each of them can show you by what they did well and what they did poorly how you might wish to conduct your own life. You'll see how they dealt with limitations and overcame them, and how they sometimes risked themselves for love or valor or some great, shining cause. Through biographies, you can see how some people don't even start setting the world on fire until they're the age when others are barbecuing at a retirement village.

You can even be inspired by biographies of improvised people. A most influential woman in my life never lived, but I thought she did until I was fifty-one. She was Mame Dennis, the flamboyant *Auntie Mame* of Patrick Dennis's 1955 book that inspired subsequent plays and films. I made my way into Mame's world as a child, through the movie *Auntie Mame* starring Rosalind Russell. I managed to see it seventeen times, which (in the days before videos and DVDs) was quite an accomplishment. From the moment I met her on screen, I wanted her in my life. I loved her spunk and her style, her courage and her loyalty, her bohemian proclivities and her complete lack of guile. She grew old during the film but she never got old. Mame was ageless.

A few years ago, I read in a New York City guidebook that I could actually walk past her Beekman Place address. It was like visiting a shrine. Later, to be near my daughter's school, we moved to Mame's part of town. We now pass her block when we take Aspen, our noble mutt, to the canine playground. I wonder about the happenstance of admiring a character for over forty years and then ending up on her island and in her neighborhood.

Shortly after moving here, I learned that Patrick Dennis never had an Auntie Mame. She was a composite, a fabrication. At first I felt dejected. Whose townhouse was I ogling anyway? Then I realized it didn't matter. Auntie Mame helped shape my life the way my mother and my childhood caretaker and my favorite teacher did. They did it by living on earth. She did it through living in the mind of a writer, and I like to think that a part of her lives in me.

Find your *Auntie Mame,* or dozens of them. Step outside your life a little by focusing on someone else's. Incorporate what you learn into your dual process of growing younger and maturing as a person of note.

REJUVENATE YOURSELF WITH ACTION: *Read or watch the biography of someone you admire. Don't see this as an assignment or worry about what you're getting from it. Just enjoy the book or the film and the person it commemorates.*

Seven Eating Habits of Highly Youthful People

Opinions on what makes a good diet diverge widely. The following seven habits are common among people who look and feel younger than they are and who have top-notch odds for living both long and well. When contradictory strains of nutritional information make you want to scream for ice cream, return to these simple suggestions. They won't steer you wrong.

- *Eat more colors than were in Joseph's coat.* The phytochemicals believed to protect against aging and degenerative disease usually show up in food as some vivid color. Different colors mean different phytochemicals, so eat red cherries, green beans, yellow squash, purple cabbage. In fashion, you start with neutrals and add some color; in nutrition, start with color and add the neutrals.

- *Have a great big salad every day, and some days have two.* A great big salad is one that takes the whole bowl to toss. Avoid iceberg lettuce in favor of greener greens: a mesclun blend, romaine, spinach. Add color with tomatoes, grated carrot, radicchio. A little dressing goes a long way if you do enough tossing.

- *Sometimes make the salad the meal.* Add something substantive to give a salad staying power: garbanzo beans, kidney beans, edamame (green soybeans); pumpkin seeds, walnuts, avocado; chunks of tuna or braised tofu; roasted potatoes, peppers, and eggplant; or raisins, chopped dates, or figs for a surprising sweet-and-sour taste when teamed with balsamic vinaigrette.

- *Have fruit where you can see it*—in a big bowl on your dining table, in a little bowl on your desk, in hanging baskets in your kitchen. What you see is often what you eat, so have the best choices in plain sight. Choose fruit that's ripe, in season, and so delicious it's better than ice cream. (Even have it with a little ice cream sometimes; just make the fruit the star.)

- *Make every meal a pleasure.* Healthy eating has to be enjoyable or almost none of us would keep it up. Perfect a few recipes and take advantage of the benefits of culinary herbs. Basil, cayenne, ginger, cinnamon, rosemary, and sage add delicious nuances to your meals *and* contain cancer-fighting polyphenols.

- *Drive past the drive-thru.* Although some fast-food places have added healthier fare, there still isn't much there to make you younger and there's quite a bit to impede your efforts. When your options are fast food or fast-ing, go for the elite of fast food, quick and casual places that didn't make their reputation from burgers and fries or fried chicken and fried wedges. In a pinch, go for a salad, a baked potato with double the broccoli, a bean burrito (with lettuce filling in for the cheese), a veggie burger (or wrap or sub), and getting where you're going as quickly as you safely can.

- *Bring back dining.* Make every meal at least a little special. Sit down. Have a place-setting. Even if you have lunch at your desk, produce a cloth napkin or a pottery mug to remind yourself that you deserve the best.

REJUVENATE YOURSELF WITH ACTION: *Copy the italicized portions of the tips listed here and post them on your refrigerator.*

JUNE 18

Schedule a Facial at the Change of Every Season

If you can, schedule a facial at the beginning of summer, fall, winter, and spring. A professional facial is first a diagnostic procedure, because your esthetician will examine your skin, determine its state of dryness, oiliness, and sensitivity, and proceed accordingly. With this information, she can also advise you on how best to care for your skin to improve the state it's in.

Although salons feature many specialized face treatments, I'm speaking here of your garden-variety, hands-to-face facial, in which the esthetician cleanses your skin with the kind of cleanser she's determined suits it best, and then uses a very gentle steaming device to open the pores and make your skin more receptive to the coming treatments. (While steaming over a pot of hot water at home can cause broken capillaries and play havoc with sensitive skin, the mild steam used by a good facialist should be tolerable by anyone.) She then exfoliates, usually with a slightly abrasive scrub right for your skin type, to remove dead cells and reveal the softer skin beneath.

The facial massage that traditionally follows is less prized in North America than in Europe, where it has long been practiced to help maintain muscle tone in the face. After the massage, your moisturized skin will be treated to a facial masque, usually of mud or clay, to draw out any remaining impurities. After the masque comes off and your skin is smooth to the touch, your esthetician will apply a moisturizer and suggest that you drink lots of water and refrain from wearing makeup for the rest of the day.

I find the entire experience relaxing and revitalizing, and it does calm my sensitive skin and give me a younger appearance. If you're going for a high-tech facial that calls for sophisticated equipment, I suggest splurging on a high-end salon or even going to a "medical spa," a new hybrid that combines the services of dermatologists and estheticians. For a basic facial, you're looking only for a sharp eye and skilled hands, a combination that needn't be expensive.

REJUVENATE YOURSELF WITH ACTION: *Schedule a facial early this summer, and note on your calendar to schedule one in late September and another in mid-December or just after the first of the year.*

JUNE 19

Contemplate Coincidence

Coincidences are gifts from life. They are event juxtapositions placed "just so" for a pair of charming purposes: first, to provide you with some unexpected delight; second, to flag an occurrence, the way you would flag an important document in a file, alerting you to the fact that this is something worth noting. Watching for coincidences turns back the clock on aging, because coincidences bring with them a little surge of youth-inviting effervescence. They also ease your stress load because you come to see that, coexisting with life's apparent chaos, there is a plan.

In the way that birdwatchers notice birds and stargazers see constellations, you can train yourself in the ways of coincidence. First, expect it. Next, observe it. Then, remark on it. Finally, be grateful for it. Do this enough, and more of it will come into your life.

Watch for the curious ways your path intersects other people's. Anticipate meeting someone who has the answer to a question that's been troubling you. Presume that you'll run into the person or the information that will make your life easier at a particular moment. Know that when you phone a friend who says, "I was just thinking about you," you're right on target with the rhythm and flow of all that is. And when the coincidence has a little joke built in, feel free to chuckle.

Let coincidence amuse and guide you. At times it could be mere happenstance. At others, it is divine appointment.

REVITALIZE YOUR LIFE WITH WORDS: *I am a connoisseur of coincidence: I expect it. I observe it. I comment on it. I am grateful for it.*

JUNE 20

Potassium

It's a balancing act: sodium and potassium. The body wants a one-to-two ratio of these, but the standard salt-rich/vegetable-poor diet most people consume stands in the way. Potassium acts as a gentle, natural, ever-in-balance diuretic. When you have enough of it, excess fluids won't hang around causing bloating and swollen feet and ankles. Getting ample potassium also means healthy blood vessels, proper flow of oxygen and nutrients to your cells, and protection against high blood pressure, heart attack, and stroke.

Eat a potassium-rich diet emphasizing salads, cooked greens, cabbage family vegetables, sprouts, carrots, fish, soy products, avocados, nuts, fresh fruits (the classic banana-a-day doctors recommend when potassium is an issue), and dried fruits (especially apricots). Avoiding salty snacks, processed foods, and most canned vegetables will also help this crucial balance stay in balance.

REJUVENATE YOURSELF WITH ACTION: *Take a look at the way you're eating. If you're emphasizing natural foods and using a light hand with the saltshaker, you're likely to be giving your cells plenty of fluid-clearing potassium.*

JUNE 21

Summer Solstice

Most of us don't get three months off like we once did, but we can go into summer vacation mode and still show up for work. It's a matter of attitude, encouraged by bare legs and sandals, light reading and extra hours of daylight.

We've traded a bit of the feel of summer for the comfort of air-conditioning. It takes something out of the season to need a sweater and scarf in restaurants and office buildings in mid-July. Before a/c, people responded to summer by moving more slowly and doing less. Women wore cotton sundresses and carried paper fans. Families who could got away to the mountains or the seaside; those who couldn't slept on screened porches or even outdoors. Everybody knew it was time to eat peaches and plums and melons, and to make ice cream and lemonade.

Don't get me wrong: I wilt on any humid day over eighty and depend on air-conditioning more than my environmentally aware side cares to admit. Nevertheless, I know that summer's gifts come only to those who shift into summer's gear, slow and easy. Some ways to do that follow:

- Take advantage of early morning coolness and choose this time to spend outside.

- Play tourist every weekend in your own hometown and in places that are easy day-trips away.

- Visit a farmers' market every Saturday morning.

- Get a short summer haircut.

- Restock your sun-block arsenal at home and at the office.

- Keep your makeup down to sheer lipstick and a dot or two of foundation to even out your skin tones.

- Swim—with the carefreeness of a child who is focused on the thrill of the dive, not how she looks in her swimsuit.

REVITALIZE YOUR LIFE WITH WORDS: *It's summer—whoopee!*

JUNE 22

Protect Your Hearing

Hearing loss can be hereditary, but far more is environmental: when loud noises bombard the delicate structures of the inner ear time and time again, they give up and give out. Audiologist Dr. Jane Thebo gave me this analogy: You can walk across the same stretch of lawn twice a day all summer and the blades of grass will bounce back. But if you have a party and fifty people walk across that grass, it's down like a crop circle. The little hair cells in your inner ear operate similarly.

Although there's no undoing past damage, it's never too late to develop a hands-to-ears reflex action anytime you hear a siren or other loud sound. If you have to be somewhere noisy, limit the time you spend there; just going out for short breaks can help your ears recover. Keep earplugs in your purse and wear them anytime you're subjected to loud noise—socializing in a bar, working in a factory, participating in choreographed exercise classes, going to the movies (the ads and the trailers can be louder than the feature). Wear them for flying, too, and request to be seated near the front of the cabin, away from the engine noise. Quiet your home environment by replacing metal garbage cans with plastic ones, installing triple-pane windows if you face a noisy avenue, or setting aside one room as quiet space—no TV, radio, or telephone.

Another way to protect your hearing is to ask your doctor and pharmacist if any medications you're on are ototoxic—i.e., bad for the ears—as a long list of medicines are. In some people, even the innocent aspirin can cause or exacerbate tinnitus, ear ringing, often a precursor to hearing loss. Caffeine can do the same.

It's a good idea to get a baseline hearing test around age forty and every ten years after that. Keep your own copy of these records; the doctor's office can legally dispose of them after seven years, and a hearing check loses much of its value without a point of comparison. Should you need a hearing aid, now or in the future, don't panic. Hearing aids have become teeny-tiny things: some hide completely behind your ear with only a clear tube—nearly invisible—going into the ear itself.

I'm telling you this from experience: I've had one since my early forties. Mine isn't exactly a hearing aid: it's a masker for tinnitus, a condition I developed from flying with an ear infection. (I know I shouldn't have, but I was sick in France, my ten-year-old had gone back to the States, and I'd run out of child-care options.) When I need to wear it I hide it under my trademark haircut and no one is the wiser (except you, since I'm telling you). While we're at it, if you or someone you know suffers from tinnitus, a common disorder in midlife, a masker can be a great help. The continual white noise erases the ringing and can convince your brain that the ringing isn't there. At this point, I often go six months or longer without needing to wear mine. That's when I know that silence is—gosh, what's better than golden? Platinum!—with emeralds and rubies and fairy dust.

REJUVENATE YOURSELF WITH ACTION: *You have a double assignment today: (1) Buy earplugs to carry with you at all times. (2) Make an appointment for a baseline hearing exam if you've never had one or if you're due.*

<hr>

|UNE 23

Coenzyme Q-10

Coenzyme Q-10 sounds like a condiment in the galley of the starship *Enterprise*. It is rather a protein present in every cell of our bodies—but there may not be enough of it there. The production of coQ-10 slows down sometime in our twenties, so when we need it most to help keep our hearts and arteries healthy, our blood pressure down, our energy up, and our brains working brilliantly, we're likely to be running low. Some coQ-10 is found in seafood and nuts, but research suggests that taking even a modest supplementary dose of 30 milligrams a day (an oil-based form in a gelcap is apparently the best absorbed) can help outwit aging on numerous fronts. There is promising research suggesting coQ-10 as an important component in fighting cancer, and it is known to be a valiant adversary against free radicals. It strengthens blood vessel walls, and when taken internally or used as a component of face creams, it may even delay signs of aging in the skin.

REJUVENATE YOURSELF WITH ACTION: *We've talked about a lot of dietary supplements thus far, and I'll be mentioning others as the year progresses. It's important that you don't feel bogged down by all this information. Eat well, take a multivitamin, and add other supplements that make sense to you. If you're feeling overwhelmed, contact the largest natural food store in your area and see if they have a staff nutritionist. Often this person is available for customer consultations at no cost and can help you come up with a simple, realistic supplementation program.*

JUNE 24

Don't Be a Yes Woman

Yes is a terrific word to hear and to say. There's nothing like saying yes to opportunities and adventures. But yes can get you in trouble, too. It opens the door to entanglements you don't need and commitments you don't have time for. The antidote to over-yessing is the simple phrase, "No, thank you."

The good news is that saying no is probably easier now than it was ten or fifteen years ago. According to Patti Breitman, coauthor of *How to Say No Without Feeling Guilty*, age forty is when a lot of women start getting some muscle around saying no. Unlike other muscles, this one gets even bigger and stronger at fifty, when we see that life is fleeting and we respond to that realization by bringing long-submerged priorities to the surface. Sometimes gradually, sometimes all at once, women in midlife come to realize that living on other people's agendas isn't nearly as satisfying as answering to their own.

Nurturing the ability to politely but resolutely say no to anything that doesn't speak to your heart's desire increases your vitality—that aspect of youth we're really after—because it compels you to be true to yourself. Breitman says that children from two to eight are the ideal role models for being true to ourselves: "If they feel like dancing or acting like a fairy princess or wearing stripes and plaids together, they do. Allowing yourself to become more authentic in this way comes from saying no to the voices and influences that may have shaped you but no longer serve you."

Practice saying no in small ways first. You can say no, if you feel like it, to going to the bank with your husband; he doesn't need you to identify the safe deposit box. You can say no to meeting your sister for lunch at the same restaurant you've gone to the first Wednesday of every month for the past three years. Give her, and yourself, the opportunity to say yes to new decor and flavors and experiences.

Don't worry that saying no will take you out of the realm of "nice person." You can still be nice, but you're old enough now that you no longer have to be "sweet"—a word that is applicable to cupcakes but not to a grown woman who came to this world with a job to do. Being nice comes from adding the "thank you" to the "no." Being sweet is going along with the wishes of others when it's at the expense of your own destiny.

To that end, the most important "no" probably needs to be said to the rules and excuses in your own head. If you've wanted for years to get your degree or audition for a musical or go to Europe by yourself, but always found some reason to nix the idea, surprise that cocky reason with a big, fat "No!" Saying it just might feel better than anything else you've done lately.

REJUVENATE YOURSELF WITH ACTION: *Watch your yeses and nos today. Make a point of saying no when your heart is shouting it but habit is pushing you to say, "Sure, and what else can I do for you?" Write in your journal how this goes.*

More Fun Tomorrow

I was once told of an engaging aunt, charged with the care of her nephew, who tucked him in every night with, "More fun tomorrow." What an attitude to grow up with! And what an attitude to adopt on the twenty-fifth of June!

The best way to develop a more-fun-tomorrow outlook is to be sure you have some fun today. Tomorrow is out of your direct control, but you can do something about the present. When you do, you can then tuck yourself in with "More fun tomorrow" and believe what you say. Moreover, any suggestion you give yourself right before bed snuggles into your psyche, where it plants the seeds of its own fruition. Knowing this, you owe it to yourself to remind yourself at bedtime that there will more fun tomorrow. You might then assure yourself that the answer to a dilemma will show up, too, and that you'll feel good and have lots of get-up-and-go for wherever you'll be getting up and going.

Take advantage of the receptive state you're in just before sleep to give yourself the message that tomorrow will have more fun, more health, or more of whatever you're after. When you do, you'll always be eager to wake up in the morning and turn the suggestion into reality.

REVITALIZE YOUR LIFE WITH WORDS: *More fun tomorrow.*

Making Time

One of the serendipitous aspects of adopting good habits is that the abandonment of old ones is built in. *Voila!* You instantly have more time for aging in reverse. If there still aren't enough hours in the day, trust that you'll find ways to make them. For instance, to get the hour and a half a day I wanted for exercise and meditation, I streamlined my personal e-mail. I put a notation on my signature line that

I do not check e-mail daily, and I do a blanket deletion of anything from unrecognized correspondents or anything marked "Fwd." And I no longer answer e-mails that don't require answers. I almost had to sit on my hands to keep from typing, "Thank you" or "Sounds good," until I concluded that I'm doing no one a favor in obligating them to write back, "You're welcome" or "I'm glad you like it."

The e-mail restrictions got me an hour. The other thirty minutes came from watching only planned TV. I look at the TV listings in the Sunday paper, decide which shows I want to watch that week, and refrain from using television to kill time. (Who would want to kill something so precious anyway?)

Aside from making minor cuts like these, you don't need to chart your schedule with mathematical rectitude. You needn't be in "balance" every day, or even every decade. When your children are young, you might appear to overbalance on mothering; if you start a business, you'll overbalance on work; if you take some time every day for becoming younger, you may feel that you're overbalancing on yourself and worry that that particular tilting can't possibly be allowed. It is. In fact, it's all this overbalancing that evens things out in the long term.

There is time, and it is safe to take yours. Use it well, not because you're afraid you won't have enough, but because time well spent is the most delectable of all.

REJUVENATE YOURSELF WITH ACTION: *Put a little extra time today toward some aspect of the younger-by-the-day program that you especially fancy or that you especially need. Maybe you can exercise a little more, schedule a beauty treatment, or give meditation another try.*

JUNE 27

Hot Springs and Mineral Baths

In Europe or Japan, no rejuvenation program worth doing would exclude *balneotherapy*, hot-spring or mineral-water bathing. Physicians there use it for conditions including arthritis, diabetes, obesity, and chronic skin diseases like psoriasis and eczema, as well as for building up general health and immunity. In the 1800s, and up until the mid-twentieth century when fast-acting drugs for arthritis relief came on the scene, "taking the waters" was a vastly popular therapeutic and rejuvenative technique in North America as well. In those days, "spa" kept its original meaning: a place for bathing in what Nathaniel Altman calls in his book by that name, *Healing Springs*.

Today there are some two hundred commercial mineral springs on this continent and many more around the world. Some are expensive vacation spots with luxury hotels attached, but the majority are simple and affordable. Often, adjunctive treatments such as massages, mud packs, and aromatherapy are offered in conjunction with bathing. A course of therapy in Europe is usually one to two weeks, while one- or two-day beauty programs are typically featured at American spas.

You can get some semblance of these benefits with mineral-water bathing in your own tub. Survey the shelves of bath additives at a large natural food store. Some of the products there are dried minerals from the world's famous spas. These minerals are absorbed into the skin in tiny amounts and are believed to assist in body processes such as healing the skin, relieving muscle aches, and strengthening immunity. Better still, if there is a mineral-water spa in your area—the website www.healingwaters.com is a quick reference—incorporate monthly or quarterly trips there into your rejuvenation program.

And if it even *might* be conceivable, consider a spa vacation sometime during your year of growing younger. If you're involved in a growing-younger circle, consider a group trip. Saratoga Springs, New York; Hot Springs, Arkansas; Sierra Hot Springs, Sierraville, California; and the Canadian Rockies Hot Springs in western Canada, are just the beginning of a long list of possibilities. Honestly: it's a trip you'll remember all your life, and it's a sure bet you'll feel younger for having taken it.

REJUVENATE YOURSELF WITH ACTION: *Do two bits of homework, please: (1) Look up natural hot springs and mineral springs online or in the book* Healing Springs *by Nathaniel Altman. See what's close for a day-trip or what's intriguing for a big trip. (2) Shop at a natural food store for some natural minerals for your bath.*

Reduce Your Exposure to
Electromagnetic Fields

For the past one hundred years or so, for the first time in human history, electromagnetic fields (EMFs) have been bombarding human bodies night and day. The body itself is a kind of electrical system and was not designed to compete with the fields bouncing off transformers and power stations and every electrical device we've come to depend on. EMFs appear to speed aging by disrupting the endocrine system. There are also studies that suggest, although by no means prove, that EMFs could be a causative factor in childhood leukemia and perhaps lymphoma, breast cancer, Alzheimer's, and ALS (Lou Gehrig's disease).

It appears to be most important to cut down on EMF exposure at night, when the body is attempting to engage in intense physiological regeneration. Some people unplug everything electrical in the bedroom at night, but you can decrease your exposure by simply sleeping farther away from electrical and electronic equipment. The effects of both the AC electric field and the AC magnetic field decrease markedly with distance.

Other ways to cut down on nighttime EMF exposure include:

- Unplug anything with a transformer on it. (When the plug that goes into the socket is a black or white box, that's a transformer. Anytime it's plugged in, there's current running through it.)

- Plug-in clocks are major offenders for AC magnetic and electric fields; replace them with battery-powered models.

- If you have upstairs bedrooms, turn off the lights in the ceilings beneath them.

- Replace electric blankets with toasty-warm bedding, preferably of untreated, organic materials (wool batting is warmest), and use a hot-water bottle instead of an electric heating pad.

- Charge cellular phones in a room where no one sleeps.

Daytime exposure is not as critical, but still turn off anything electrical when you're not using it, and when it's on, back off. Sit at least six feet from the TV. (If you find that your far vision is better than your near vision these days, this will be easy.) When you use a blow-dryer, hold it as far from your head as you can to get the job done—it's better for your hair anyway. Use this backing-off philosophy anytime you're around anything electrical—the copy machine at work, a microwave oven, your computer.

And choose a regular phone rather than a cordless. In addition to saving yourself from EMFs, a phone with a cord will work during a power outage and get you incidental exercise when you walk over to answer it.

REJUVENATE YOURSELF WITH ACTION: *If it's only buying a clock that doesn't plug in, or unplugging your computer at night, or moving the humidifier farther from your bed, do something today to decrease your exposure to electromagnetic fields. To learn more, there is a helpful section on EMFs in the book* The Healing Home, *by Gina Lazenby.*

JUNE 29

Live Your Fantasy One Way or Another

I met a youthful pediatrician, Dr. Judy Goldstein, at a dinner party. Knowing that I was writing this book, she asked, "What's the secret?" I started talking about diet and nutrients when she interjected: "I don't think that's it. I think it's living the life you've imagined for yourself, no matter what it takes." Immediately I knew she'd hit upon an underlying aspect of living young, even when you're not. If you're leading the life of your dreams, you are no longer subject to the aging effects of the daily grind, and you'll do everything necessary in a practical way to prolong this happy state of affairs.

When I say "live your fantasy," I mean in the most literal sense *your* fantasy, not what you think your fantasy ought to be. The heavy media influence in our lives can suggest that if you're not phenomenally rich and preferably a household name, you couldn't be living your fantasy. Poppycock. Your fantasy is your heart's desire. Chances are some version of it has been with you since you were a little girl. Your fantasy, when it's the true calling of your heart, is your destiny speaking to you, telling you why you won the prize of a lifetime: having a life to live.

If your life today doesn't look like your dream come true, look to the essence, not the trappings. What is important to you? Why do you think you're here? How close have you come so far to fulfilling your mission? You may be nearer than you think, even if, like most of us, you still have a ways to go. Think today about how you can come even closer to fulfilling your destiny and living your dream. It will make you younger—and I got that from a doctor.

REVITALIZE YOUR LIFE WITH WORDS: *I live the life of my dreams.*

JUNE 30

Play Day!

July

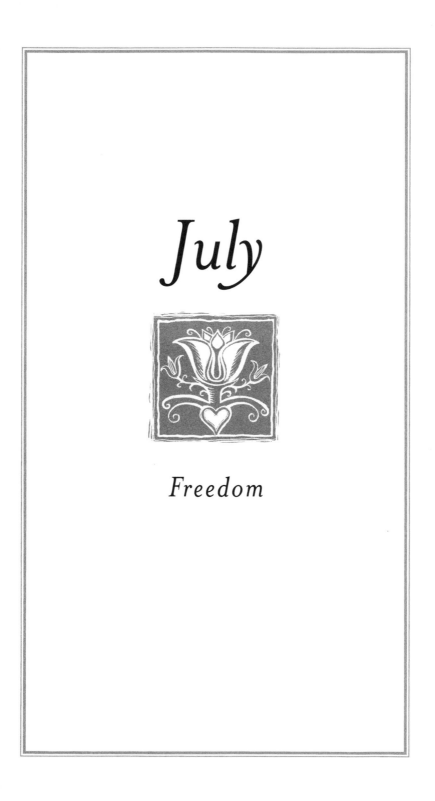

Freedom

Free to Be

The human soul so longs for freedom that people around the world have died for it—a millennium ago, a century ago, and this morning. What a strange paradox that, despite the powerful urge within us to live freely and be who we are, we too often erect invisible prisons for ourselves. Addictions are prisons. So is being tied to a belief that no longer serves us, or a system that may suit other people but that clashes with something in our personality or physiology or with the way we need to operate in the world. Fear is a prison: "I can't quit this job. No one else would hire me." Self-criticism locks us up, too: "I'm too fat to be seen at that wedding."

The tyranny that holds back so many women these days is that of effortless perfection. Most of us have bought the belief that we're supposed to have all our ducks—and pigs, chickens, and aardvarks—in a meticulous row. We think that *normal* is to always look our best and always have a totally tidy house. The car should be clean, inside and out. We need to be smart, educated, and continuingly-educated. We should be model employees and model partners. When it comes to mothering, we need to be supermodels. We have to be there for our friends, but that shouldn't keep us from looking out for number one. We mustn't age, of course, or ever get sick, and here's the clincher: *All this perfection needs to look as if it simply happened.* "She's really amazing!" we want to overhear about ourselves. And we should hear that because we are amazing, but we're not machines, and we'll never be free if we expect to operate like one.

Few of us are immune to this despotism, and that includes me, but awareness is the first step to freedom. In my country, we'll celebrate freedom a few days from now. Wherever you live, I encourage you to think about freedom this month and celebrate it every day this year. Commit to your rejuvenation as an act of freedom, not a condition of imprisonment. It's just a subtle shift in attitude: "Getting older is awful—I'm going to work hard to stay young so things won't be so bad" is a prisoner's attitude. "I love living long, feeling well, and looking radiant" is an attitude of freedom. It's yours for the taking.

REVITALIZE YOUR LIFE WITH WORDS: *I love living long, feeling well, and looking radiant.*

JULY 2

Spend a Day as If You Saw Everything Differently

Do something revolutionary with this day: spend it as if you saw everything differently. This means that, just today, nothing will be irritating and nothing will be ordinary. When you take your shower this morning, for instance, it won't be just a shower; it will be an experience that cleanses your soul and frees you to spend this day seeing everything differently. The houses and cars and yards you see on your way to work today will have some beauty or some quirkiness to color your morning. You'll see the people who are pleasant to you during the day as saints and angels, and those who aren't as precious beings who must themselves be having a bad day (or a run of them).

As you proceed through this day seeing everything differently, let your other senses in on the fun. Taste every morsel as if you had never in your life had vanilla yogurt or fresh guacamole. Feel textures. Listen closely. Don't just stop and smell the flowers: stick your head in a cathedral and smell the frankincense; pop into a candle shop and smell the cinnamon and sandalwood and bayberry. Make this a day of extrasensory perception, not in the supernatural sense, but by making extra use of the senses you've got.

"The contentment we seek," writes Sam Horn, author of *ConZentrate*, "is available anytime, anywhere . . . for a moment's notice. And age becomes immaterial when you're immersed in appreciation." Give yourself a day of this kind of immersion, and repeat it anytime you like.

REJUVENATE YOURSELF WITH ACTION: *Spend today as if you saw everything differently.*

Dining Without Dieting

Dieting should be classed with cheerleading. It is something to try early in life but, once experienced, not revisited. Many of us, however, watched our mothers diet and got the misshapen impression that this is the natural female relationship to food, even though people who lose weight for life almost never do it by dieting. Instead, they get in touch with an inner sense of what's enough. "Enough," wrote John Heywood in the sixteenth century, "is as good as a feast." It still is.

You learn about enough by sometimes having too much and not berating yourself, and sometimes having too little and not being afraid you'll starve to death. Getting comfortable with enough is an interior and largely silent occupation. There is no saying, "This isn't on my diet" because you're not on a diet, or "I really shouldn't," because if you really shouldn't, you really won't.

You see, the diet mentality in any of its interpretations is flawed, because no one can live on a diet. If you want to grow younger today and stay youthful all your life, you need to eat in a way that's sustainable, so you can do it on a trip to New Guinea or while spending a week in a hospital when a sick family member needs you there. You have to be able to go to work, go to restaurants, and live in the world while still nourishing yourself in the best possible fashion. This isn't sexy. You won't be able to brag to your friends that you've gone two weeks without a carb or a fat or whatever is anathema at the moment. There is no drama or suffering. You just eat and enjoy it, look healthier and brighter, and lose weight if you have some to lose.

Underneath it all, the fruits and vegetables you're eating will up your intake of antioxidants to defray the aging effects of molecules gone bad. In fresh fruits and salads, you'll get enzymes to help digest your food without robbing your own enzyme reserves. The fiber in these and in whole grains, beans, and other vegetables will both help you feel full and make your elimination work like a charm.

Being "clean" on the inside will show up in a luminous complexion and high energy levels. These changes take place with no rules and no regimen, just eating the food the good earth gives you and being all the better for it.

REVITALIZE YOUR LIFE WITH WORDS: *Everything I eat makes me lean and healthy.*

JULY 4

Creative Sun Protection

Finding a gentle, effective sun-block and using it properly (see May 2) certainly needs to be part of your sun protection strategy, but it can't do the job alone. We know that a good UVA/UVB block (you can keep the rays straight by thinking UVAging and UVBurning) is first-line defense against sunburn, dermal aging, and squamous cell carcinoma, one of the largely curable types of skin cancer. The research is less clear as to how much protection currently available sun-blocks provide against basal cell carcinoma (the other highly curable skin cancer) or against melanoma, which accounts for 77 percent of all skin cancer deaths.

Therefore, you need hats, gloves, sleeves, and self-control as well as sun-block. The lighter your skin, the more vigilant you must be, but even dark skin can get sun damage, including skin cancer. Retinol and alpha-hydroxy anti-wrinkle products can make your skin more susceptible to harm from the sun; if you use these, double-protect.

In addition to your faithful application of sun-block, include the following tactics:

- *Don't stay out long between the hours of ten and four.* That's when the sun's rays are most direct.

- *Wear a hat with a brim spring, summer, and fall.* Better yet, have a wardrobe of them. Women who learn to carry off hats have it over mere mortals anyhow. A hat will protect your hair (especially if it's colored) as well as your skin.

- *Help bring gloves back into fashion.* Someone needs to make the white cotton gloves women used to wear in summer a fashion statement again. It may as well be you and I. Also, wear golfing, tennis, and biking gloves if you do those sports, and driving gloves whenever you're at the wheel. Otherwise, driving is like putting your hands under a sunlamp; it's just asking for brown spots, discoloration, and hands that look a whole lot older than you feel.

- *Should you be out in some serious sun (the beach, the desert, a tropical isle), consider sun protection clothing.* Online companies and some swimwear shops offer everything from swimsuits to hats, gloves, shirts, and "driving sleeves" specially designed to shield you from UVA and UVB rays. Ordinary clothes offer protection, too: the tighter the weave, the more it blocks; all else being equal, white lets in more rays than colors, and blue is said to block best of all.

Skin that is rich and dark by nature is exquisite. The rest of us have to be exquisite some other way. If you love a bronzed look, learn to apply bronzer skillfully to those places the sun would give you color—your nose, cheeks, chin. Self-tanners, too, are much improved over the early versions. If you're patient and careful, they can look surprisingly authentic.

REJUVENATE YOURSELF WITH ACTION: *If you don't have them already, shop for a brimmed hat and driving gloves. Put your purchases into immediate service.*

JULY 5

Orthotics

To grow younger from the ground up, consider orthotic inserts for all your shoes, or, minimally, for your walking and workout shoes. Orthotics are arch supports. That sounds, and they look, simple enough. The wonder of them, though, is that they support more than your arches. They keep your ankles from turning inward (the term is "pronating," and most women's ankles do it). In making a slight alteration of the angle at which your feet meet the ground, orthotics can help your entire lower body work more efficiently. Walking and exercise become more comfortable; you can do more without fatigue; and knees, hips, and lower back can all feel better as a result.

Rigid orthotics, made of hard plastic, control motion to help alleviate discomfort in the lower extremities. Soft ones, crafted from foam or leather, act as shock absorbers and feel wonderful to arthritic feet or those with minimal padding. Some soft orthotics are slim enough to wear with dress shoes, even sling-backs and sandals.

At the elite end of the orthotic spectrum are those custom-built for your feet only, as determined by a mold made of them by a podiatrist or chiropractor. There are also inexpensive, over-the-counter orthotics sold at drugstores, athletic shops, and shoe repair places. If you're on your feet a lot, or if you have aches and pains you've been blaming on age instead of alignment, I suggest you give orthotics a try. In addition, if you're embarking on a new exercise program that will ask you to hit the ground running—or dancing or walking fast—these supportive insoles just might make your venture safer, more comfortable, and more a lifelong commitment than a flash on the track.

REJUVENATE YOURSELF WITH ACTION: *If you've never worn orthotics and are simply curious, get an over-the-counter pair and see what you think. If you have ankle, knee, hip, or low back trouble, speak with a health-care provider about customized orthotic inserts.*

<hr>

JULY 6

Smoke and Mirrors

There are two sides to almost everything: taking vitamins, eating meat, drinking wine, going gray or coloring. There is only one side to smoking: stop if you do it, and refuse to breathe anyone else's smoke if you don't. This is not to diminish how difficult quitting can be. I was never a smoker—my grandmother's calling cigarettes "coffin nails" kept replaying in my head—but someone I admire who overcame both alcohol and drug addiction told me that putting down cigarettes was tougher than either of those. Knowing this, there seems to be too little compassion shown to smokers who want to quit, as surveys suggest that four out of five do. While we understand that alcoholics and addicts need eight weeks in rehab and meetings all their lives, many of us expect smokers to give up their habit with a little willpower on the first try.

If you are a smoker attempting to stop, keep at it until you make it, and show yourself some of the compassion the people around you may be short on. If you started smoking in your teens or twenties, you were a different person then. You don't even have the same cells in your body. In one sense, you're stuck with the formidable task of overcoming an addiction somebody else got you into. Reconnect with that girl or that young woman. Why did she start? Was smoking the cool thing to do? A way to rebel against parental rules? A way to lose weight, feel accepted, or deal with nervousness or self-consciousness? Through counseling or spiritual practice or daily journal writing, help that girl who still lingers invisibly inside you to feel strong and safe and taken care of, and let the energy of the girl who picked up that first pack help you put down your last one.

You know how much is riding on this—your life, for starters. We all know that smoking causes lung cancer, emphysema, coronary heart disease, birth defects, and respiratory distress. It can also play havoc with the way you look. It breaks down the collagen in your skin—the stuff people are paying to have injected into their faces—and creates a host of free radicals to damage your complexion. If you quit, or if you never started, you'll have healthier color in your face, fewer lines around your eyes and mouth, and less chance of black-heads and breakouts. Even better: after three years, an ex-smoker's lungs can look like those of someone who never smoked.

Stop with a buddy; join a support group; get gum or patches or hypnotherapy or whatever it takes. If you fail, start over. If you fail again, start over again. You have to win this one. When you do, expect to be around to convince your grandchildren and great-grandchildren that they shouldn't smoke.

As for other people's cigarettes, it is not obnoxious to ask a smoker to smoke somewhere that you're not breathing. Just as a smoker is entitled to compassionate quitting, a nonsmoker—that's you, or the person you're soon to be—deserves to be able to breathe deeply, age slowly, and stand up for herself.

JULY 7

Healing Your Childhood Before Your Old Age

If you haven't dealt with the past, do that now. If you can't get over dealing with the past, do that now, too.

We are all on the receiving end of the dubious Chinese toast, "May you live in interesting times." In the interesting times since my youth, seeing a therapist has gone from shameful to standard. Doing away with the stigma of getting help is a great thing; being in counseling forever because Dad drank and Mom enabled (or whatever made one's particular childhood rough) is excessive.

We know that our early years affect us long after they've passed, and that if childhood experiences still color our lives today in ways we don't want, therapy or some other focused work addressing those effects is absolutely necessary. In doing that work, however, we need to be wary of getting caught in the snares of the past, a danger that is curiously inherent both in ignoring our history and in its opposite, taking up residence there.

While a few people had nightmarish childhoods and a few others had idyllic ones, most of us spent our early years somewhere in the middle. We had parents or other caregivers who did the best they could but who often failed us because the best a human being can do falls somewhere shy of perfect much of the time. If you have children and they're grown or nearly so, you get to see this from front and back: your parents did their best and frequently missed the mark, and so did you. So have all of us.

Get some help, if childhood specters haunt your life today, for the simple reason that going forward is arduous when you're lugging the burdens of the past along. Get this help with the commitment that understanding what happened long ago is not an end in itself, interesting though it may be. Instead, this delving into what went before has a purpose: to make for a better present and a better future. If you're seeing a therapist who would like to keep you wandering around in your childhood for the next ten years, consider a different therapist. The purpose of dredging up the past is to grow beyond it. Then you're free.

REJUVENATE YOURSELF WITH ACTION: *Write in your journal today about where you stand regarding your childhood. If it was necessary to do psychological or spiritual work on what took place in your early years, have you done that sufficiently? Is there more work to do? Or have you been working so long and hard on events of the past that it has you bogged down? What can you do to live more in the present?*

JULY 8

Break the Comparison Habit

It can be worse than high school. Then we compared ourselves to our friends and to the in-crowd if our friends weren't it. Now we're comparing ourselves to models with one-in-a-million bodies and actresses with million-dollar wardrobes. They have hair and makeup people at their beck and call, but we look at their pictures, and then look in the mirror and chide ourselves for coming up short. Most of us would also come up short if we compared our pay stubs to theirs; we just don't often do that. It's too ingrained in the cultural ethos that women are to rank themselves first on how they rate visually compared to other women. We also get to compare our mothering, grandmothering, lovemaking, money-making, people-pleasing, and problem-solving skills, but the face/hair/body comparison is primary.

And it's not just between us and the glitterati. Many of us are still concerned about how we rate compared to the "other girls," but we're better off all the way around if we just stop comparing. Even when we come out looking good, it's human nature to keep comparing until we find somebody up against whom we can feel comfortably inferior. Gosh, it's just like high school! If you recognize yourself here, I suggest that you make two promises to yourself today:

1. *I will not compare myself to famous women, younger women, or my peers.* You make this promise to elevate your self-esteem, celebrate your individuality, and embrace the reality that all you know of another woman's life is what *you* see, not what *she* feels.

2. I will not compare myself to myself when I was a lot (or a little) younger. You make this promise to ground yourself in this day and compel yourself to appreciate your present beauty—it's real—and not some past beauty that is only a memory.

There is tremendous freedom in the post-comparison life. For one thing, you'll have more friends. So what if one has fewer wrinkles and another has more jewelry? You'll like going to the movies better, too, because you'll be able to pay attention to the story and not the state of a stranger's abs. Escaping from the comparison trap means that you can go forward knowing that the best you can be, for today, is the way you *are* today. And that's just fine.

REVITALIZE YOUR LIFE WITH WORDS: *I am incomparable, just as I am.*

JULY 9

Revamp Your Pantry and Fridge

The food you eat will fuel your rejuvenation. Revamping your pantry and fridge will hasten the process. You can take it slowly or make changes all at once. The goal is to make healthy eating easy and mindless eating difficult.

If you live alone, or if you hold sway over the kitchen and can make changes there without a family uprising, do away with its less laudable denizens:

- Refined sugar, artificial sweeteners, soda pop, and packaged sweets (cookies, cakes, etc.)

- Chips and hyper-salted snacks

- Most white-flour products (a nice semolina pasta is okay; gooey white bread you're better off without)

- Shortening and bottled oils except for olive and canola (if you did this April 22 you're ahead of the game)

- Any items in your cupboards or fridge that are so colored, processed, or artificial that extraterrestrials would never take them for products of earth

After making this clean sweep, you'll have room for:

- Seasonal, organic produce (your crisper should always be full of vegetables, and a bowl of fresh fruit is lovely on a kitchen table)

- Whole-grain breads and cereals (oats, millet, brown rice)

- Whole-wheat flour if you bake bread and whole-wheat pastry flour for muffins and cakes (alternatively, rice, garbanzo, spelt, and/or potato flour if you avoid wheat)

- A variety of legumes—lentils, split peas, black beans, garbanzos

- Frozen vegetables and unsweetened frozen fruits and berries

- Select dried fruits and your favorite natural sweetener (such as raw, local honey, pure maple syrup, or barley malt)

- Soy milk and tofu made from soybeans that have not been genetically modified

- Extra-virgin olive oil for cooking and salads, organic canola oil for baking, flax oil (kept refrigerated) for omega-3 fatty acids, and either ghee (the clarified butter prized in Ayurveda) or a natural margarine that contains no trans-fatty acids

- Herbs and spices, organic when available, in small amounts to keep their freshness

- And, if you wish, unprocessed meats, very fresh or freshly frozen fish, free-range eggs, and dairy products from cows who were fed organic feed and not given questionable drugs such as BGH (Bovine Growth Hormone)

When you're stocked up, move on to the cookbooks. With the exception of a couple to which you have some sentimental attachment, see that your cookbooks emphasize well-being. A word like "light," "healthy," or "whole" in the title or subtitle suggests that the creators of these recipes care as much about your arteries and your pants size as about the compliments you'll get from preparing their dishes.

REJUVENATE YOURSELF WITH ACTION: *Make an appointment with yourself to do a fridge and pantry revamp on your first day off.*

Revamp the Rest of Your Kitchen

Yesterday we talked about the pantry and the fridge—in other words, the food in your kitchen and the cookbooks that tell you what to do with it. Today let's look at the kitchen itself. This isn't about remodeling or replacing major appliances, just about making the room, which is in large measure your revitalization laboratory, inviting and efficient. Is yours cheerful and bright? Do you like spending time there? If you answer yes to these questions, you have a head start. If not, arrange to do something to perk up the space. You might make weekend plans to wash the windows and hang clean, crisp curtains, or put up new potholders and tea towels, or give the woodwork a sparkling coat of white paint.

Then look to your cookware. Ideally, you'll have high-quality pots and pans of stainless steel, baked enamel, or cast iron. Tough nonstick coating is helpful on frying pans, sauté pans, and bakeware to minimize your use of oil. Have a steaming trivet for cooking vegetables with a minimal loss of vitamins. Get your knives professionally sharpened every year or two; they're going to be doing lots of peeling and slicing.

Your food processor and blender will come in handy for chopping veggies and making healthy drinks, spreads, and sauces. Having a juicer means you'll drink more juice, and certain juicers, such as the Champion, can make sorbet from frozen fruit and soft-serve "ice cream" from frozen bananas. If your crockpot didn't end up in a garage sale years ago, it can be the next best thing to a private chef, simmering grains and beans all day so dinner is waiting when you get home. An electric rice cooker takes away any intimidation brown rice (or any rice, for that matter) may hold, since the rice always turns out perfectly. (Some rice cookers are also steamers that can be used for preparing fish and vegetables. They're surprisingly inexpensive.)

Microwaves are controversial. They do make it possible to heat foods without the addition of fats or oils, but no one could argue that we were designed to eat food that has been zapped with microwaves or, as it's sometimes called, "nuked." I suggest you consider using the microwave only for reheating and do your real cooking via conventional means.

A kitchen revamp is an ongoing affair. You won't do everything today, but by this time next year, expect to have transformed this vital room. For now, make even one adjustment. Then expect to start feeling as healthy as your cupboards look.

REJUVENATE YOURSELF WITH ACTION: *If you're at home now, walk into your kitchen; if you're somewhere else, visualize the room. What easy, inexpensive changes could you make there to either create a more pleasant space or make your kitchen more conducive to preparing the healthiest foods you know of?*

JULY 11

What Would Your Life Be Like If You Approved of Yourself Every Day?

Sometimes I think there are two of me in the outward, physical sense. There is basic me—showered and covered but not much more—stopping at the Organic Harvest Café after my Pilates class. Then there is my other self, the one who's dressed well, wears makeup, and goes out into the world beyond my neighborhood. Of course we're the same person, just different presentations of that person. I'm sure you're familiar with what I'm talking about, because you have different presentations, too.

The key to integrating these divergent aspects of our visible selves is, I think, to accept ourselves both ways. This means no more feeling embarrassed when, as basic self, we run into someone who knows us as adorned self. You know the scenario: "I was only going out for a loaf of bread. If I'd known I'd be running into [fill in the blank: Prince Charles, Prince Charming, the woman who's out to get my job], I would have looked better." But basic, as long as you're neat and smell pleasant, is no less presentable than dressed to kill, and at times is even more appropriate. Going out without makeup and knockout clothes is the way some very famous women protect their privacy: fans are so shocked to see them *a cappella* that they're less likely to approach. It's like a sign that says, "This is my day off." You and I deserve days off, too, when a pony tail and lip gloss are enough doing up, no matter whom we meet.

This is not an excuse for letting yourself go, just for sometimes letting yourself be, and approving of what that looks like.

REVITALIZE YOUR LIFE WITH WORDS: *I am who I am, when I'm all decked out and when I'm only in sweats and sun-block.*

JULY 12

Avoiding the Nostalgia Trap

Nobody sounds older than someone waxing poetic about the good old days, whether those days were five years ago or fifty. True, thinking about days gone by is a great excuse not to do the work inherent in today, but it's a poor mindset for growing younger.

I get nostalgia-prone when I remember growing up in an exciting city now muted by suburban sprawl. Or when the computer confounds me and I remember doing just fine with a pen and a typewriter. Nostalgia marches alongside me when I trudge through a voice-mail jungle and recall the sweet service performed by receptionists and switchboard operators. It's a cunning trap, because speaking to a receptionist *was* more pleasant than receiving commands from a disembodied voice that, chances are, doesn't even belong to a human being. But in memory exempt of varnish or revision, sometimes those receptionists said things like, "We can't give credit to a single woman," or "I'm sorry, that job has been filled," when you knew those words were code for "You're the wrong sex" or "Your skin is the wrong color." The past was, to paraphrase Dickens, the best and the worst of times.

A powerful exercise for avoiding the nostalgia trap and valuing yourself as you are today is to make a photographic timeline of your life to date. To do this you need to get out your albums and assemble a photo montage. It needs to include a baby picture of yourself and images of you as a toddler or preschooler, an elementary schoolgirl, a preteen, a teenager, and one photo per decade in your twenties, thirties, and so on, right up to a very recent shot. Print it if it's digital. Then spread the images out before you on the table or floor.

With your photos in front of you, study each one and think about what was going on in your life at the time it was taken. In the case of the baby pictures, you'll be recalling what you heard from your parents or older siblings. Because life is always a mixture of what we label good and what we label bad, it may be that you were a very wanted child but your father was out of work, your mother wasn't well, and the joy of having a beautiful baby was sometimes eclipsed by the strain of late mortgage payments and unpaid doctor bills. What about those school pictures? You were smiling, but was long division baffling you, or were you worried about your big brother who had gone to a far-off place to fight a far-off war? Come up with all the details you can about yourself and your circumstances at each of these photographed times of your life. Then ask yourself this question: When, in all these times, was life the best?

I've done this exercise with hundreds of women, and the answer to this question falls into a fifty-fifty pattern. Nearly half the women say that it's not a matter of best and worst, that their lives have almost always been a blend. Most of the other half say, "Now. *This* is the best time. If life is a game, I've finally figured out how to play it." Ironically, this kind of looking backward saves you from looking back at times when you need to be facing full frontal forward. When you can see your life in retrospect, the romanticism of how good things once were gives way to the reality that positives and negatives comprise every day and every decade.

REVITALIZE YOUR LIFE WITH WORDS: *These are the good old days.*

This Is the Moment

I spent seven years working for a society magazine where I wrote about weddings and debutantes and parties to which I would otherwise not have been invited. Once I spoke with a seventy-five-year-old bride who, like her new husband, had been widowed the preceding year. "There are plenty of people who think we didn't wait a respectable amount of time," she told me, "but at our age, if you wait, who knows if you'll get the chance?"

Without being fatalistic, it is safe to say that after you reach forty, what was once reasonable—waiting to marry until you finished school, waiting to have a child until your career was established, waiting to travel until you'd saved the down payment for a house—becomes less reasonable. It's time to shift your thinking, as a general rule, toward sooner rather than later. This is a strategic move that will help you establish priorities, put first things first, and never have to say, when you're seriously senior, "I always wanted to [fill in the blank], but I never got around to it."

You can start this shift today with the smallest of choices. Maybe you've been wanting to go to the new sushi place on the other side of town. Go. If every year you've wanted to splurge at the Big Fancy Store's midsummer sale but it's never seemed practical, head for the Big and Fancy. Perhaps you get a hankering every semester to enroll in a university course, but time or money or intimidation has kept you away. Your commitment to doing it now will take care of the intimidation; once that's out of the way, you'll figure out the time and the money.

Taking action is, to coin a much-needed word, *youthening*. Indecision and immobility are aging. This is the moment: take it.

REJUVENATE YOURSELF WITH ACTION: *Think of something you really want to do but have been putting off. If it's doable today—sushi for lunch, for instance—do it. If you're looking at something more momentous, take one action today to get the wheels in motion. This can be as simple as a phone call to request information, a visit to some websites, or writing in your journal about what you intend to do. Make notes on your calendar to follow up on these actions weekly or monthly until you've brought your vision into being.*

When You're Just Not Doing Great

Sometimes we hit roadblocks: fatigue, discouragement, or the powerful desire to assert our inalienable right to impersonate a vegetable. As a result, we slack off, cut corners, get lazy, and then whine about why things aren't better. We'd be happier people if we didn't do that, but asking to be flogged in the village square isn't going to help. Besides, we always do the best we can. If you let things go that you'd really like to be doing, chances are you're exhausted, or some problem has you down, or someone close to you is in trouble and your caretaking energy is on round-the-clock call. You can still get younger, though, as long as you maintain your membership in your own fan club.

We love our kids, even when they come in late and dye their hair bizarre colors. We love the dog, even when she snaps at the poodle next door or throws up on the carpet. We love our friends when they make the same mistake the thirty-second time; we tell them we understand and we *know* there won't be a number thirty-three. We have to love ourselves like this, too. The only way you can mess up becoming younger by the day is by giving up entirely. So don't do that. When you feel overwhelmed, concentrate on the ways you can rejuvenate that take minimal effort: play enlivening music; stand tall; toss a bottle of water into your bag. If you haven't been keeping up with this book every single day, what does it matter? Double up now or give yourself extra time—whatever makes this work for you.

When it's difficult to get everything together, resist the temptation to believe there is something inherently wrong with you. There isn't. Everything in life is cyclic. If we can accept that there are bright days and dreary ones, hot days and cold ones, good times and bad, why is it so incomprehensible that similar cycles would affect us? When your cycle is at a low spot, avoid throwing in the legendary towel and instead take this opportunity to learn to treat yourself with at least as much kindness as you show your dog.

You are the same person when your day's dietary intake could be a sidebar in *Better Lives and Bodies* and on days when the major food group represented was cellophane. In the latter case, you just don't feel as well. You're no more valuable to the world and the people who love you when you stop at the gym on your way to work than when you stop at the doughnut shop, but you feel more valuable and you have a better day. You're not a slob when you care for yourself less and a saint when you care for yourself more. You just deserve to be cared for all the time.

REJUVENATE YOURSELF WITH ACTION: *Assess how you're doing up to this point. (If you're just beginning the younger-by-the-day program, assess your overall level of self-care at this time in your life.) Where would you like to do better? Take a look at your priorities and be sure your energy is going where it's of most use to you.*

JULY 15

Play Day!

JULY 16

Make Peace with Change

You know how it is when a concept really grabs you and you remember forever where you were when you first heard it? I was on a train in northwest China watching with my daughter a children's video about Buddhism on a tiny, in-camera screen. "In Buddhism," the female narrator explained, "change is seen as the most constant force in life. To the Buddhist, enlightenment is being perfectly at peace with change." I pushed "rewind" and listened again. It was so simple and made such good sense.

I don't foresee enlightenment any time soon, but I know that if I fight change, I lose and the changes keep right on coming. Midlife is one of the most changeable times of all. We may have children becoming adults and parents becoming aged. We're advised to get medical tests we thought were for people older than us. We might look in the mirror and catch a glimpse of our mothers instead of ourselves. Some of us stop saving for retirement and actually retire, and even we who figure we'll work till we're ninety receive by mail—in the United States anyway—a provisionary membership card from the AARP as a fiftieth-birthday greeting. When a friend of mine had her fiftieth-birthday party, the invitations said, "You are invited for the signing of the card."

Although change may seem to have accelerated recently, it is, as the voice in the video said, the most constant fact of life. Look at the seasons, the tides, and the stars. Everything is moving, changing. Even inside our bodies, cells are dying and being born, so that after seven years you can't even find the physical stuff that made up the person you once were. Circumstances shift more reliably than the weather in Chicago. Peace comes in accepting that when you went to the recruiting office to apply for life on earth, you signed up for one wild ride. You can't do a thing about that except fasten your seat belt, hold on tight, and remind yourself that people have lots of fun on roller-coasters, in race cars, and in tiny little airplanes.

REVITALIZE YOUR LIFE WITH WORDS: *I'm up for change. I go with it and flow with it.*

JULY 17

Chromium

Chromium renders insulin more efficient at dealing with sugar, and many women opt to take a chromium supplement for this reason. It has been used clinically in the treatment of diabetes, and there is evidence that it may protect against type II (adult-onset) diabetes. A unique endowment of chromium is its ability to balance blood sugar, whether it is high or low.

Chromium has also been shown to increase lean body mass. (This is why it is sometimes touted as a slimming supplement.) We know this trace mineral is able to ramp up the body's manufacture of DHEA, a hormone that young bodies create in abundance and older bodies often lack. DHEA may check memory loss, enhance immune response, strengthen bones, and even play a role in preventing cancer.

Although chromium is found in some foods, notably nutritional yeast, broccoli, eggs, and shellfish, it is not believed to be well absorbed from food. Our levels of chromium decline with age, and eating sweets ups our need for it. Although the dose prescribed by a health professional is sometimes higher, it appears to be safe and reasonable to supplement 100 to 200 micrograms daily. The preferred form of the mineral is chromium picolinate.

REJUVENATE YOURSELF WITH ACTION: *Speaking of sweets, how are you handling your sweet tooth this summer? Strive to keep it satisfied with the season's juicy fruits and go easy on refined-sugar treats.*

JULY 18

Create a World in Which You Can Age as You Like

"Create a world" may sound like a tall order for a daily reading, but we largely create our own worlds anyway; I'm just asking that you devise a personal world that will let you age as you like. Women have always lived in different spheres as far as aging is concerned, but these were more often imposed on them than created by them. For example, an academic was traditionally allowed to age differently than an actress. The former wore silver hair and bifocals as signs of experience and tenure, while the latter sought to hold on to a youthful appearance as long as she could.

In your life today, if you like focusing on physical appearance and spending money and energy on looking younger, you have every right to be part of the salon, spa, and even surgery set and enjoy it. If that seems like a waste to you, or it's alien to your values, create a different world for yourself. You can be an artist, an intellectual, an activist, an eccentric, or something I can't even think of because it's your life and your world. You can combine worlds, too, and be an artistic eccentric with regular salon and spa appointments. This is *your* creation.

When you create a personal world like this, there is reinforcement and reassurance all around you. Certainly there will be times when you'll interact with people who move in different circles, but if you're firmly ensconced in the life you've created, they'll respect and admire your differentness, the way French wine and Russian ballet are especially appreciated when exported.

REJUVENATE YOURSELF WITH ACTION: *Contemplate today how much effort you expend trying to be part of some world that isn't "you." Sometimes this is unavoidable—the requirement to be part of an office culture, for instance—but in those parts of your life over which you have control, how much are you conforming to please others? Are you being forced to adjust the way you're maturing to keep up with standards that are not your own? How can you create a world in which you have more autonomy?*

JULY 19

The Learned Skill of Letting Go

Letting go is both an art and a skill. The more you practice, the more competent at it you'll become. You cannot successfully conduct your life's second half without developing this capacity.

In this half, you will be called upon to let go of chronological youth and that heady feeling of having an endless span of time before you to do just about anything. The way the timing often works, you may have to let go of the ability to have children around the same time you're letting go of the children you birthed. You'll have to let go of having periods, and you may be shocked to discover that this erstwhile nuisance is all of a sudden a lovely thing, your connection to womanliness and the tides and the moon. You may be asked to let go of the home where you collected blue-ribbon memories, or the job that defined you, or being the wife of a professional this or that when your husband retires. Then there is the hardest letting go of all, letting go of people who pass away, as more and more will the longer you live.

Thank goodness all this letting go doesn't happen at once and you can increase your aptitude for it over time. Start by loosening your grip on little things. Unless you have a bona fide collection, don't collect, and other than the truly meaningful, don't hang on to a lot of memorabilia and souvenirs. Enjoy experiences for their time and let them go. Let go of past events and past identities. Allow the people around you to grow and change and move to Minneapolis. They will, with or without your blessing. Giving it just makes it easier for you.

Once you understand that nothing is yours to keep—not your youth, or your job title, or even your baby—you put yourself in the position of enjoying all these, and every other benefaction you've been given, to the fullest. You'll have more energy because you won't be grasping at what's going or gone. You lose one thing; you gain another. When you learn the skill of letting go, you're first in line for receiving what's next.

REVITALIZE YOUR LIFE WITH WORDS: *I live with open hands, letting go when it is time to let go and gratefully receiving the next wonder.*

JULY 20

Become an Adept

You become an adept when you are really—*really*—good at something. It could be litigating in a courtroom or teaching in a classroom, playing piano or playing poker, growing investments or growing day lilies. Being an adept is better than just being a professional, and you can become adept at something that is not your profession. Either way, it means you have fulfilled your potential in at least one area of life.

A while back, in a shopping mall in Springfield, Missouri, I stopped for a ten-minute trial of a reclining chair with a massaging mechanism inside. I told the man at the booth, "I'm familiar with your company. My mother worked for the Kansas City franchise when I was a little girl."

He squinted at me a second. "You wouldn't be speaking of Gladys Marshall, would you?"

"Well, yes," I said. "That's my mom."

"They still talk about her!" he exclaimed. "She's a legend—one of the best salesmen this company ever had." I was impressed—especially considering that when she did it, her colleagues and competitors were almost all salesmen. That's the level of adeptness we're after.

Think today about what you do best. Can you become still better at it, go all the way to adept? Or does something intrigue you that you would love to try, something at which you believe you have the potential to become adept? Either way, commit yourself to this thing—ideally something you love. It takes time and effort and close association with a job or a hobby or an art form to become adept at it. You'll be far happier if you're adept at something you adore.

REJUVENATE YOURSELF WITH ACTION: *At what are you adept (or nearly so)? At what would you love to become adept? Take one solid step today toward developing this expertise. Write what you did in your journal.*

JULY 21

Never Apologize for Being the Age You Are

Whatever your age, make it a point of pride, not shame. This is hard for middle-aged women in a society like ours. Being able to say, "I'm twenty-seven," gets a woman points because it states that she's young and desirable and "right." Not long after that, though, she can start feeling "too old" if she lets herself. I first felt this at thirty-two when, pregnant with Adair, I saw that my chart in the OB's office was stamped in red: ELDERLY PRIMAGRAVIDA. That's medical jargon for "woman over thirty having her first baby," but "elderly"? Come on.

Decide today to be proud of the years you've lived, whatever their number. You don't have to tell people your age unless you want to, but don't apologize for it, whether it's voiced or not. You are no less valuable than you were at twenty-seven. In fact, you're more valuable. There's more to you, and I don't mean pounds. You are your basic spiritual self—that's already a miracle—plus all the experiences of your life. If you're going to apologize for anything, make it that you're only fifty-six, a mere shadow of the personage you'll be with another three decades under your belt.

REVITALIZE YOUR LIFE WITH WORDS: *I am exactly the right age.*

Take a Hard Stand on Soft Drinks

The Center for Science in the Public Interest has called soft drinks "liquid candy." I agree. But soda is worse than candy because it goes down so easy. Nobody is eating six hundred twelve-ounce servings of candy a year, but that's the amount of soda drunk by the average American. If you're still "average" in this way, I challenge you to become exceptional.

Here are the problems: A single can of regular soda has nearly ten teaspoons of sugar—that's all the added sugar a mature woman should get in a day, according to the American Institute for Cancer Research. All this sugar can lead to weight gain, type II diabetes, and more time in the dentist's chair than anyone wants to spend there. If you drink diet soda, you're ingesting a lot of aspartame, a possible cause of some ninety disorders, from headaches and muscle spasms to joint pain, ear ringing, and blurred vision. Colas and some other soft drinks contain high levels of caffeine, an excess of which can irritate the stomach and cause disorders of the nervous system and adrenal glands, and many sodas contain phosphoric acid, which can irritate the stomach and weaken the bones.

Anytime you buy a drink in a bottle or can, read the label. Some that are called "juice" or even "water" are really soft drinks, carbonated or not, and full of high-fructose corn syrup (September 29) or artificial sweetener, and perhaps various chemical additives.

To wean yourself away from these less-than-salutary beverages:

- *Make your own "sodas" from sparkling mineral water and fruit juice, or drink the sparkling water alone with lemon or lime.* Carbonation seems relatively harmless. The only caveats I've come across are: some people find that it gives them gas; Chinese medicine suggests that eliminating carbonated beverages might do away with some joint pains; and singers and speakers are advised to avoid carbonation on performance days.

- *Keep a pitcher of tea, regular or herbal, in the fridge in summer.* Black tea does contain caffeine, but quite a bit less than cola, and you can control the amount by how strong you make the tea.

- *Drink plenty of water and eat fresh fruits and raw vegetables.* This will help keep you well hydrated.

- *Avoid salty snack foods.* These beg to be eaten in the company of soda, inviting trouble.

REVITALIZE YOUR LIFE WITH WORDS: *I am as particular about beverages as I am about food.*

JULY 23

Don't Let Them Get You Down

This world is full of naysayers, crêpe hangers, and prophets of doom, especially on the topic of maturity. You've got to watch what you read about aging (and what you believe of what you read). Much of what's out there is scarier than the evening news and more depressing than a bear market's stock report. For example, not long ago I visited a respected website to get some information about menopause. It read like a litany of decay: Your bones will weaken. Your muscles will atrophy. You'll lose control of your bladder. You'll open yourself up for getting Alzheimer's. It wasn't phrased to imply that *some* of these *could* happen, but rather that *all* of them *would*. There wasn't a word about this transition's being the gateway to wisdom and self-acceptance. There was nothing about this as a key time for coming into your own. I just shut down the computer and turned on the TV. After that site, even the news looked hopeful.

I am not suggesting that we fail to educate ourselves about what we're up against, medically, economically, socially, and all the rest, just that it is essential to get your information in ways that won't make you want to hitch a ride on the nearest hearse. Not letting "them"—negative messages, whether they're from modern media or old wives' tales—get you down is also a socially responsible action. When you refuse to be drawn into ain't-it-awful scenarios, you make maturing less horrific for those coming later. Baby-boomers tend to think we changed the world every time we burned a bra or took a

Pill. Well, here's another chance. We've already altered the image of aging; there is no question that fifty *looks* younger than it used to. Now we have the opportunity to revolutionize the reality behind the image by taking the fear out of the post-forty decades and emphasizing instead their pluses and their potential.

Do this first by paying close attention to the tone and content of the information you allow in and to how you process that information once you have it. Then pay equally close attention to what you pass along to others, striving to be a bearer of good tidings whenever possible. In so doing, you create an immediate world in which things are generally looking up, and "looking up" is a state conducive to health, happiness, and longevity.

REJUVENATE YOURSELF WITH ACTION: *Set your antennae to detect negative messages and send them back where they came from.*

<hr>

JULY 24

Financing Your Transformation

While many of the suggestions in this book involve spending money—"Go for a facial"; "Buy something to wear that looks like you"; "Get a great haircut"; "Eat organically grown food"—growing younger needn't be beyond anyone's means. The basics are either free (valuing yourself, seeing yourself as youthful and vital, having a viable spiritual life) or cheap (eating simple, natural foods, exercising, and grooming yourself like someone who deserves to be well cared for).

One way to finance those parts of your transformation that do require cash is to funnel the money saved from giving up bad habits into an earmarked fund for self-care and growing younger. Ex-smokers get the best deal here: they end up with substantial extra money in addition to extra years to live. But no longer buying junk food and soda saves money, too. Walking more and driving or taking cabs less is a frugality move. Shopping carefully and buying only clothes you love saves money in the long run.

In addition, most people can find the wherewithal for transformation if they look at their spending patterns and plug the leaks. Using cash often and credit seldom is a great start, and writing down every dollar and cent you spend, at least for awhile, can be an enlightening exercise. At the end of the month, codify the amounts you've jotted down into categories: "Auto," "Rent," "Groceries," "Eating Out," "Cosmetics," "Clothing," "Cards and Gifts," etc. Once you have a reasonable picture of where your money is going, you may see that you're putting a fortune into something that gives back very little—weekday restaurant lunches, for instance. You could find that brown-bagging twice a week would give you the means for a pedicure or a half-hour massage.

Ultimately, we all decide, consciously or unconsciously, where our money goes. Decide today that a little more of it needs to go toward keeping you young, vital, and full of life.

REJUVENATE YOURSELF WITH ACTION: *If you've never tracked your spending, do it for a month, starting tomorrow. Carry a little notebook with you and jot down the cash you spend. Checks and debit-card transactions are already in your checkbook. After thirty days, total what you've spent in the various categories. This way you see where your money is going and how you can put more of it toward rejuvenation. If you'd like additional details on keeping financial records, I recommend* How to Get Out of Debt, Stay Out of Debt, and Live Prosperously, *by Jerrold Mundis.*

JULY 25

Pharmaceuticals

Modern medicine is one of the reasons we're living so long and doing so well. Still, it's often misused. It's nothing for a woman in midlife to be taking daily medications for diabetes, depression, hypertension, nasal allergies, nail fungus, insomnia, and hormonal imbalance. That's a lot of chemicals.

The medication your doctor prescribes may improve your life or even save it, but it is nevertheless essential that you keep track of your pharmaceutical profile. Do this by meeting periodically with your doctor and/or pharmacist (in this case, *and* is better than *or*) to review it. You may be taking two drugs that should not be used together. This is a particular problem when you have prescriptions from different physicians, but it can happen with just one doctor, too. In addition, with the healthy lifestyle you're adopting as you read this book, you may be taking some medication in a dose that is no longer right for you. You may even be taking some drug you no longer need; your doctor can ascertain your status on your next visit.

I must admit, I felt proud when I was taking no prescribed medicine except bio-identical hormones, but pride comes before a fall and I fell—into an excruciating condition called *adhesive capsulitis*, a.k.a. "frozen shoulder," an alias that doesn't begin to describe the intense pain and life-altering immobility it causes its victims, generally women between forty and sixty. Although it is neither life-threatening nor permanent, the time it does last, eighteen to twenty-four months on average, feels like forever. I got through the first two months before turning to over-the-counter pain relievers (which came from over a counter but didn't relieve the pain) and later filling the prescription for painkillers that I had received on diagnosis.

It was humbling: Ms. Natural, with something stamped "controlled substance" on my shelf between the vitamins and the nutritional yeast, but it was an opportunity to learn. Now, better educated and post-smug, here's what I know about pharmaceuticals:

- *This is no place for improvisation.* Once you agree to taking a prescribed medication, take it the way it is prescribed for you, no doubling up or cutting back without a professional okay.

- *Drugs don't make a beeline to your headache or your heartburn or whatever it is you're taking them for.* They affect your entire body. Therefore, when you and your doctor agree that a drug can be avoided, avoid it. In a way, all drugs are addictive. That is, you start to take some medication and you might need another for a side effect, and before you know it, you have your own pharmacy of little brown bottles. Find a doctor who understands alternatives and who will tell it to you straight when you really do need medication.

- *There are knowledgeable pharmacists who will take the time to talk to you.* There are also drugstores with cross-referencing computer programs to be sure you don't get incompatible medications. Look for people and places like these.

- *If some medication makes the world look too rosy, be on your guard.* Addiction can sneak up on people. If a drug you are taking turns life into the shiny perfection of a 1950s musical, chances are it is too good to be true—or too good to be safe anyway.

Bottom line: listen to your doctor. Bottom-bottom line: listen to yourself.

REVITALIZE YOUR LIFE WITH WORDS: *I assist my body's healing in the wisest, safest ways.*

|ULY 26

Living Foods

At lunch with my friend Lisa, the discussion turned to the various ways people choose to eat to enhance their health. I mentioned someone I know, a man in his forties who, for the past three years, has eaten only fresh, uncooked foods from the plant kingdom. "It's odd, but every time I see him, he gets more and more . . ."—I was searching for the right word when Lisa interjected, "Gorgeous?" "That's it," I said. "Gorgeous." And younger. And brighter. And more alive.

For the people suited to it, this Edenic dietary style apparently works wonders. Certainly not everyone is cut out for such a departure from the norm, but we could all stand to include in our meals more foods that are absolutely fresh and that come to us precisely as nature provided them. It is a curious fact that only humans and our domesticated animals eat cooked food. Perhaps we can learn something from every other species on earth.

Fresh vegetables and fruits keep the digestive system moving: if digestion is sluggish, the material that should be expelled stays with us to ferment. Having to deal with a backlog of undigested food is a drain on our energy—energy we could be using for exercise or creativity or growing younger. There is also the enzyme issue: assimilating food requires digestive enzymes, and every cellular function uses metabolic enzymes as catalysts. We have a wealth of enzymes in our bodies at birth, but according to Stephen Parker, editor of the newsletter *Raw Dish!*, we borrow from them to help us digest cooked foods and thereby deplete our supply. Raw foods don't need our enzymes since they have their own.

With summer in its glory, this is a great time to eat more living foods: salads, sprouts, crudités, fresh fruits, and unroasted nuts and seeds (ideally soaked from several hours to overnight to deactivate their enzyme inhibitors, nature's defense against premature sprouting). If you're healthy and not on a special diet from your doctor, you might do this for ten days as a detox, or one day a week during the warm months, or one meal a day as long as it feels right. When I do a week or two of living foods, my skin is clearer (no redness or blotches), I have a lot of pep, and I don't miss washing pots and pans one bit.

Living foods can be utter simplicity or an adventure into a unique cuisine to tempt the curious diner. I've had raw plant foods prepared to taste like everything from meatballs to salmon, and "live" desserts that are, well, *to live for*. Some large cities have raw food restaurants, and booksellers and health food stores stock "cookless books." A couple I've enjoyed are *Living in the Raw* by Rose Lee Calabro, and *Raw*, by Charlie Trotter and Roxanne Klein. Or you could just bite into a ripe summer peach.

REJUVENATE YOURSELF WITH ACTION: *Take advantage of the bounty of the season by eating more fresh, uncooked food this summer.*

JULY 27

Limiting Limitations

It can seem that life presents more limitations, liabilities, and drawbacks when we're older, but maybe they just get more sophisticated. In your quest to look and feel more youthful, there may exist one seemingly insurmountable circumstance that stands in the way of seeing yourself in possession of many of the best characteristics of youth, whatever your chronological age. Maybe it's weight ("Didn't losing ten pounds used to be easy?"), or sun-damaged skin ("Sure there's laser, but for my whole body?"), or some health problem that may or may not be life-threatening but that sounds depressingly elderly either way.

The limitation may have material evidence: a walking stick, a hearing aid, visible bifocals. Or it may not show to other people but always be present in your mind's eye. When I had frozen shoulder, I had to sleep with special pillows and get my groceries in double paper bags that I could carry cradled like a baby. I felt like a picky old lady with days of so little consequence that I had to make a federal case out of how I wanted my groceries bagged.

Then it hit me that "picky old lady" was an image I had chosen—no one else. Since I invented it, I could change it. My need for special bagging would no longer make me elderly and limited. I could choose something else. How about privileged and entitled? I've noticed that women of means demand all sorts of favors and do it really well. In a café, one of them might ask, or rather state, "You're not using that chair, are you?" with such certainty of the answer that even if the chair is holding a coat, hat, laptop, and birthday gifts for triplets, the other customer says, "Oh, no, help yourself." I decided to be like that self-assured woman, easily deserving of two paper bags.

You can do the same thing about any obstacle that is interfering with your growing-younger process. Take it in stride. Work around it. Frame it differently. This is the way stretch marks become battle scars. It's how a middle-aged shape stops being something to resent and becomes instead evidence of six well-spent decades and three awesome offspring. It's one way that a health concern, whether a challenge to overcome or a cross to bear, ceases to define you.

Some women will feel they're growing younger only if a friend who's been away sees them and says, "My God, you must have married a plastic surgeon!" Those who grasp the essence of renewal will know they're there when they wake up in the morning and sense, cohabiting peacefully with the stretch marks and the softening jawline, an irrepressible eagerness to seize this day.

REVITALIZE YOUR LIFE WITH WORDS: *I am entitled to all good things.*

JULY 28

Revisit Feminism from a New Perspective

At a bookstore café not long ago, I overheard two men about my age discussing post-divorce dating. "I try not to date American women," one of them said. "They have too many rights." That's the kind of statement that reminds me that feminism, on both a personal and a political level, is as relevant as it ever was.

It stuns me to think that my mother was alive when women weren't allowed to vote or have bank accounts. Even as an adult in the 1940s she was once refused gasoline at a rural service station because she was wearing pants—something that in her mother's lifetime had actually been illegal. It is because of women who were willing to espouse feminism—both first round, prior to 1920, and second round, 1970s—that our daughters take their equal-to-men status as a matter of course. But this happy state isn't etched in stone, whether we're talking about political issues or personal ones. I've heard women in their twenties say things like, "The man should pay when you go out," and "My boyfriend comes over to fix things and I make him dinner." And when I dropped my pen in that café, the man who wouldn't date an American instantly swooped down to retrieve it from under an adjacent table. Part of me wanted to say, "I'll get my own pen: crawling under that table is my *right*," but another part of me was touched by the chivalry, so I just said thanks and kept on writing.

On a long summer day like this one, you might want to revisit feminism, in your mind or in your journal. How do you feel about the status of women in general and the milieu in which you're maturing and your daughters and granddaughters are growing up? What still needs to be done, for young women and older ones? Do you feel a conflict if some of your opinions seem like feminist ones and others don't? Can you respect and value yourself as a complex individual who can hold divergent views? The right to have a dissenting opinion is, after all, a vital part of being free.

REJUVENATE YOURSELF WITH ACTION: *Revisit feminism today, in your mind or in your journal.*

JULY 29

The Microscope or the Telescope?

If you've devoted most of your adult life to family, career, or both, you've exerted a lot of energy. Now you're likely to have either a heartfelt desire for peace and quiet and slowing down, or an equally fervent longing to make a great big splash. Both are valid. Most people choose the former and society encourages it. If you or people you know are looking for more peace and tranquility, you, or they, should have it, and find within it a beauty not visible from the outside.

I find as I speak to groups of women, though, that a growing number are in the other camp, chomping at the bit to get out there and do something extraordinary. New passions are taking hold, to start a business or end an injustice. There is an urgency within, perhaps what Samuel Beckett meant when he wrote, "Maybe my best years really are behind me, but I wouldn't want them back, not with the fire in me now."

It's interesting that early-retirement offers seem to be sending fewer women out to the proverbial pasture and more into entrepreneurial and philanthropic ventures that, when combined, have the potential to change history. Listening to your deepest self may never before have been as important as it is now. What are you going to do with the rest of your life? You can model either the microbiologist or the astronomer. One finds captivating worlds in tiny things. The other looks out to the vastness of the heavens. Both spheres are magnificent. Take your pick. Just be sure that what you choose is your own heart's desire.

REJUVENATE YOURSELF WITH ACTION: *Write in your journal about where you fit in this picture. Do you want to create a bit of bliss in what appears to be a small way? Or do you need to go after something big by any reckoning? Either way is just right. Also, write about how your plan jives with that of your life partner (if you have one). If one of you fancies the microscope and the other the telescope, what can be done to see that you both get what you need?*

JULY 30

Play Day!

Become Very Clear as to What You're About

At forty-three, I bought my first house. I'd wanted one like crazy. A house meant family, a happy childhood for my little girl and for the little girl self inside me. A house meant stability and legitimacy and respect. I was still a single mom, but I would be a homeowner, and that carried weight. Well, I got the house, but signing those papers was like signing my life away. I was soon to be overwhelmed by the upkeep and overcome by the yardwork. I missed the safe feeling of our apartment. Even my daughter longed for the old block, the old days. In the bright light of closing, it was obvious: it was never a house I wanted; it was what a house symbolized to me.

As you go forward with your life, become so clear as to what you're about that you never again do what I did and make the mistake of going for what you only *think* you want. This isn't to say that our errors, like a software program's, are "permanent and fatal," but let's face it: around the midpoint of our allotted span, who wants to waste time learning lessons the long way? Instead, come to know yourself well through your journal writing, meditation, and commiserating with friends who will tell you the truth. If you don't have friends like this, engage a counselor or a life coach: better truth for hire than no truth at all.

This knowing what you're about also pertains to your becoming younger by the day. If looking young is important to you because of the work you do, the crowd you're in, or simply because it's important and it's nobody's business why, you'll work toward that. If looks mean very little to you, but vitality and energy mean a lot, that's where you'll put your focus. If growing older fascinates you because of the freedom it can afford for being yourself, or because of its spiritual depths ripe for uncovering, concentrate your efforts on freedom or spirituality. Whatever you yourself find compelling *is* what you're about. Get very clear on it. It's you. It's correct. And you deserve the best of it.

REVITALIZE YOUR LIFE WITH WORDS: *I know what I want from life. I am open to receiving this or something even better.*

August

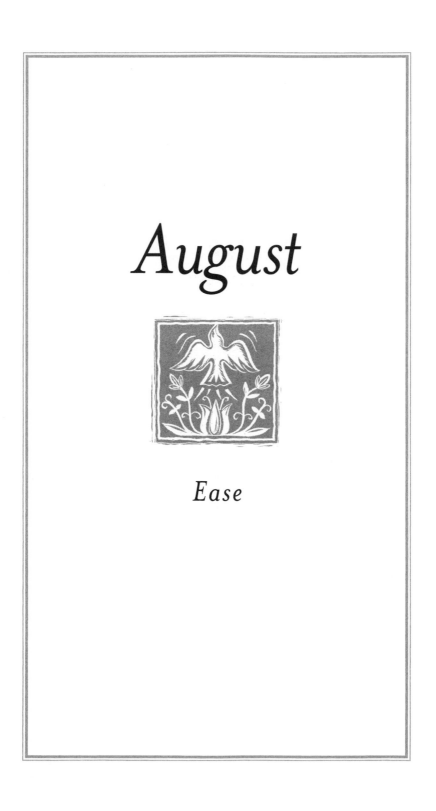

Ease

The Art of Allowing

Most of us were taught that the way to get ahead was to go out there and make things happen. Even as you proceed through *Younger by the Day*, you're taking certain actions with the expectation that they will yield certain results. No problem here.

What can be a problem, however, is when we overbalance on the side of making things happen to the exclusion of *allowing* them to happen. The art of allowing is the way you let the upward progression of the universe into your personal life and draw yourself upward with it. Of course you need to do your part, but sometimes your part is to step aside and allow previous efforts to come to fruition. Sometimes it's seeing that, in a particular circumstance, there is no work for you to do. Your role is simply to be present and allow life to take its course.

The long, lazy days of August are all about ease, moving slowly, doing a little less than usual as you gear up for fall, when you're likely to do a little more than usual. As you proceed through August, do everything you need to do, of course, but see if you can do it with a bit more ease. Find the efficiency paradoxically inherent in expending less effort. Trust the process and the purpose of your life. "Believe," as the poet and novelist Rainer Maria Rilke wrote, "in a love that is being stored up for you like an inheritance, and trust that in this love there is a strength and a blessing, out beyond which you do not have to step in order to go very far."

REVITALIZE YOUR LIFE WITH WORDS: *I allow life to mold me and shape me in beautiful ways.*

You and Your Dentist

Nowadays, having terrific teeth doesn't have to hurt. Take advantage of that with this advice from Lorna Flamer-Caldera, DDS:

- *Show up at the dentist's office for your exam and cleaning every six months like clockwork.* That way some problems can be prevented and little problems can be caught before they become big ones.

- *Insist on composite (white) fillings rather than mercury amalgam.* The latter may be at the root of an array of physical and emotional disorders. Some people opt to have old mercury fillings removed and replaced with composite. (If you have "silver" fillings, know that these are some 50 percent mercury.)

- *Protect your gums and bone.* The hormonal fluctuations of perimenopause and the precipitous drop at menopause can exacerbate early periodontal disease and dramatically accelerate bone loss. Head this off with conscientious home care, frequent professional cleanings, and a special deep-cleaning procedure called *scaling and root planing* that can work wonders.

- *If your dentist knows about nutrition, you've struck gold.* Teeth and gums need adequate calcium, magnesium, zinc, vitamin C, vitamin E, and selenium. Too much meat can negatively affect your bone density. Sugars (especially sticky sweets, hard candies, and cough drops), as well as refined carbs like white flour and white rice, create the acid medium favored by the bacteria that cause tooth decay and gum disease. Go easy on acidic substances (citrus fruits, apple juice, and cola, even diet) to protect tooth enamel.

- *"Who cares if Dad had dentures?"* Your dentist does; let her know about your dental family history.

- *Your dentist should also know what medications you're taking.* Many common drugs affect the state of your teeth. For instance, both antidepressants and high blood pressure medication can decrease saliva and lead to a subsequent increase in cavities.

- *The nightly grind.* Grinding or clenching your teeth while you sleep can grind away enamel, cause or exacerbate temporal mandibular joint disorder (TMJ), and even loosen teeth. A night guard will provide protection and may discourage the practice; biofeedback or acupuncture may help you stop grinding altogether.

- *An oral microbiology test.* Testing multiple saliva samples can show if there is a nutritional problem to be addressed, or if unusual bacteria are at work in your mouth that need to be treated in a more assertive fashion than keep-'em-clean-and-floss.

- *The big guns.* If warranted, your general dentist may send you to a periodontist, a specialist in gum disease, or an endodontist, who specializes in performing surgery on the roots of teeth. With this kind of team, and dogged determination on your part, you can get yourself a younger mouth.

REJUVENATE YOURSELF WITH ACTION: *If it's been more than six months since you've seen a dentist, make an appointment for a clean-and-check.*

AUGUST 3

Opening Your Mind

Being stodgy, "set in your ways," and closed-minded are mental precipitators of physical aging. You may be in danger of these if you've heard yourself saying things like "We've always done it that way," or "This is how I see it and this is how it is." Another warning sign is criticizing people who are different or who seem to be expressing themselves a little too freely: "I would never have let my kids dress that way." "You mean she changed jobs/churches/political parties/hair color just like that? I always knew there was something not right about her." And maybe there is. But there is also something "not right" about being so tied to our own view of things that we forget that other people are looking at life through their lenses, not ours.

All this considered, I think we close our minds to keep ourselves safe. If only one prescribed way of thinking and acting is satisfactory, we never have to take risks, make mistakes, embarrass ourselves, or start over. That's dandy for anybody who doesn't want to grow anymore, but a three-letter word for no more growth is O-L-D.

Ways to keep your mind open and ready to accept new things—not all new things, but some of them—include:

- *Judge less—or at least later.* When you hear something that sounds outrageous, let it settle in before you rush to judgment.

- *Give new ideas and images a chance.* While the very young latch on to things simply because they're new, the not so young tend to dismiss them just as readily. Find the golden mean.

- *Understand that everyone has his own truth or her own truth.* This truth is the star each person needs to follow to be authentic and fulfilled. The orb that your neighbor looks to may not be your star; it might come from another galaxy. That's okay. You have a star of your own.

- *Remember: you are not married to any belief, opinion, or ideology.* We expect people to change in their twenties; that's part of why they're so lively. There is no age limit for changing, though. You're entitled to a new favorite food, favorite color, and favored philosophy anytime the spirit moves you. Your sister is equally entitled. So is your ex-husband.

- *Expect to discover something delicious every day.* Same old, same old makes you rapidly grow old, grow old. Opening your mind is like opening your hands to receive the gifts you're offered.

Getting Hair Care Down to a Science

Some women have enviable hair all their lives. My friend Dolores has thick, wavy hair and although she's in her mid-fifties, she has yet to produce a gray strand. But then, her mother has only a few at ninety-one. In the genetic lottery, Dolores and her mom got great hair; you may have that or some other boon. Either way, we're all supposed to take care of what we've got.

If you're over fifty and if your mother had thin hair or your father was bald, chances are you have less hair than you once did. There are prescription and over-the-counter preparations that do grow hair for some people, although they're not without possible side effects (i.e., hair growing where you'd rather not have it). If thinning hair is a big problem for you, see a dermatologist. Otherwise, hair-thickening products (shampoos, conditioners, leave-in treatments) work surprisingly well, and their effect is cumulative.

Coloring your hair also makes it thicker, since color coats the hair shaft, giving it extra volume. If you color, protect your hair and your investment by using only shampoos and conditioners for color-treated hair. (There are some that both add texture and protect color.) You can shield your hair from the bleaching propensity of the chlorine in tap water with a chlorine-filtering shower head, available at large natural food stores or through natural living catalogs and websites. Whether you have virgin or tinted hair, condition it with an appropriate conditioner.

If you blow-dry or do heat-styling every day, give your mane the advantage of a thermal protectant, a leave-in conditioner formulated to defend hair against heat damage. Get your hair halfway dry before you blow it by using an extra-absorbent towel (available in cosmetic shops and some drugstores). Choose the medium and low settings on your blow-dryer, and since hair is damaged most in the final minutes of bombarding it with hot air, stop before it's bone-dry.

Perming and relaxing are anathema from your hair's point of view, but if it takes one of these to make you feel your best, be sure you're dealing with top-quality products in top-notch hands. Always treat your hair gently—no yanking or pulling. Use brushes and combs that have smooth teeth and bristles. Don't wear a pony tail every day, and use a covered band when you do.

Wearing a hat will defend your hair against drying and fading from the sun. Help it from the inside with B vitamins (in whole grains, beans, nuts, and seeds), protein, and the high-quality oils found in avocado, nuts, flax seeds, and olives. Like the rest of your body, your hair appreciates ample rest and sleep, wants you to drink lots of water, and hates it when you're stressed. Stress is, in fact, right up there with hormones and heredity as a major cause of hair loss.

Your hair should be a pleasure, not a problem. It might frizz in humidity and fly when the weather is dry, fall when it rains or flatten under a hat. It's just hair. It has good days and not-so-great ones, just like we do. Keep a spirit of play around it. Take good care of your hair and the rest of yourself.

REJUVENATE YOURSELF WITH ACTION: *Inventory your hair-care products. If they're not the type you need to be using now, eighty-six them and start over with those that will protect your color, give your hair more body, or do whatever it is your hair needs to look its best. You don't have to spend a lot, but you do want products that smell nice and make you feel that you're treating yourself like a million bucks.*

AUGUST 5

Keep Busy, Just Not Frantic

When keeping busy means staying energetically involved with life, it's a youthful trait. When busy goes overboard, it turns into frantic and goes from youthful to stressful.

Ideally, you have plenty to do but you're seldom double-booked or overwrought. There is downtime built in for taking care of yourself and enjoying your life. In observing myself and my peers, I think more premature aging comes from hyperactivity than from more obvious errors like too much sun or too little exercise. We competed through high school and college, in the job market and the dating market. Even having it all meant juggling it all, fitting thirty-six hours of commitments into twenty-four-hour days. This can't help but take its toll on a body.

You know you're too busy if you routinely miss out on the basics. These include sleeping, eating (sitting down), exercise, recreation, being with the people you love and being available for what matters to them, and doing work that means something, either because it's making the world better or because it's sustaining a person—you—who makes the world better by simply being in it.

If you're out of touch with any of these basics, it's time to cease and desist. There may be extraordinary circumstances, times when you have to work an extra job, or care for both your parents and your children, but living a nonstop emergency would do Superwoman in. Admittedly, I don't know the facts facing you today or what is being asked of you right now. But if you're busier than you know is good for you, please do what you can with what leeway you have to get from crazy-busy back to regular-busy. It could mean living longer and doing even more.

REJUVENATE YOURSELF WITH ACTION: *Assess your current level of busyness. Are you (1) bored and empty, (2) pleasantly busy with fulfilling activities, or (3) running from one thing to another, missing out on the basics more often than not? You know the right answer. What would it take for you to get there?*

AUGUST 6

Give Your Lymph a Leg Up

Other than having some vague notion that my lymph glands swelled when I had a cold, I had no conception of the nature of the lymphatic system or its importance to health and youthfulness until I met Cheryl Morgan, PhD, founder of the American Society of Lymphology. Trained in Europe, where the importance of the lymphatic system in health and disease has been more thoroughly appreciated than in the United States, Dr. Morgan taught me that the lymphatic system operates with the venous system to maintain fluid and nutrient balance in the body's tissues. In addition, as a vital part of our immune apparatus, it produces antibodies, destroys bacteria, and fights cancer cells.

While the circulatory system has the heart as its pump, the lymphatic system is on its own and can use a little help from us. One way we can support it is to increase our activity level. It doesn't have to be excessive: tai chi, Pilates mat exercises, and the mild forms of yoga work just fine. Drinking lots of water helps, too, as do the nutrients rutin and bioflavonoids, found in comprehensive vitamin C supplements. Conscientious skin care also does the lymphatics a good turn since healthy skin acts as a barrier to infection.

In addition, there is a special kind of gentle massage called *manual lymphatic drainage* (MLD). This is particularly indicated after a mastectomy or radiation therapy, and is also useful in cases of fibromyalgia, fibrocystic breast disease, and lymph stagnation (i.e., a full sensation in the armpits that a doctor cannot tie to any pathology). I like to go for MLD a few times a year even when I'm feeling fine. It's a pleasant experience and a way to say thanks to an often overlooked part of my physiology.

REJUVENATE YOURSELF WITH ACTION: *Ask yourself: Am I being active? Drinking plenty of water? Does my multivitamin or vitamin C supplement include rutin and bioflavonoids? If you'd like more information, visit the website of the American Society of Lymphology, www.lymphology.com.*

AUGUST 7

Turn Ordinary Tasks into Spiritual Practice

The chores that are yours to do and the routines that comprise your day can either age you or do the opposite. It depends on the attitude you have toward them. Dreariness, resignation, and especially resentment favor aging; acceptance, appreciation, and losing yourself in a task support youthening.

Nearly every job you do has a social, sensory, or intellectual inducement. If you wash dishes with another family member, for instance, it's more like a party than a chore—i.e., there's a social payoff. If you're doing the same task by yourself, you get to feel the warmth of the water, play with the slippery suds, and smell the lemon in the dish detergent—all sensory rewards. And although dishwashing may not do much for your intellect, balancing the checkbook can, or helping a child with homework, or reading the manual before you assemble the new purchase that you didn't realize came in thirty-seven pieces.

Look for the social, sensory, or intellectual pleasure in all your labors. When you come to a task that has no redeeming feature in any category, give it to God (or spiritual power by whatever name you choose). If you went to Catholic school, you probably remember the phrase, "Offer it up." When something is a drag and a drain and you'd rather not do it but it's yours to do, offer it up. Offer it for the good of the whole or the good of your household or whatever good is applicable.

To grow younger, we can ill afford to feel put upon, bored, or trapped every time we have to clean out a file or put the trash on the curb. Certainly none of us should be the fall guy for every unpleasant job at the office or at home. If that's the case, put some of your mature assertiveness into getting things more equitably assigned. Even in the best of circumstances, though, we're all sometimes left with the files or the trash. When you turn it into spiritual practice, you don't have to judge it any longer. You may even enjoy it.

REVITALIZE YOUR LIFE WITH WORDS: *My life is a spiritual adventure, and every task is spiritual practice.*

AUGUST 8

Essential Fatty Acids

A lack of essential fatty acids (EFAs), or an imbalance of these, is believed to affect up to 80 percent of Americans. It is linked to diabetes, cancer, and heart disease, and it could be making the transition at menopause harder than it has to be. Ordinary margarine, anything deep-fried, and processed foods containing partially hydrogenated oils block the absorption of EFAs. Eating white-flour products means we're missing the EFA-rich germ of the wheat. Meat and other animal products, as well as cooking oils other than olive and canola, are overbalanced in favor of one EFA (omega-6) and low on another (omega-3), an arrangement that does not please your cardiovascular system.

Sources of omega-3s include cold-water fish (salmon, cod, trout, mackerel), English walnuts, and flax seeds or flax oil. You can also take supplementary EFAs in capsule form (fish oil or, for vegetarians, EFAs that are algae-derived). EFAs deteriorate rapidly and are sensitive to light and oxygen as well as heat. Too much exposure to any of these changes the oil's molecular structure from natural and health-promoting to deranged and toxic. Therefore, buy flax oil in opaque bottles, keep it refrigerated, never use it for cooking, and dispose of any unused oil by the expiration date; use similar precautions with EFA capsules. If you opt for flax seeds rather than oil, grind them in a little electric coffee mill immediately prior to use and sprinkle one or two tablespoons of the pleasant, nutty-tasting powder on cereal or fruit. (Flax seed has a laxative action, so make two tablespoons your max.)

Although EFAs are most often prescribed to prevent coronary heart disease, other conditions we're quick to blame on age—dry skin and hair, brittle nails, fatigue, arthritis, loss of memory, slow digestion—have also been shown to respond favorably to them. Note that these are essential *fatty* acids and, like all fats, they have twice the calories of either proteins or carbohydrates. By all means get them; just understand that unless that two daily tablespoons of flax oil replaces two tablespoons of some other fat in your diet, you'll be chalking up an extra fourteen hundred calories a week.

REJUVENATE YOURSELF WITH ACTION: *Start today to get the omega-3 fatty acids you may be missing in your diet.*

AUGUST 9

Discipline and Routine

Today let's hone in on the *essence* of rejuvenation, habits to adopt so that the years will be exceptionally good to you. This requires some discipline, the willingness to stick to a routine that creates health, beauty, and the kind of infectious happiness that years can't diminish. Discipline and routine may seem at odds with ease, the keynote we've assigned to August, but they're really a component of it. Once you come to terms with them, your life gets easier.

Here are the bare-bones basics you'll need to delay the negative aspects of aging and help you take full advantage of the positive ones. Physically, you'll want to:

- Eat real food.

- Drink plenty of water.

- Use your body vigorously and often.

- Care for your skin and protect it from the sun.

- Get plenty of rest and sleep.

- Have people on your side, from your internist to your yoga teacher, who can help.

Mentally:

- Think well of yourself.

- Think well of your age.

- Live fully in the moment.

- Look expectantly toward the future.

- Practice gratitude and stay long on good humor.

Spiritually:

- See yourself as part of something greater.

- Spend some time each day in quiet contact with the best that's inside you.

- Promise yourself that you'll come alive every day.

- Empathize so fully with other beings that generosity and kindness, even self-sacrifice when necessary, become second-nature.

With the essentials capsulized like this, you can see that growing into your future with health and grace and beauty doesn't have to take all your time. It rather requires a dedication to caring for yourself as if you were rare and precious, which you are, and regarding all life around you as equally so, which it is.

REJUVENATE YOURSELF WITH ACTION: *Make a plan for yourself of a practical, sustainable, growing-younger lifestyle. What can you realistically do every day? Every week? Every month? Write your plan in your journal.*

AUGUST 10

Veggies and Dip

This is veggies-and-dip season. You can put them out for company and take them to potluck suppers. Dips keep raw vegetables from seeming diet-like. My standard (and virtually instant) dip is half a pound of drained tofu blended with half a tablespoon each of lemon juice and extra-virgin olive oil, and dried dill weed and sea salt to taste. You can serve it immediately as a dip, or use it as a spread for crackers after it thickens in the fridge for a couple of hours. A slightly more enterprising dip—if you're having a party, maybe—is this one from Jennifer Raymond's *The Peaceful Palate:*

Creamy Cucumber Dip

2 cucumbers
$1/4$ cup finely sliced red onion
1 pound firm tofu
$3 1/2$ tablespoons lemon juice
2 garlic cloves, peeled
$1/2$ teaspoon salt
$1/4$ teaspoon coriander
$1/4$ teaspoon cumin
pinch cayenne

Peel, seed, and grate the cucumbers. Let stand ten minutes, then squeeze to remove any excess liquid. Place in a mixing bowl with the red onion. In a blender, combine the tofu, lemon juice, garlic, salt, coriander, cumin, and cayenne.

Blend until completely smooth, then pour over the cucumbers and mix well. Transfer to a serving dish and chill two to three hours. Serves six (64 calories, 6 grams protein, 6 grams carbs, and 2 grams fat per serving).

REVITALIZE YOUR LIFE WITH WORDS: *Veggies and dip taste yummy; that they're good for me is just a bonus.*

AUGUST 11

When You're Out of Your Element

It's one thing to provide yourself with the best of everything when you're in your own home eating your own food and living on your own schedule. When you travel on business, or you're on vacation, or you're somebody's houseguest, you lose some of that autonomy. The idea here is to lose as little as possible.

If you've been on the rejuvenation track for awhile, you're starting to see what is essential and where you can sometimes take it easy. You may, for example, work out less when you're traveling, but as long as you don't give it up altogether, you'll still be on track when you return. I've gotten temporary health club memberships everywhere from Taipei to Frankfurt, and in Paris where the hotel health club was beyond my budget, I walked the halls and climbed the stairs. So improvise. Rent a bike. Go for discovery walks by yourself and take walking tours with fellow sightseers. If you're in shape to do it, climb the hill, take the stairs up the tower, make it to the top of the dome. You get the idea.

To balance exercise with rest, call on the bedtime ritual you've established at home (April 8). Since a different bed and time zone can wreak havoc with your sleep cycle, take a few of your familiar slumber triggers with you when you travel. How about your journal, some lavender oil, and your trusted skin-care products, so you can see, smell, and take part in your expected pre-sleep routine? And a hot bath, of course, is soporific anywhere on earth.

If you do a morning warm oil massage (January 14), take your sesame oil along, guaranteeing its safe arrival by putting packing tape over the lid of the plastic bottle and placing the whole thing in a zip-tight plastic bag. Fit in meditation wherever you are by simply getting up earlier. (I awaken without a clock at home, but I take a travel alarm when I'm on the road to compensate for strange beds, strange time zones, and hotel clock-radios, which I unplug. I've been roused at 5:00 A.M. by high-volume used car commercials too many times to trust the OFF button.) I used to pack a snapshot of the little altar in my bedroom: I could prop it up anywhere and feel right at home. Once you're a seasoned meditator, just closing your eyes and taking a breath will do the same thing.

Help keep up with your supplements when you're away by purchasing a container that holds eight days' worth; they go for less than a dollar at a vitamin shop. I keep mine packed at all times so that when I leave town, which I do a lot, it's always ready.

The easiest way to eat well when you're away may be to eat well when you're not. Once feeding yourself in superior fashion becomes a habit, you'll make sure you do it, wherever you are. Seek out natural food restaurants, Thai and Japanese and Indian places, and salad bars. If I'm a guest in someone's home, I eat what my hosts are serving. Since I am a vegetarian I do let them know that in advance, but otherwise I don't make a fuss. There is a fine line between eating superbly and staying young, and being so particular you come off as an old crank. Sometimes you'll eat something that you know isn't the gold standard of nutrition, but if you make the best choices when the choice is yours, your body can deal with something less stellar when the choice is out of your hands.

REJUVENATE YOURSELF WITH ACTION: *Make a travel plan by writing in your journal which growing-younger habits are important enough to you that they deserve to be made portable.*

AUGUST 12

Don't Go Too Far Too Fast

Self-improvement. For some it's a hobby, for others an obsession. I see it more as the nature of life, motivation for getting up in the morning. What you want to avoid, as you're every day in every way getting better and better, is going too far too fast.

Whenever you set out to change a practice, your brain decides what your body should do: "I will work out, eat better, calm down." But your brain and your body are hogtied if your emotions don't approve of this new deal. That's why grand intentions so often bite the dust: the emotions, left out in the cold, raise heck. To bring them along and ensure success in what you're trying to do, go slowly. Maybe you've decided that you'd be better off without sugar, let's say. This is a big change for a lot of people—especially for someone for whom it's enough of a problem that she wants to cut it out altogether. Don't do this at the same time you decide to give up coffee and break up with your fella. That's way too much change for the emotions to handle.

It's also important to nurture your emotional self through any transition. Get support from other people and use the tools at your disposal—meditation, journal writing, affirmations. Give yourself lots of pleasure, physical and esthetic, to fill in for the pleasure you used to get from sweets (to stay with our example) or whatever else you're letting go of.

Remember the axiom, "Slow and steady win the race"? These traits may not always win, but they definitely finish, and that's what's important.

REJUVENATE YOURSELF WITH ACTION: *Evaluate your self-improvement efforts at this time. Are you keeping up with all you want to do? Are you comfortable with the level of will and energy you're asking yourself to put forth? How are your results to date? Would it help to slow down just a little?*

AUGUST 13

Lessen the Stress That Looks Like Aging

When stress crosses the line from exhilarating to enervating, your adrenal glands, pushed to produce adrenaline yet again, are saying, "What's with this woman? She has to fight or flee all the time." That such uncontrolled stress leads to exhaustion, even disease, has been common knowledge for decades. More recently we've realized that it's a first-class pro-ager as well. Manhattan plastic surgeon

Darrick Antell, MD, discovered in working with identical twins that when one twin looked a great deal older than the other, smoking, sun exposure, and/or stress were the primary culprits. The theoretical explanation for the role stress plays is that the shot of adrenaline the fight-or-flight response triggers causes blood to be shunted from the periphery to the internal organs. As a result, the periphery—i.e., your skin—is deprived and ages more quickly. Not only that: stress hormones called glucocorticoids can, when they're in constant circulation, impair the immune system and even weaken the bones.

Stress management has been around long enough that we can all recite a stock list of stress-busters: *Pound pillows. Make a call. Take a bath. Get a massage. Write. Exercise. Tidy up. B-R-E-A-T-H-E.* Funny, we know all this but a lot of us are still stressed. The reason is that tips like these do work *for intermittent stress.* Talking about a problem is therapeutic for women, whether or not it solves the problem. Railing on paper gets the strain out of your mind and your muscles, and lets your adrenals off the hook. Exercise works out tension in the body and causes the brain to release calming, coping chemicals. Organizing your environment can make you feel more capable and in charge. And slow, deep breathing counteracts the stress response of taking rapid, shallow breaths, thereby restoring composure. It's an impressive showing, and applying one of two of these suggestions may be all you need to make your stress level manageable.

If stress is your way of life, however, you'll need more than a chat and some oxygen—something more akin to a lifestyle makeover featuring more time for yourself, more rest, and more recreation. If you can't figure out how to get it with your level of commitments, consult a therapist or a coach or an incredibly balanced friend. Let her look at your schedule the way a financial planner would look at a spreadsheet and say, "Do this." Take the advice, even if you'll miss the stimulation that comes from having so much to do and so little time to do it. It's the rest of your life we're talking about. You don't want to burn out before you get to the best of it.

REVITALIZE YOUR LIFE WITH WORDS: *I no longer equate stress with success.*

Listen to Your Parents' and Your Children's Music

Appreciating the music of many times and places is a flexibility exercise that keeps people young. You don't have to like all of it. Just listen. When you listen to your parents' and your children's music, you gain a commonality with generations outside your own. You won't be stuck in a musical comfort zone rigidly bound by time and taste. You'll increase your ability to appreciate diverse musical styles, and that could lead to the youth-enhancing ability to appreciate diversity in other ways. When you can intelligently discuss popular music, your children or grandchildren won't think you're totally uncool. And you won't be: the lyrics of popular songs sing volumes about popular culture. Whether or not you *approve* of what they're saying, you'll at least *know* what they're saying.

My daughter was the one who reintroduced me to the music of my parents' day, music I'd decided years and years ago was, I don't know—I probably used a word like "yucky." I was aghast when Adair came home with a Frank Sinatra CD. I wasn't going to listen to it, but simply overhearing it was an entrée into a kind of music I adore today, music I'd denied myself for years based on a teenage decision.

So expand your musical scope: today's music, yesterday's music, and day-before-yesterday's music. You can expand it further with world music that includes timing and beats and instruments with which your ears may be totally unfamiliar. Musical flexibility leads to all 'round flexibility, and that's a good thing.

REJUVENATE YOURSELF WITH ACTION: *This week, spend some time listening to today's music—with a young guide, if there's one available. Also, listen to the music your parents loved back before you were thought about. Let these experiences expand you and loosen you up.*

Play Day!

Do Right by Your Joints

Osteoarthritis, the arthritis that comes from wear and tear, affects some forty-two million Americans, predominantly men and women over forty. The longer you live, the more likely you are to notice it. Still, you can give it an ounce of prevention. First, lose a few pounds if you have them to spare. It's estimated that if the average American lost eleven pounds, the incidence of osteoarthritis would decrease by 50 percent. In addition, choose low-impact ways to exercise, cross-train so you're not always stressing the same joints in the same way, and work out with weights to build muscle that will cushion nearby joints. Strengthening the quadriceps muscle through weighted leg lifts, for example, is known to decrease arthritic knee pain.

If you're already noticing stiffness or discomfort in your joints, you might try eliminating from your diet foods from the nightshade family—tomatoes, bell peppers, white potatoes, and eggplant. Some people get substantial relief this way, and you'll easily know in a month's time if you're one of them. Also investigate the following supplements:

- *Glucosamine* may alleviate symptoms by providing an important chemical building block of joint cartilage. Research indicates that 1500 milligrams of glucosamine daily helps rebuild cartilage in the knee and hip, and revitalize the cartilage that's there. (*Chondroitin sulfate* is often included in glucosamine capsules and powders; the combination appears to afford additional dietary support for joints and bones.)

- MSM (methyl sulfonyl methane) provides the nutrient sulfur, necessary for joint cartilage and mobility. Some studies indicate that it may even reduce the pain of rheumatoid arthritis, an autoimmune condition that can strike at younger ages and is usually more severe than osteoarthritis.

- *Essential fatty acids* (August 8) offer additional support for the joints. They can use both the omega-3 fatty acids found in fish, walnuts, and flax, and a particular omega-6 fatty acid, GLA (gamma-linolenic acid), which can be taken in supplement form as borage or evening primrose oil capsules.

- A *variety of vitamins*—the antioxidant three: A, C, and E—may reduce joint inflammation as they scarf up free radicals, and pantothenic acid, one of B-complex, has been shown to alleviate some stiffness and pain.

Obviously, you don't want to be swallowing pills all day. I suggest that you add one or two of these supplements to those you already take and give them a good six months to see if you notice a difference. If you do, stay with them. If not, try something else.

REJUVENATE YOURSELF WITH ACTION: *As you bathe or do your self-massage, pay special attention to your joints. Tell them they're appreciated. As goofy as that might sound, we are made up of living cells and living atoms. My bet is that they're listening.*

AUGUST 17

Food from the Neighborhood

If you have a vegetable garden, you have access to the freshest food possible. That from farms in your locale comes in a close second. Foods that were grown or raised nearby share a climate and an environment with you, making them uniquely suited to your needs. If you live in a city or a sprawling suburb, the term "local farmer" sounds like an oxymoron. It isn't. I live in Manhattan, and yet there are farms within an hour of here. These farmers and those from a bit farther afield offer their bounty at open-air markets and through

Community Supported Agriculture programs. (With the latter, you sign up and purchase a tiny percentage of "your" farm's crops for the season.) In addition, farmers have arrangements with supermarkets and natural food stores in their region. Often there are signs to let you know that this lettuce or those eggs came from—almost—the neighborhood.

When you choose locally grown produce, you get to eat it closer to the time it was harvested, when it hasn't lost so many nutrients. Fruits and vegetables consumed within forty-eight hours of being picked are *living* foods, abundant in life force. After that time, they're still good food, but not as life-promoting as something that's fresh and homegrown. One study found that 25 percent of some vitamins were lost when fruits and vegetables sat in the market for only two days. Add to that the shipping time and the stretch in the fridge after you buy it, and you'll see that "fresh" isn't always fresh. If produce is local, it's days younger.

In addition, when produce is sold where it's grown, it can ripen before being picked, allowing its nutrients and flavor to develop fully. This isn't to say that I'm opposed to luscious delicacies from the tropics, but when I'm not going for a pineapple or mango or papaya, I try to stay close to home. When you do that, you're supporting a local farmer and making a contribution to the community with every meal.

REJUVENATE YOURSELF WITH ACTION: *Do some checking to see if there is a Community Supported Agriculture program in your area. (Ask at a health food store or farmers' market.) If you're feeling energetic, consider actually going to a farm—a pick-your-own-produce place where you can get a real sense of where food comes from and the skill it takes to harvest a raspberry.*

AUGUST 18
_____

Great Legs

"The legs are the last to go." My nana used to say that, and I'm finding that she was right. With a little exercise, you can have attractive, shapely calves when you're ninety-five. Exercise can firm your thighs; limiting caffeine and alcohol and drinking lots of water can decrease cellulite; and those firming lotions do work, but only a little. Still, other than for swimming or getting a little weekend sun, how much thigh does a mature woman have to show anyway? Every alluring woman over thirty-five has learned to balance what she wishes to reveal with what she chooses to camouflage.

Something most of us prefer not to reveal, in North America anyway, is leg hair. For some women, hairy legs make a statement about self-acceptance or feminism or living naturally. I respect that view but I don't share it. Culturally brainwashed though I may be, I feel cleaner and better groomed when my legs are smooth. Interestingly enough, if you're postmenopausal and don't take hormones, you'll probably have less hair on your legs than you used to. Regardless of how much you have, you need to decide what to do with it. If you're not invested in leaving it alone, your choices are shaving, waxing, or laser hair removal.

Shaving is cheap and efficient, and if you're careful and use enough pre-shave preparation, you won't lacerate yourself. Laser is permanent but pricey. (Do you notice how twenty-five-year-olds in entry-level jobs manage to pay for services like this, while we have other demands on our money? Different times, different motivations.)

Waxing works for me. It makes legs silky-smooth, and you can go up to six weeks between waxes if you follow this formula: get your legs waxed the first time; go back in two weeks and again two weeks after that. Because these little hairs are growing at different rates, it takes a few closely spaced waxes to get all of them and establish an even playing field. After that, wax every three weeks, then every four. With any luck, you'll eventually be waxing only every five or six weeks, and the hair you do grow back will be finer and less noticeable. Consistent waxing also gives hair follicles the message, "You may as well give up; you'll never compete with this," and many of them believe it.

On a more serious matter, if varicose veins are an issue, they can be dealt with surgically. Little broken "spider veins" can be erased in a doctor's office, although the word on the street is that other ones spring up with more frequency than the doctors let on. To help prevent future vein problems and palliate existing ones, exercise, exercise, exercise. Walking and other activities that get the blood flowing in your legs can help ward off varicosities in women genetically prone to them. A high-fiber diet (lots of fruits, vegetables, beans, whole grains, and bran) is also recommended. Avoid anything that constricts blood flow—knee-highs, thigh-highs, tight socks, crossing your legs, and sitting or standing for too long in any one position. Support pantyhose can make you more comfortable (they're not ugly anymore) and putting your feet up can, too. You deserve to do that anyhow.

REVITALIZE YOUR LIFE WITH WORDS: *It's a fact: I've got great legs.*

AUGUST 19

Living in Real Time

You'll live longer, based on your own perception of time, by living more slowly. When you "don't know where the day went," it's as if you didn't get that day. Time seems to go faster the more of it you experience anyway. Remember how long summer lasted when you were a child? And how interminable a year once seemed from birthday to birthday? A smidgen of that is what we're after.

Time's going faster is not entirely without merit: everyone knows it flies when you're having fun. By the age you are now, you probably have more say over what you're doing than you used to. You may have worked your way up to a job that has visible impact and minimal busywork. Or you may have worked your way out of a job altogether and become a full-time mother, artist, entrepreneur, or volunteer.

But a lot of us, whether or not we love what we do, forego great chunks of our lives by dashing from this thing to that, trying to do everything and do it perfectly, keep up with women years younger than ourselves, and make enough money, preferably *today*, for a child's education, our retirement fund, a parent's retirement home, and a facelift for the house or a facelift for us. We have valid reasons for working overtime at the office, at home, and for causes that matter, but if we don't pace ourselves we lose ground, both to physical exhaustion and to the spiritual paucity that comes from going so fast we miss out on *now*.

None of us knows how many years will comprise our lives, but we know how many hours comprise our days. Sleep takes a third of them, work a third, and the third that are left have to cover self-care and self-actualization, relationships and recreation, getting from place to place and tending to the errands you just can't do while at the office or in bed. When you look at it this way—and most time-management systems do—it's pretty discouraging. The pursuits most worthy of time often get the least of it.

But there is more than one way to wind a clock. You know how we're thinking about food these days, less in terms of carbs and calories than in terms of color, vivacity, and life force? We can do the same with time. Then it's no longer about having enough of it but about infusing color and vivacity and life force into every moment.

It's putting your time toward valuable work and valuable pleasure, doing a good deed or saying something kind when something snippy would have been more satisfying in the short run. It's turning something ordinary into something beautiful or, when you catch something beautiful out of the corner of your eye, stopping to look at it square-on. Pay attention to the minute as well as the major aspects of your life, because minutia is more plentiful, and some of it is lovely.

REJUVENATE YOURSELF WITH ACTION: *Assert yourself with time today by valuing your own priorities at least as much as anybody else's.*

AUGUST 20

Just Say No to Vicarious Aging

Some things are hard to overcome. Genetics certainly. Bursitis, tendinitis, and arthritis that flare concurrently at the very mention of exercise. Sun damage acquired by lifeguarding seven summers. A dietary pattern of meat and potatoes, preferably fried and followed by pie, going back seven generations. Today's work is easy, though: Just say no to vicarious aging.

Vicarious aging is pro-aging stress inflicted upon you from external sources. Culprits here, depending on the individual, include violent or depressing films, the fear-mongering that can pass for "news" (March 6), and more exposure to the seamy side of life than you can handle in one sitting. When these ideas and images flood your consciousness, they can take your mood down with them and leave you feeling shaken, sad, helpless, or in need of an hour-long shower. Sometimes it can take days to shake the gloom.

Even if its basis is fictional, like that scary or depressing movie, your body doesn't know that. It responds to the fear signals or the depressed signals it gets from your brain as if you yourself were in danger or despair. The physiological response is the same as if you were the one being pursued by the ax murderer. Who needs to invite in vicarious stress just to be sure her adrenals are working?

As in all things, know yourself. If you find crime novels or horror movies a way to escape for awhile and have a grand time, enjoy every thrilling page and every chilling frame. If this stuff gets inside you, though, just say no.

REJUVENATE YOURSELF WITH ACTION: *Use your power of choice today, tonight, and this weekend. Don't let yourself be aged by a violent movie, a depressing TV show, or a media pundit who loves turning events into disasters.*

AUGUST 21

Become the Shoulder Massage Lady

Most people carry the lion's share of tension in the trapezius muscles spanning the upper back and shoulders. Having that tension kneaded out with massage means less tension and instant youthening.

Reading, writing, keyboarding, leaning over, looking down, and slouching all contribute to shoulder tension. Yoga, full-body massage and other body work, meditation, and decreasing mental stress before it shows up in your body are all good ways to keep your shoulders from taking permanent residence half an inch from your earlobes. Even so, tension heads for shoulders the way a white cat heads for a black skirt. If some kind person were to step up behind you at this second and start to work the kinks out of your shoulders and upper back, you would probably purr as surely as that cat.

If there is no shoulder massage lady (or gentleman) you know you can call on, become one yourself. Ready clients include your honey, your children, your friends. Here's how to do it: Have the lucky person sit in a reasonably straight chair. Tell him to relax, enjoy, and let you know if anything is at all uncomfortable. Then stand behind him for a moment and hold the intention to help and soothe this person. Once you're centered, place your hands on his shoulders and use your thumbs and fingers to work into the muscles of his shoulders, back, and arms. Start gently and ask if he'd like more pressure. As long as you stay off the vertebrae of the back and neck, you can safely improvise, sometimes kneading back and shoulder muscles with your fists or your elbow. Grateful "oohs" and "ahs" will let you know when you're doing something very, very right. With permission, you can rub his head, moving the scalp in tiny circles with your fingers, and gently massage his face, avoiding the eyes if there's any chance he's wearing contacts. At the end, place your hands back on his shoulders and give him a silent blessing.

In a perfect world, such an act would always result in reciprocation. In the world we've got, you can count on a 67.2 percent return of the favor (that's my rough estimate). If you ask in advance to *trade* massages, your odds will rise to nearly 100 percent. This isn't self-indulgence. There are too many tense people in the world. Consider it your obligation to be sure there's one less.

REJUVENATE YOURSELF WITH ACTION: *Get a shoulder massage today. Offering to give one is the best way to get one.*

AUGUST 22

Leave Doing What's Expected to the Young and Insecure

Just because you're grown up and then some doesn't mean settling into the doldrums of predictability. Surprise people. Surprise yourself.

I'm not suggesting that you cease being dependable, but rather that you sometimes alter a habit that is in danger of becoming etched in stone. If you're careful with your money, good for you, but every once a while, splurge on yourself or your husband or a friend who's not even first tier. If you're the listening ear for everyone on the block, get yourself listened to. On the other hand, if you could display a bumper-sticker that says "It's All About Me" and not a soul would say, "No way," pull out your inner philanthropist and volunteer on a grand scale: commit to becoming some child's Big Sister, or help build a house with Habitat for Humanity, or teach somebody to read.

While you're at it, you don't have to be predictably "middle-aged." You can get away with a flippy skirt and a flirty sweater, provided they're becoming and the right size. You don't have to give up skydiving and take up comparing liniments. Break some rules or make your own. A book seldom far from my bedside table is Leslie Levine's *Ice Cream for Breakfast: If You Follow All the Rules, You Miss Half the Fun.* She suggests such unexpected acts as being the one who dawdles, or plays in the dirt, or talks back. Levine says, "Altering the rules leads to ideas that ultimately can reshape the way we see ourselves." I think it means we'll start to see ourselves as bright-eyed and whimsical and right at home anywhere except in a rut.

REVITALIZE YOUR LIFE WITH WORDS: *Sometimes I do what's expected and sometimes I don't. I get to choose, and I like that.*

AUGUST 23

The Price Is Right

The secret to looking fabulous without spending a lot on clothing is developing an eye for quality.

Rather than having jam-packed closets, most well-dressed women have instead a carefully selected wardrobe in which everything is becoming and works with everything else. These women know how to shop for one remarkable piece and fill in with simple, well-fitting extras, even if they're from the sale table or the outlet store. The right jacket, for instance, can play top half with skirts, pants, a sleeveless dress, or jeans. It can go over a turtleneck, a lace blouse, a simple camisole, or, if you're daring, nothing but a string of pearls. If it's well made, it will last you years and be well worth having relined at some point, and receiving whatever other mainte-nance a favorite deserves. With this kind of innate longevity, your purchase pays for itself, even if it uses most of your clothing budget for the season or the year.

Be an eclectic shopper. There is a lot between couture and the rum-mage sale. Explore it all. Approach an end-of-season sale like an archaeological dig: you're out to find treasure. Don't always judge a shop by its windows. In some of the teen places I've been with my daughter and stepdaughter, places where 80 percent of the stock would look obscene on someone my age, I've found in the other 20 percent terrific buys on T-shirts, sweaters, and gym clothes. The best rain boots I've ever owned came from a camping store in Arkansas, and the Chinese crimson jacket I currently have my eye on is in the shop of a Manhattan museum where I went not for a jacket, but for a lecture about East Indian dance. When I go home to Kansas City, I make a beeline for the Junior League Thrift Store. I can't imagine buying new jeans when I can get soft, comfy, pre-owned ones for ten dollars.

Use whatever fashionable fringe benefits are part of being you. If you're able to sew, you can make (or remake) things the rest of us can only dream about. If you travel, you can avail yourself of back-street boutiques, unfamiliar department stores, and Salvation Army thrift shops. Look at fashion magazines as textbooks as well as pleas-ure reads. Their purpose is not to tell you that you should be eigh-teen and have dangerously protruding hip bones, but rather to show that this shade of peach and that shade of taupe are smashing together, and that flowered stockings between a long black skirt and a simple black pump could make the difference between a ho-hum look and a beguiling one.

Give yourself a day for "just looking." Go to stores you might never have ventured into before. Look in the designer department for quality and the junior department for the next trend. It's okay: you're just looking. Go to vintage boutiques and secondhand stores and import shops. Visit fabric shops even if you don't sew; touch the cloth and look at the buttons and trims. Educate your eyes and your fingertips. When you next go shopping for real, you'll find some sen-sational things.

REJUVENATE YOURSELF WITH ACTION: *Make an appointment with yourself for your "just looking" date. Write it on your calendar.*

A Postcard from Paris

I don't think it was accidental that I ended up in Paris just as I was trying to learn to make the most of being fifty. The French make art out of life, an art easily observable to anyone looking. They effortlessly turn simplicity into style, and look fabulous despite all those buttered baguettes and chocolate croissants. There are theories aplenty about how they can do this and largely avoid obesity and heart disease. I side with the appreciation theory. The French appreciate beauty: the beauty of art, architecture, a fresh-faced *mademoiselle*, an elegant mature woman, or a fine meal.

When it comes to dining, it is about taking time, seeing the food, smelling it, savoring it. This means putting your knife and fork down between bites so you can feel the textures in your mouth and discern the flavors on your tongue. It means never again consuming anything while standing up or on the run, because you're worth more than that. So is the person who prepared the food and the time spent doing it.

It is refraining from inferior food because quality is a key value in your life as a whole. In food, quality shows itself in produce that's fresh and crisp and bright, bread that was kneaded by human hands and baked this morning, and entrées skillfully prepared and presented. In dining like a French woman, you eat sensible portions, because quality satisfies in a way quantity never could. You rarely eat between meals—why spoil your appetite?—or while watching TV—why dilute your attention?

This attitude can carry over into every aspect of life: a few wonderful pieces of clothing, tailored to fit and painstakingly cared for; rooms that may be cozy or elegant but invite you in either way; days evenly invested in work, love, and leisure, with love and leisure seldom slighted for the sake of success.

For most of us, such a change in sensibilities is no small undertaking, but it can be done, and you don't have to move to Paris. If you're so overly scheduled that you not only eat on the run but put on your makeup, return calls, and write thank-you notes that way, too, slash your schedule. The sky won't fall and your star will surely rise.

REJUVENATE YOURSELF WITH ACTION: *You have just received a postcard from Paris. Take it to heart. Whether you're at home or out, dine. Treat yourself to fresh flowers and the good china, even when you're all by yourself.*

AUGUST 25

Let Life Flow

I love the title of the play *Your Arms Are Too Short to Box with God.* We all have short arms when trying to manipulate life to suit us.

Life has its rhythm and we have ours. They're designed to coexist in harmony, so that when we do what is ours to do and otherwise let life be, we garner acceptance and serenity. Certainly we're supposed to envision what we want and work toward that, but we'll stress ourselves into the geriatric ward early if we think we can control the nuances, detours, and timing along the way. Even the ultimate outcome is out of our hands, and that's not necessarily a bad thing. What we want just might get us into no end of trouble, or it could keep us from something better, or from learning some truth we've waited a lifetime to discover.

Perhaps you remember the hippies' mantra, "Go with the flow." They had a point. Obsessing over the way things proceed just makes you worried, and fighting against it just makes you weary. Instead, stand back and look as a neutral observer at the twists and turns life takes, all the while putting one foot in front of the other and doing what is before you to do. When you aren't getting in life's way, it does all it can to help you out.

REVITALIZE YOUR LIFE WITH WORDS: *I flow with the current of life. I am secure and content.*

AUGUST 26

The Upright Advantage

Modern life breeds thrusting chins, rounded shoulders, sunken chests, and protruding abdomens. Think about it: we started school when we were little more than toddlers; we leaned over desks, carried books, and for relaxation slumped into easy chairs to watch TV. We're still leaning over desks, carrying burdens of various sorts, and slumping into easy chairs. Using a computer, especially a laptop, encourages us to look down for much of the day as well. Even the casual clothes that most of us wear most of the time encourage casual posture. Say what you will about corsets and girdles: their built-in discomfort was at least a reminder to sit and stand tall.

Combined with lack of exercise, slumping and scrunching weaken our skeletal foundation and musculature, molding us into the stereotypical image of *old*. Fortunately, except in cases of advanced osteoporosis or a structural malady like untreated scoliosis, we can, with some practice and perseverance, turn this around. Here are some techniques:

- *Let your mind create the template.* Our bodies are obedient to a fault. They respond to what we think. Visualize yourself as graceful, erect, holding yourself beautifully, and gliding as you walk. Think: Grace Kelly, Audrey Hepburn, Fred Astaire.

- *Take a class.* The physical education most of us got in school didn't educate our bodies in ways we could use later. Start over. The Alexander Technique is specifically designed to help you use your body in the most efficient and balanced way, without struggle or strain. Yoga, Pilates, and ballet—there are adult classes—support lovely carriage as well.

- *Strengthen your abdominal muscles and your back.* The strong abs you're building with crunches and curls (May 17) support your whole torso, protect your lower back, and help maintain your balance. Strong upper- and mid-back muscles enable you to comfortably sit straight for extended periods. To strengthen these, simply sit near the edge of your chair with your back straight when you're working, conversing, riding the bus. This is more challenging than it sounds. If you get tired after a few minutes, rest, but do it again several times a day.

- *Stand with your hands behind you.* Do this when you're standing in line at the post office or the supermarket, or while you're waiting for the pot to boil or the document to print. In other words, stand with your hands behind your back every chance you get. This compensates for the bending, leaning, and carrying you do the rest of the time.

- *Look straight ahead.* Simply look straight ahead when you're walking, contemplating, or otherwise have no pressing reason for looking down. When your chin is parallel to the ground or the floor, you'll have better posture and you'll see a lot more.

REJUVENATE YOURSELF WITH ACTION: *If you're not already involved in a program such as Pilates or the Alexander Technique, make some calls this week to see what's available in your area. In the meantime, do the easy exercises from this chapter.*

AUGUST 27

Beta-carotene

With the late summer vegetables coming into season and taking us into fall, this is a fitting time to look at beta-carotene, the vitamin A precursor that shows itself as the yellow pigment in carrots, cantaloupe, apricots, pumpkin, yams and sweet potatoes, and that is also found in—you guessed it—dark leafy greens.

The body uses beta-carotene to make vitamin A as it's needed for doing its job of assisting in white blood cell formation, increasing resistance to infection and carcinogens, maintaining a well-functioning respiratory tract, and keeping skin healthy and youthful-looking. Beta-carotene is a major antioxidant and free-radical foe, playing an important role in the fight against cancer, heart disease, and stroke. It also protects the eyes from macular degeneration and cataracts. A supplementary dose of 10 to 20 milligrams appears to be a very good idea. For optimal absorption, take with a meal that contains some fat.

AUGUST 28

Our Souls, Ourselves

We come here, I believe, to give our Creator the opportunity for material expression. In so doing, we get to experience this life and learn all sorts of things—first and foremost, how to put love into practice. We do this in physical bodies that, according to quantum physics and certain spiritual teachings, *should* be as ageless as the souls that inhabit them. In time, human beings may solve the mystery, and eternal youth may become a reality. For now, we can live healthfully, take advantage of whatever cosmetic and medical enhancements appeal, and otherwise direct our attention to our souls, ourselves.

Because we tend to become what we identify with, the key is to focus on our eternal selves, to identify with the timeless light inside us, regardless of the face we see in the mirror. We do this by seeing life as a journey, a wondrous adventure in a faithful vehicle that, despite the best care, is subject to showing the passage of time. But the adventurer on the journey is removed from such things. She is as fresh and expectant as the day she arrived here, and looked around, and decided to stay.

REVITALIZE YOUR LIFE WITH WORDS: *I am an ageless being on an adventure trip.*

AUGUST 29

Beware of Dietary Dogmatism

Certainly smart food choices are essential for long life, good health, and getting younger by the day, but even the best food choices can be aging if you get orthodox about them. A woman recently told me, "Fruit has too much sugar, and grains have too much starch. Meat is acid-forming and nuts are too high in fat. Dairy gives me mucus and beans give me gas." There was an air of finality to her soliloquy, as if it should have ended with, "So there!" "You just eat salads and algae, then?" I asked. "No," she replied in utter serious- ness. "Since everything is bad, I eat whatever I want."

I know you're not like that, and although I got pretty strange about food in my weight-obsessed youth, I don't believe I was ever *that* strange. Surely there are things I eat rarely and others I don't eat at all; that's a choice each of us is free to make. Still, the specter of extremism looms large in a society that has plenty of food and just as much subconscious guilt about it, causing us to make meal- time less a simple joy and more a complex ordeal.

The upshot of all this? Eat well. Eat better than you ever have. Regard your body as a temple and your food as an offering to it. But don't go overboard. See your meals as lovely times and lovely gifts. You're not eating to harm yourself or adhere to a system or impress anybody. You're eating to get stronger and feel younger, and live richly and do great things.

REJUVENATE YOURSELF WITH ACTION: *Watch for dietary dogma in your friends and in the media. Be thankful that you aren't buying into it.*

AUGUST 30

Play Day!

AUGUST 31

An Eye-Opening Experience

At a museum exhibition about cosmetic surgery, I looked at dozens of before-and-after images of people who had had eye lifts. Each time, I thought, "She looks as if she's had a brow arch." That's how dramatic the results of a professional tweezing or waxing of the eyebrows can be. Every time I get one, I'm astonished at how much a face can improve after this simple, usually inexpensive, and not terribly uncomfortable procedure. After having your brows done, your eyes will seem more open and you'll appear more rested. The result: you'll look younger, and it will have taken only ten minutes.

Most brow arches use wax with a tweezer follow-up to get stray hairs the wax missed. Some purists use tweezers only; this takes longer and smarts a bit, but the payoff is precision. With either technique, the idea is to eradicate the stragglers, hairs that grow beneath and beyond the basic brow line, and give the brow a shape that is most becoming to your eyes and face.

You don't want to tweeze from the top or over-tweeze; it was a great look for Garbo, but times have changed. After menopause, you may find that your brows get sparser anyway, and you don't want to risk losing well-placed hairs you'd rather keep. I get a brow arch from a bona fide brow artist about three times a year and keep it up myself with tweezers in between. (Tweeze after a shower—you'll feel it lots less.)

If your brows are sparse or too light, the adept use of a brow pencil or powder will help a lot. Learn this adeptness from a makeup artist to avoid the kewpie-doll look that comes when an untrained hand gets hold of a brow pencil.

REJUVENATE YOURSELF WITH ACTION: *Book an appointment to get your eyebrows done by someone skilled at the procedure. Then buy some quality tweezers (drugstore tweezers are fine, just not the cheapest ones) to eradicate hairs that show up to spoil the effect.*

September

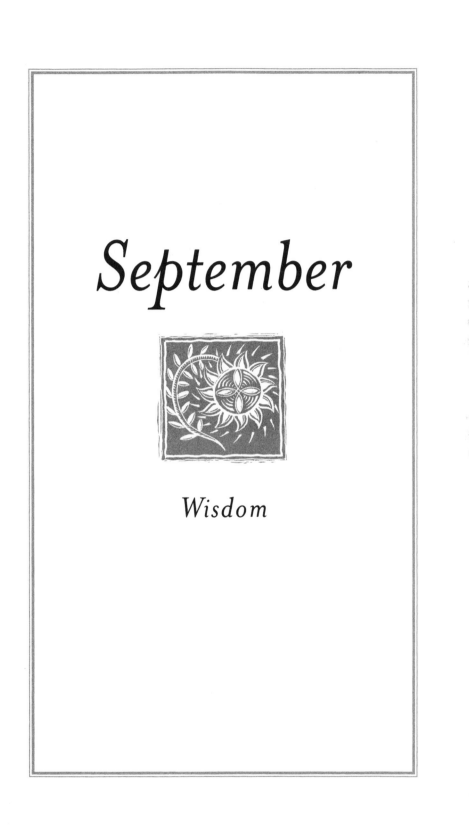

Wisdom

I'm Older: Why Aren't I Wiser?

Knowledge comes from education, whether formal or self-directed. Wisdom, on the other hand, takes living life. By forty, living life has granted most of us an Ivy League degree. Give yourself credit for that during this month of back-to-school, when the very air seems to smell of new textbooks and new shoes. This wisdom piece can be a mixed blessing, however, on days when we feel lacking in the insight department. Let the truth of mature wisdom be told: we do become wiser over time, but we don't always have split-second access to our sagacity. That's why we can sound so brilliant when we talk to a friend—and *be* so brilliant in advising her—yet feel clueless when we're in trouble and need to play tribal elder for ourselves.

When problems crop up all at once, there is no time to ponder your years of experience and there are no *Cliffs Notes* to summarize them. You can't pull out impromptu wisdom for every situation, but you do pull out impromptu wisdom about two dozen times a day. You find lost items and fix broken ones. You've probably even found a few lost people and fixed them, at least a little. You make decisions, take risks, and come up with solutions without breaking a sweat. But when you're in over your head, or fears rise up and make you feel more like a little girl than a wise woman, it's easy to forget how much majesty you carry within yourself. At times like these, you get to be human. You're allowed to be imperfect. You can even take some time off from being strong. In fact, it's not only permissible; it's required.

REVITALIZE YOUR LIFE WITH WORDS: *I am wise but not omniscient, so there's still a job for God.*

Read a Book from Your Youth, or One You Missed

One of the joys of living in New York City is looking at what people read on the subway. I see men and women who don't look like students reading Shakespeare, those who don't look like intellectuals reading Sartre, and those who don't look like teenagers reading *A Tale of Two Cities* or *Catcher in the Rye*. Some of these people are discovering anew books they loved long ago—or books they were forced to read then and want to revisit without coercion now.

A book from your youth can take you back to your youth and touch you in whole new ways. Heathcliff is a different character than he was when you were fifteen. And if you've heard of Rousseau and Goethe and James Joyce but never read them, read them now. If you missed the poems of Sylvia Plath, the novels of Edith Wharton, or the short stories of Dorothy Parker, they're at the library, and in low-cost soft-cover editions you can own and underline and scribble on in the margins. And there are audiobooks to listen to when you're driving or putting in miles on the treadmill.

Much of what used to be homework is now a kind of heart work, a way to understand the human condition, life and love, the way things were that are different now, and the ways things are that never change. Reading books like these lets you add an author's perspective to your own, giving you an inner life that gets deeper and richer and more enthralling by the page.

REJUVENATE YOURSELF WITH ACTION: *Reread a book from your youth, or read one you missed.*

A Compatible Club

If you get most of your formal exercise at a health club, find one that is compatible with you. Unless you're so dedicated that an uncomfortable environment or uncaring people won't faze you, the gym you choose could mean the difference between fitness and failure.

Gyms have personalities, just as people do. Some are young and hip. Others are rough and tough. There are gyms that are more for hooking up than shaping up, and those that are so social the members do more chatting than sweating. Women-only health clubs, as is said of women-only colleges, frequently offer a level of encouragement not routinely found in a coed setting. Whatever you're looking for, find a club where you fit in and feel comfortable, one that's close to your home or workplace, and one whose philosophy jives with yours. Do you want "the toughest trainers in Seattle" or "the most yoga classes in the city"? The club's hours need to be your hours: if the Y looks great but closes at four o'clock three days a week, when will you go? And if you want to take group classes, when are these offered? Are several of them geared to people at your fitness level?

I chose the gym I belong to now because it was offering a class in the "five Tibetan rites." These are exercises purportedly brought out of Tibet in the 1930s, delivered via a mysterious British colonel to one Peter Kelder, who shares them in his intriguing bestseller, *Ancient Secrets of the Fountain of Youth*. Whether or not they hold the secret of Shangri-la, I'm not sure. I just knew I wanted to belong to a health club that was open-minded enough to offer a class on something that peculiar. I am a funky person; I need a funky gym.

And you, if you choose to belong to a gym, need one that reflects your style, too. If it feels like home, you'll go; if not, nothing's certain. Since getting out of a contract with a health club can be as difficult as divorcing a guy in the mob, be sure you're compatible before you sign.

REJUVENATE YOURSELF WITH ACTION: *If you're in the market for a gym, do some research today. If you belong to a gym, get there today. If you think gyms are silly, you can feel self-satisfied when you exercise today that you're getting yours free and the rest of us are paying for it.*

Your Burgeoning Intuition

Intuition is what you know without having learned it, or without looking it up or asking Jeeves. Intuition expert Lynn Robinson, author of *Compass of the Soul*, gives a two-part definition of this widely misunderstood component of the human mind. The first is "quick and ready insight"; then "a source of wisdom to guide your life." Who wouldn't want that?

Everybody is intuitive; it's a matter of degree. A woman in midlife can expect a rise in her intuitive faculties almost as surely as she can expect a drop in her estrogen levels. This may be part of the compensation package life offers when we leave chronological youth behind, or perhaps it is a natural component of maturity, the birth of the wise woman within us.

Certainly intuition has been with us all along. As Rilke wrote, "The future enters into us in order to transform us long before it happens." We don't benefit from it as much as we might because, in Robinson's view, "We can spend years allowing our intuition to be dismissed by the voices of judgment in our heads that clamor, 'I can't do that,' or 'What would people think?' As we ignore those voices and let them fade away, we're free to sharpen our intuitive skills." We render our intuition useful when we become quiet enough to hear it. Intuitive inklings may be softer than a whisper, and more subtle than a breeze that might lift a downy feather but leave an iris petal on the ground.

This "still small voice," in fact, needn't be a voice at all. It can be a feeling of the emotional sort, or one that's physical, the well-known "gut reaction." It can come as an image or in a dream, or you might find this internal quality stirred by external stimuli: a sunset, an aria, a small boy at play, or a girl just his age but in need of food or comfort, entering your home on TV. Any of these or a thousand other triggers might activate your intuitive current, the way flipping a breaker lets electricity flow to a dishwasher or a chandelier. Then you know that your next life assignment is to phone a faraway friend, take flowers from your garden to that little boy's mother, or keep your old sofa awhile longer and send the money you'd stashed away for a new one to help the girl, or one like her, half a world away.

However it comes to you, your intuition is part of your standard operating equipment, no less necessary and no less genuine than your physical senses, your mental prowess, or your talent for sewing or singing or selling. Developing it doesn't mean we should all hang out signs that say, "Psychic Readings, $20." It does mean we need to pay attention to our intuition and use it with discernment and gratitude. Any woman who resents her age or attempts to deny her present reality diminishes her intuitive potential because, as a spiritual quality, your intuition can find you only when you're living your real life and accepting your real circumstances. What it can then do for you is grace those circumstances with an extra light.

Develop your intuitive sense patiently, expectantly, and with the childlike sense that you're unearthing a cache of riches, because you are. You're learning something new, but you don't have to study or take quizzes or be graded on the curve. You simply need to remind yourself to be a little more open, a little more aware, a little more in awe than you were yesterday. And that, my intuition tells me, will help you feel a little younger tomorrow.

REVITALIZE YOUR LIFE WITH WORDS: *I am highly intuitive, fully rational, and very wise.*

SEPTEMBER 5

Calculations, Crosswords, and a No-Longer-Foreign Language

I know a woman in her twenties who refuses to use a calculator. "When I'm old," she says, "I'll be famous as the only person left who knows how to add." She may be right. She's definitely on track for keeping her brainpower up to snuff. This is one case in which "use it or lose it" applies without question. Whether it's keeping track of your finances with a pencil instead of a program, figuring the tip at the restaurant in your head, or playing with numeric mind-teasers, your brain stays sharp with exercise.

Reading an intelligent newspaper and books that take some concentration, going to museums and lectures, and even memorizing phone numbers will do the job. (When my cell phone gave up the ghost, along with all its stored numbers, I realized that the only ones I had memorized anymore were my husband's office, my daughter's mobile, and 911. After that, I committed to memorizing a phone number a week.)

Not as pragmatic as becoming a human telephone directory, playing strategic games and squaring off against the crossword puzzle are choice exercises for cerebral fitness. I do the *New York Times* crossword with my husband. He knows things like "Southeastern Conference mascot" and I know things like "Hindu goddess of destruction." What neither of us knows straightaway we get to figure out (and in the process revitalize our brains).

Learning a language is excellent as well. When I picked up French after thirty years, what I used to know came back easily, while everything new was harder. It took me weeks to get down the word for computer: *l'ordinateur, l'ordinateur, l'ordinateur*. It may be my imagination, but when I study French I can *feel* my brain working. Conjugating imported verbs is like running mental laps. I'm not forgetting words in English the way I was some time back, and I haven't put my keys in the refrigerator in the longest time.

REJUVENATE YOURSELF WITH ACTION: *Try a variety of brain exercises—word games, number games, puzzles, riddles, crosswords, brushing up on a language. When you find something you enjoy, turn it into a hobby.*

SEPTEMBER 6

In Sickness and in Health

Getting older does not necessarily mean enduring lots of illness. Even so, if a genetic predisposition is going to turn into something, or if the stresses or poor choices of earlier years are going to cause trouble, they usually wait until after menopause to do it.

So what do you do if you have to deal with illness? You start when you're still well to build the resources that will carry you through anything, resources you can put to good use in other ways should you live in perfect health to 103 and die peacefully in your sleep. Some of these are inner resources: an interest in other people and in the world around you strong enough to take your mind off yourself; and faith that things happen for a reason and that you're up to playing whatever cards you're dealt. The outer resources include friends and family who will be there for you, and, prosaic though they may be, financial reserves and good insurance. If you feel short on any of these material or spiritual resources, start today to put more of both into your life. Then you won't have to worry about what will happen in the future and you can focus on living well now.

If you're dealing with a health challenge, *know that you have options.* You're worth a second opinion and a third. If you need to travel, travel. If you have to take a second mortgage in order to do it, take one. Somewhere out there in the realm of the experimental, or in a procedure that they've used for years in other countries but that hasn't yet been approved here, or within the wide world of alternative therapies, there is something to help just about anything. This has to be a team effort, though: you, your doctors, your nephew who can find anything online, and everybody who loves you or even knows you.

See yourself healthy, no matter how you feel. Think about what you'll do as soon as you're able, and envision yourself doing all those things. Speak the Truth to yourself in the form of affirmations, even when the facts of discomfort or debility loom large. Fill doubtful spaces with hopeful thoughts and, when you can, look at your situation as if you were another person, observing yourself from the outside. In this state of the neutral observer, surprising insights can come about as to what you may need to do or learn in order to get through this dark night of the body and soul. And get yourself prayed for, whether you've been a praying person or not. Even scientific studies show that prayer can encourage healing.

Although avoiding it is ideal, illness can be a wake-up call, a way that life gets your attention so you make changes you wouldn't make otherwise. And getting well can be a rebirth. When you're able to do simple tasks again and you think, "Wow, this is incredible!" you're living more sublimely than most people do most of the time.

REVITALIZE YOUR LIFE WITH WORDS: *My true nature is life and health and joy. I express that nature right here, right now.*

Give Some Attention to Popular Culture, Just Not Too Much

In my early childhood, I spent a lot of time in the beauty salons where my mother worked. I noticed certain customers who avidly read movie magazines. They seemed less sophisticated than the other clients—they chewed gum and often asked to go home with curlers still in their hair—but they always knew the latest on Elizabeth Taylor and Marilyn Monroe. Nowadays, celebrity-watchers are no longer a curious cultural subgroup: almost everybody has become one. The most reliable topic for small talk is the goings-on of stars, whether they're rising or falling, and whether or not a particular story about them is truth or fiction. This is way out of balance. It invades the privacy of men and women who didn't give up being human when they became famous, and it negates the meaning inherent in our own lives.

There is a fine line to walk here. To become younger, most of us need to know something about popular culture. In keeping current with trends and personalities, today's buzz and tomorrow's scuttlebutt, we extend our prime. Without a basic familiarity with these things, we're out of the loop, particularly when we try to relate to people younger than ourselves. Basic familiarity, however, is what you can get reading any good newspaper. Hours in front of the TV to follow some celebrity's divorce or run-in with the law are hours of living passively instead of actively. It's almost like not living at all.

According to its own PR, pop culture has supplanted every other culture. This is a lie with many believers, one that leads to more adulation of stars and their stuff than is healthy for an individual or a society. Despite the pitfalls, though, popular culture is a colorful carousel that can be fun to ride, as long as you refrain from purchasing the all-day ticket.

REJUVENATE YOURSELF WITH ACTION: *Look at your life in relation to the popular culture. Are you out of touch, too much in touch, or successfully taking the middle road?*

Breakfast, Lunch, and Dinner

I'm sure you've read that grazing—eating six or eight small meals a day—is superior to the traditional three meals, especially for losing weight. Longevity studies, however, tell us that people who eat breakfast, lunch, and dinner, with nothing between except perhaps some fruit, have the edge. My experience bears this out. When I eat, I want enough that my body and brain realize we've eaten. In other words, I want a meal. I spent the first thirty years of my life either gaining or losing weight. When I started eating three moderate meals a day (and working on the inner issues that were behind my recurrent pattern of eating with wild abandon), I lost weight and didn't need to regain it.

Every time you eat something, you have to put the brakes on. It's easier to do this three times than six. Because the world is set up for breakfast, lunch, and dinner, there are pauses in the day for these when you can sit down and focus on the meal and the ambience surrounding it. Snacking is more an on-the-run activity, and snack foods are generally less nutritious than mealtime foods.

Unless you have a medical condition that requires you to eat more often, see how you do on three meals a day. This isn't a marriage or a religion: if you experience a late-day dip and "afternoon tea" brings you back, or if dinner is going to be delayed an hour, or your stomach is growling and you know you won't sleep, have a piece of fruit or a glass of milk or whatever makes sense to you at the time. As a general rule, though, stick with three meals and living in between.

REJUVENATE YOURSELF WITH ACTION: *Unless you have a health condition that requires frequent eating, see how you do on three meals a day. Have a piece of fruit or a glass of freshly squeezed vegetable juice in between if you're hungry.*

Old Sayings

Clichés got to be that way because people valued their guidance, said them a lot, wrote them down, and passed them on. "If at first you don't succeed, try, try again." "An ounce of prevention is worth a pound of cure." "Early to bed, early to rise, makes a man healthy, wealthy, and wise." Of course you've heard these a thousand times, but did you go to bed early last night?

This is why truisms are not just true but ubiquitous: we forget their advice and have to hear them again. Not all "old sayings" are this hackneyed. You can pick up maxims you haven't heard before—those that come from other cultures, perhaps, or other people's grandmothers—that express timeless truths in novel fashion.

Still, the timeworn aphorisms that are part of your personal repertoire have the greater value, because they're deep inside you already, contributing to your values and your character. The next time one comes into your mind or out of your mouth, or when you read or hear one that is almost wearily familiar, give it at least a moment's thought. It might be, "Do unto others as you would that others do unto you," or "God doesn't give you more than you can handle." You wouldn't have thought it or said it or heard it if it didn't have a message for you right now. Don't let its overexposure negate that message.

And pass the old sayings of your family, your faith, and your fancy along to your children and grandchildren, even if they're at times met with a meticulously practiced rolling of the eyes. This is how your great-grandchildren and those who come after them will get something from you beyond a genetic link. They'll get to apply to their lives something you've used in yours. I think that's pretty special.

REVITALIZE YOUR LIFE WITH WORDS: *Repeat your favorite old saying several times today.*

Selenium

Selenium is a trace mineral shown to prolong youthfulness due to its own antioxidant properties and as a component in the body's production of the enzyme glutathione, known to counter free radicals. Selenium appears to fight cancer, promote immunity, relieve depression and anxiety, and maintain skin elasticity and mitigate sun damage, especially when taken with vitamin E.

This mighty mineral is found in whole grains, nuts (especially Brazil nuts) and seeds, and fish and meat. After reading Jean Carper's *Stop Aging Now!* and learning that eating two Brazil nuts is the equivalent of taking a selenium supplement, I started shaving a couple of Brazils (along with the English walnuts, for omega-3s) into my morning oatmeal. According to Carper, Brazil nuts purchased in their shells have more selenium than those that are imported shelled.

If you prefer to take a supplement, a stand-alone pill with 100 to 200 micrograms of selenium is the recommended dose. There isn't likely to be this much in your multivitamin, but take a look at the label; going over 200 micrograms could lead to toxicity.

REJUVENATE YOURSELF WITH ACTION: *Pick up a bag of Brazil nuts and eat one or two a day.*

Act from Anything but Fear

It is a curious phenomenon I'm sure you've noticed: two people can do the same thing—cut out junk food, take up jogging, adopt a skin-care regimen—and one will have great results while the other's are so-so. A host of variables contributes, of course, like each person's state of health, metabolic level, and degree of commitment, but my observations tell me that the primary variable is their mental state. Someone who takes on a new good habit out of zest for life and appreciation for herself gets a great deal more from her efforts than someone who is going through the same motions because she fears distressing consequences if she doesn't. This principle goes beyond self-care to apply to every action we take in our lives.

Fear can be a legitimate early motivator—when, for example, the doctor says, "Don't smoke or you'll die"—but it's not good for the long haul. A fearful thought is unpleasant and easily buried; from underground, it's no motivator at all. Instead of taking action out of fear, then, take it out of love for yourself and other people. Take loving care of yourself because you have talents to express and a job to do that you can do best if you're healthy and vital and strong. Do the best you can in every area of your life on the off chance that, since miracles happen all the time, one could happen for you any day of the week. Go out and make a difference, for any reason you like other than fear. It's okay as the gunshot at the starting gate, but you don't want to hear shots every lap of the run.

REVITALIZE YOUR LIFE WITH WORDS: *I put good habits into place because I love feeling fabulous. I do good works because I love doing good.*

SEPTEMBER 12

Figure Shifts

Shifts happen. They happen at adolescence, they happen after childbirth, and they happen around menopause. The typical menopausal shifts include a droopier bosom (yes, even droopier than from pregnancy and nursing), less indentation at the waist, a rounded tummy (a low blow if you can do more sit-ups than your daughter with the concave abs), and, to keep my vocabulary current, "less baggage in the booty." Will exercise help? Sure it will, and sometimes a lot, but forces of nature are at work here. Short of surgical intervention and all other things being equal, you will have a somewhat different shape in your mid-fifties than you had in your mid-forties. You can work with that, let it get you down, or go for liposuction. I like what's behind door number one myself.

Working with a figure shift starts with self-acceptance. You've probably helped a daughter or granddaughter or niece accept her changing body when puberty came to town; now you have to accept your own. It means accepting the number of years you've lived in this body and praising yourself for the beauty you have now, in this phase of life. It means eating well and exercising because you deserve that kind of care, even if it takes longer for results to show on your body or if those results aren't as sensational as they would have been ten years ago. It also means being scrupulously honest about what you're doing: if you've been watching a lot of TV with a revolving bowl of ice-cream in your lap, there are factors affecting your body other than age and hormones. Advancing age and retreating hormones are a given: how we treat ourselves is something else.

REVITALIZE YOUR LIFE WITH WORDS: *I accept any shift in my body that nature deems necessary; I change whatever is in my power to change; and I do not confuse the two.*

SEPTEMBER 13

Your Mobile Phone Is Cute as Anything, but It Could Be Aging You

I didn't really want to talk to Mary about my cell phone. I finally have one that is just adorable—it's silver, almost weightless, and *it flips.* I am embarrassed to tell you this, but when I flip that phone, I feel cool. That's why I wasn't eager to bring up the subject with Mary Cordaro, a Los Angeles *Bau-biologist*—that is, someone trained in the relationship between personal environment and human health and well-being. She always tells it straight, and she did: "Cell phones age you because they put a big range of radiation around you."

"But what about earphones?" I wanted to know. "And those little stick-on things they sell in the phone stores that are supposed to protect you from radiation?" It seems that the sticky things *may* do a little something by strengthening your own energy field, but any help you're getting from them isn't measurable. An earpiece definitely cuts down on the thermal radiation that literally heats up your head—and using one if you must talk while driving is just good sense. According to Cordaro, however, the wire going into the ear can transmit even more focused non-ionizing radiation closer to the brain. Non-ionizing (or non-thermal) radiation means radiation at levels below those that heat, and some studies suggest that it might damage DNA.

In fact, you get non-ionizing radiation whenever you're within several feet of a turned-on mobile phone. "You even get it when you're not on the phone but someone nearby is," says Cordaro. "It's like secondhand smoke." A study at a German university looked at cell phone radiation and found that being within several feet of an operative mobile phone caused an EEG abnormality in 70 percent of subjects—and it took some twenty hours for that effect to dissipate. How harmful this may or may not be is anybody's guess, but all of a sudden I was feeling less cool.

If enough research confirms these problems, the mobile phone companies may be forced to lower the phones' power intensity. For now, the prudent course appears to be using our clever little phones as little as possible by keeping them turned off at home and using a voice-mail message such as, "If your call goes directly to voice mail, I'm probably home; please try me there." I've taken to telling people, "Let me call you on a land line. Did you know that talking on a mobile might be aging?" It's taking some time, but I'm learning to use my traveling telephone only for directions, business calls, and quick questions. Long conversations I'm starting to save for a land line or a visit face-to-face.

REJUVENATE YOURSELF WITH ACTION: *Wean yourself from long conversations when you're away from a land line.*

SEPTEMBER 14

The Other Side of Sun Exposure

Protecting your skin from the sun is essential for both looking younger and guarding against skin cancer. Still, the sun is the reason there is life on earth. It has to have some redeeming qualities.

You have to know that something is amiss when the American Academy of Pediatrics alerts breast-feeding mothers, as it has, that their babies need supplementary vitamin D because they're doing *too* good a job at sun protection. Human beings of all ages make vitamin D as a result of sunlight on the skin. When babies and children lack it, they're at risk for rickets; when adults are short on it, calcium utilization is compromised, making the specter of osteoporosis loom larger than it would otherwise. Some foods are fortified with vitamin D, but it makes sense to get at least a portion of our quota the way nature intended.

Sunlight is also instrumental for proper immune function and keeping the pituitary hormones in balance, and it is a prescribed therapeutic agent for skin diseases including seborrhea and psoriasis. Additionally, lack of sunlight is the undisputed cause of SAD, seasonal affective disorder, the debilitating depression that affects many people during the winter or when they move from a sunny locale to a cloudy one.

While *sunshine*—tanning, and repeated exposure of the same unprotected skin—should be avoided, getting some *sunlight* is a good thing: morning and late afternoon outings, brief midday sunning for vitamin D, and using sun-block on those areas that are often uncovered but letting the sun caress usually shrouded parts like your tummy or legs. There is intriguing research that suggests that there may be a sun-protective diet as well. It indicates that limiting consumption of animal fats and unstable, refined oils may provide a little SPF from the inside out. Until more is known on this, hedge your bets by eating lots of foods that grew in the sun and being sensible about the time you spend in it.

REVITALIZE YOUR LIFE WITH WORDS: *I am sun-smart every day. I give myself enough sunlight, but never too much.*

SEPTEMBER 15

Play Day!

Respect the Limits

Parenting experts say, "Children not only need limits; they want them." So do grown-ups. At any age, honoring the limits keeps us safe, and doing so is a trait shared by the majority of attractive, successful people.

You honor the limits when you don't confuse your body's abilities with those of Wonder Woman's. You respect them when you live within your means, and when you make a to-do list that can be accomplished in a twenty-four-hour day. Ignoring or resenting limits is aging. Sometimes you'll hear it said of someone who looks older than his years, "He's done some hard living." Hard living is the kind we do that's outside those protective limits. You respect them when you nurture yourself with proper rest, movement, and calm, and when you take in for yourself as much as you give out in work or service. You heed them by listening to your body when your eyes are saying, "I've stared at this screen too long," or your stomach beseeches, "Why are you doing this to me?"

The limits are there for your benefit. Let them do their job of helping you stay youthful.

REVITALIZE YOUR LIFE WITH WORDS: *I respect the limits and I reap the rewards.*

Learn a Word a Week

One way to exercise your cerebral self is to learn a word a week. There are all sorts of places to find captivating words. My favorites are novels and the New York Times. When I look up a word that was in something I read, I know I'm not wasting my time learning some esoteric term I'll never see again and couldn't use in real life. My other source for weekly words is my own head: there are always words floating around in there with meanings I'm unclear on.

Those words are like foreign currency; both have value, but only in the proper context—the money after it's been exchanged, the words after they've been looked up.

Write your word of the week in your journal along with its definition. If you really get into this, you may want to keep a special vocabulary book. When a definition is mind-boggling—one of those "of or pertaining to that which is of or pertaining to . . ." definitions—I've found it helpful to get the basic meaning from a dictionary designed for students. Once I have a handle on the essential meaning, the more elaborate definition gives me the nuances. I suggest you treat your new word the way you did when you had vocabulary quizzes at school. Go over the definition. Use the word in sentences. Tell somebody else what it means. Write it on Post-its with an abbreviated definition and stick them where you'll see them. Anything new that you learn will help keep your brain fit. Words give you the bonus that once you know them, you get to use them.

REJUVENATE YOURSELF WITH ACTION: *Learn an enticing word every week for the rest of your life. Include it in conversation when you can. An oddball word here and there can be fun, but the ones that have the most value are those you will actually use.*

SEPTEMBER 18

Do a Little Detox

Your body is constantly detoxing, lightening its load of material that's harmful or useless. Sometimes, though, the process gets backed up and can use a little help from you. You help your body detox every time you take a steamy shower, exfoliate your skin, eat high-fiber foods, or drink fresh juices. Devoting a Saturday to detoxing involves combining several elements to give you total refreshment, body and spirit.

Prepare by eating lightly Friday night—maybe salad, brown rice, and steamed vegetables—and get to bed early. Arise naturally Saturday morning. Gently scrape your tongue with an inexpensive tongue scraper you can find in the toothbrush aisle. Excessive coating on the tongue is, in Ayurvedic terms, *ama*, metabolic debris; get rid of some of it first thing in the morning (a good idea every day, not just when you're detoxing). Next, drink hot water with lemon (January 28) and settle in for your meditation (May 21), which you can see as a detox for the mind. Follow with some yoga or stretching.

Enjoy a light breakfast of fruit salad or stewed apple and prunes. (If you think eating only fruit will leave you lightheaded, make muesli by soaking raw oats and chopped nuts in pure water overnight and serving it in the morning with fresh fruit and almond or soy milk.) If you're used to caffeine in the morning, have one cup of green tea, steeped two minutes or less; otherwise, choose an herbal tea like peppermint or hibiscus. Follow your meal with a vigorous walk outdoors. Bring water along; you'll want to be sipping constantly today. When you return, clean up with dry skin brushing (October 20) and a brisk shower where you can exfoliate your body with a loofah or grainy scrub. If you have access to a steam room, steam first—no more than fifteen minutes. (Confirmed detoxers say there's a bonus that comes with a cold splash as part of that post-steam shower.)

Lunch can consist of salad, a steamed vegetable, and clear soup with less salt than usual. Spend the afternoon doing something you enjoy that isn't too labor-intensive—sketching, writing, or easy gardening. If you can, schedule a massage, a reflexology treatment, or both for the late afternoon. Keep drinking water. If you feel hungry, have a piece of fruit.

Fit in your second meditation before an early dinner of salad, steamed vegetables, and edamame (green soybeans) or grilled tofu. After eating, either take a short walk or rest with some inspiring reading. Then indulge yourself in a candlelight bath with some lovely scented bath oil. Get to bed by nine or ten without TV. Write in your journal, do your nightly check-in (June 9), and sleep like a babe.

REJUVENATE YOURSELF WITH ACTION: *Schedule a detox for your first vacant day, and once per season after that.*

Personal Evolution

Some of us are still expressing an identity we were handed in childhood—"the helpful one," "the smart one," "the rascal"—or living out a reputation earned in college. Like the clothes we wore then, that image is probably no longer appropriate. A girl known for being pretty, unless she develops other attributes, will find growing older difficult indeed. The campus sex kitten has to cultivate a wider range of talents, lest she end up like Grisabella in the musical *Cats*, singing "Memories" in the middle of the night. Even the super-student gets the rude awakening that nobody cares about her grades anymore.

The need for renewal holds for nearly every reputation you've made for yourself. The assertiveness that got you where you are when jealous bosses tried to hold you back could be perceived as aggression now that you're the boss. "I am a mother and have finally found my role in life" can be fulfilling for years, but when your kids are making their own way in the world, you need a revised identity. Conversely, an "I am woman; I shall roar on my own" persona can be terrific, but if you find yourself adopting a baby at forty-five or getting married at sixty, you need to shift that image.

Because they're evolving so rapidly, teenagers are excellent at depicting the shifts and detours that constitute evolution. All sorts of things enthrall them, and they try myriad ways to express themselves. I got a kick out of watching my daughter develop her fashion sense. She went through a phase of wearing men's dress shirts and neckties with short skirts and chunky shoes. Then there was the vintage tuxedo jacket that she put over jeans and teamed with pink patent oxfords. Mature evolution usually involves more internal transition and less pink patent faux leather, but the motivation—the urge to grow and develop—is identical.

At every stage of life, we're challenged to know ourselves, make choices that suit us, and let other choices go. At the mid-adult stage, we have the advantage of a solid identity; otherwise, we'd just be thirteen-year-olds with gray roots. This advantage makes right now the ideal time to try new things, take risks, have adventures, and show up on occasion wearing a new color, endorsing a new cause, or engrossed in a new avocation. If we don't, we can get stuck, and a stuck place is an aging place.

REVITALIZE YOUR LIFE WITH WORDS: *I am an evolving human being: I risk; I experience; I grow.*

SEPTEMBER 20

Teach What You Know

You know a lot. This knowledge is one of the gifts of the years you've lived and the work you've done. You will own your knowledge more fully if you share it with someone else—in other words, if you teach what you know.

Mentoring at work, tutoring in the inner city, teaching adult education, and taking seriously a younger person's request that she wants to learn some skill from you are all ways to do this. People want to learn the language you speak and the craft you've perfected. They're longing for the wisdom you got from your mother that she got from hers, and the adeptness you have on the computer or in the kitchen. You might teach something formally and get paid money, or teach informally and get paid in other ways. Do teach, though—somehow, some way. Nature means for us to be teaching at this time of life, and she rewards those who cooperate.

The other way that we fulfill our instructive destiny is by living as examples of characteristics we would like to spread and share. People are watching: our children, our friends, our co-workers. When what we do is in alignment with what we believe and what we say, the lesson is complete.

REJUVENATE YOURSELF WITH ACTION: *Give some thought today to something you might teach, why you're qualified, and how you wish to do it.*

Tea Time

I find tea more romantic than champagne and more satisfying than chocolate. I'm enchanted by its hundreds of varieties, named for where they're grown, how they're harvested, and how they're scented. Jasmine, for instance, is green tea with the fragrance of jasmine blossoms; Earl Grey is black tea scented with oil of bergamot. To keep things simple, we'll look at the four basic types of tea:

- *Black tea:* mature and fully fermented; the highest caffeine content (approximately half that of coffee)

- *Oolong tea:* fermented to half the degree of black tea; the midpoint between black and green teas in terms of taste and caffeine content

- *Green tea:* dried but not fermented; half the caffeine of black tea; the subject of the most research on tea's health benefits

- *White tea:* once rare outside China, now gaining in popularity; withered and dried but neither heated nor fermented; light, delicate, and low in caffeine; rich in polyphenols (so much so that it's being included in some very effective anti-aging serums for topical application)

Caffeine stimulates the central nervous system, digestion, and metabolism. In moderation, it oxygenates the brain, acts as a mild diuretic, and promotes circulation. Sleeplessness and nervousness result from too much. How much that is varies widely from person to person, and any amount is probably too much if you're pregnant or nursing. Legions of people who get the jitters from coffee appreciate the morning boost of a cup of tea and experience no unwanted after-effects. You can also control the caffeine content of any tea by how long you steep it. According to *All the Tea in China* by Kit Chow and Ione Kramer, a five-minute infusion of black tea yields 40 to 100 milligrams, while a three-minute infusion has only 20 to 40 milligrams.

In addition to caffeine, tea leaves contain essential oils and polyphenols. The essential oils, more abundant in green tea than black, give tea its characteristic aroma; and they're believed to aid digestion and help emulsify fat. It's the polyphenols, however, that appear to inhibit the formation and growth of cancer cells, and to protect against stroke and heart attack by keeping blood vessel walls pliable and curbing absorption of cholesterol. The polyphenol GHCH in green and oolong teas may be as effective against the fat on one's thighs (and elsewhere) as the fat in her arteries. Research also suggests that tea can increase immune function and strengthen teeth and bones.

To brew green tea or white tea, heat spring water to just below the boil and steep to the desired strength (go for weaker at first; if steeped too long, green tea can taste bitter) and serve it without milk. For black or oolong tea, use rapidly boiling water, steep, and serve in the company of either lemon or, for black tea, milk (dairy, soy, or rice). For sweetening, I suggest Sucanat (dehydrated cane juice) or agave nectar, the light, sweet syrup derived from a type of cactus. Health food stores stock both of these sweeteners.

Tea of any stripe, like most of life's pleasures, is best with ceremony surrounding it. In other words, when you can, measure out loose tea, brew it in a pot warmed with a tea-cozy, and serve it in a pottery mug or china cup. This is simply one more way to treat yourself like someone who matters. When this much formality isn't practical, use a teabag, know that polyphenols don't require a pot, and remember that you matter no matter what.

REJUVENATE YOURSELF WITH ACTION: *If you're a coffee drinker, see how you fare with tea instead. If you drink black tea but haven't yet given green tea a try, do that today or tomorrow. If white tea is new to you, go out in search of it and have a little tea party, even if you are the only guest.*

SEPTEMBER 22

The Autumnal Equinox

This is my favorite change of seasons, with a nip in the air, the leaves about to turn, and that comfortable back-to-business feeling of settling down again after summer. As with the other changes of season, this is a time to take appropriate, life-revitalizing actions. Some to consider:

- *Take a class.* You went back to school every September for years. Do it again this fall by taking a course in something that fascinates you.

- *Buy something new to wear.* Sit down with a fashion magazine, catch a trend or two, and buy yourself something you'll love wearing.

- *Do what the squirrels do and stash away food for the winter.* You can take this literally and stock your pantry with healthy staples, or you can take it as metaphor and use this seasonal shift to take stock of your resources. Where is your money? How is it working for you? Do you need to make any changes there?

- *Make your environment cozier.* Summer is wide open; autumn speaks to drawing inward. Get out the afghans and the candles, whatever accoutrements carry the spirit of September and the cooler months to come.

- *Indulge your cultural side.* Theater companies and orchestras are starting their seasons. Traveling exhibitions are coming to the art museums. Give yourself a day or an evening to enjoy some of this.

- *See the fall colors.* If you live where the leaves make a bold display, plan to spend a weekend in the midst of it.

REJUVENATE YOURSELF WITH ACTION: *Make a list of everything you like about fall—soup, sweaters, leaves that crunch when you walk on them. If you're a summer gal, your list will be shorter than mine, but strive to find at least a dozen blessings that belong to this time of year.*

The Heart and Soul of Transformation

Whether you've been practicing the younger-by-the-day program for several months or only a few days, it is crucial that you understand the essence of transformation, the heart and soul of change that comes from the inside out. Sometimes you'll hear, "People don't change." This is true more often than it ought to be, but listen again: "People don't change." It says "don't," not "can't."

Your life experience up to now has surely included some remarkable transformations: from shy young girl to self-assured young woman, from unappreciated underling to well-paid supervisor, from hard-nosed cynic to open-minded seeker. If you've experienced one transformation, you know others are possible. Some people worry that their transformation isn't proceeding in the proper order. "Does the mind change first or the body? What if my body changes and my mind can't keep up? What if I have a spiritual experience and the whole world is different, but I look in the mirror and everything is the same?" A wise teacher once told me, "If transformation touches you anywhere, it touches you everywhere." In other words, don't analyze it and don't judge it. If you see your life changing on any level, know that it is changing on every level. You may have to pay extra attention to some aspect that seems to be lagging behind. You may need to get some extra help or do some extra work, but once transformation starts inside you, there's no stopping it unless the glory of it scares you and you make it stop as an act of will.

Do what you're drawn to do today. Your focus may be on the physical or the spiritual. It's fine to accentuate one of these, as long as you don't abandon the other. Trust that transformation has already begun inside you. If you let it, it can grow to encompass every aspect of your life.

REVITALIZE YOUR LIFE WITH WORDS: *I live in continual, positive transformation.*

See Through Circumstances

Things can happen that seem dreadful, and some of them are. Most of the time, though, we're simply cycling through circumstances, golden days and leaden ones, periods when we're on top of the world and others when it seems to be on top of us. It is essential that we not allow circumstances to age us unnecessarily. We have to see through them.

Just about everything that happens on earth comes to pass and not to stay. Circumstances do not deserve to have a hold on you, because they're already headed out of town and you're not going anywhere. The strong one in this picture is you, not some circumstance. Of course it's painful when the man you thought was your one and only decides he isn't. It is scary when the doctor says your Pap smear looks "suspicious," and it is discouraging to find yourself downsized at work or upsized in the fitting room. But these are circumstances to see through and go through; they do not negate who you are or where you get your power. And, more often than not, even situations we wouldn't care to revisit turn out to house treasures.

REJUVENATE YOURSELF WITH ACTION: *Be on the lookout for circumstances today and as time goes by. As they come and go—believe me, they'll do both—know them for what they are. See through them. Live through them. Grow through them. Excavate their treasures.*

Outgrow Intimidation

I used to be easily intimidated. My alphabet of threatening people included:

Accountants, athletes, and authority figures
Ballerinas and businessmen
Chic people, cool people, and clerks in chic, cool shops
Doctors

Editors

Famous folks

... all the way to Young people and Zealots. I was intimidated by anyone who could do what I couldn't, or who did what I did better than I did it, looked better while doing it, or made more money in the process. There was a payoff: as long as these people seemed big, I could stay small.

One of the more satisfying aspects of growing into ourselves in midlife, however, is coming to know our worth relative to everyone else's, and finding that it is absolutely equal. We neither have to intimidate another nor be intimidated ourselves.

Sometimes you'll run into someone who doesn't know this, someone empowered by a plastic ID badge, a job he's had two weeks, or an attitude she picked up this morning in traffic, who will try to intimidate you anyway. I feel embarrassed for this person. Should your path cross that of someone in such a pitiable state, make short work of the situation. You don't have to be right, just out of there.

REVITALIZE YOUR LIFE WITH WORDS: *I live in a world free of intimidation: none goes out and none comes in.*

SEPTEMBER 26

The Divine Feminine

Women I meet who, at middle age and far beyond it, maintain a vitality and momentum many others lose, often have a sense that they somehow reflect their Creator as much as any man does. Among these women are Jews, Christians, and Muslims, whose religious traditions are patriarchal (i.e., Yahweh, God, and Allah all get the masculine pronoun), as well as those from Hindu and Buddhist backgrounds that may recognize a pantheon of gods and goddesses. Others have discovered the ancient nature traditions that revered the Goddess (or several goddesses and gods).

When you talk to these sophisticated, modern women, they don't tell you that they believe in an old man with a white beard, or a hallowed convention of superhuman beings holding court in the sky. Instead, they see the Divine of their understanding more as Oversoul (Emerson's term), which cannot be contained in a gender but must hold the best elements of both male and female. "When I realized that Goddess was as valid a word as God," one of them told me, "I felt for the first time that in this life and this body, I was in that image and likeness, too."

I've spoken with women who have found the divine feminine in the Virgin Mary, in a female guru, and in Mother Earth, who gives birth to all of nature. Whatever your religious beliefs, and with all due respect to them, finding yourself as you are, yourself as a woman, within your concept of divinity, may do more to raise your opinion of yourself than any other single act. When you believe you reflect what is holy and good, you can see more that is good in every stage of your life.

REJUVENATE YOURSELF WITH ACTION: *In a way that fits with your belief system, ponder the divine feminine today. Strive to see yourself in the image and likeness of divinity. Books to explore include* The Feminine Face of God, *by Sherry Anderson and Patricia Hopkins, and* At the Root of This Longing: Reconciling a Spiritual Hunger with a Feminist Thirst, *by Carol L. Flinders.*

SEPTEMBER 27

Push Yourself into Life If You Have To

If you're repeatedly morose and fatigued and nothing seems to pull you out, see your health-care provider. There could be a physical cause. Low thyroid function, for example, is more common in middle age than before, and can cause debilitating tiredness. Or you could be suffering from depression. Depression is to sadness what double pneumonia is to the sniffles; it needs a doctor. But if your situation is only pain and not pathology, push yourself into life.

Some mornings getting out of bed, not to mention living with enough ardor and self-regard to turn back the clock, can be inconceivable. There are times you probably *shouldn't* get out of bed. This is why God made weekends and some enlightened human resources manager came up with personal days. But you can't stay in bed forever.

Should you do the duvet-and-DVD thing for twenty-four hours (or double that) and still feel as if life is just too much, push yourself into it, whether you think you have any push left or not. You do this by playing your messages, washing your hair, seeing the movie, taking the class. This informs your brain that you're choosing life.

You see, we think the brain tells us how things are. If it says, "You're sad [tired, discouraged, etc.]; go to bed," we tend to accept that conclusion and take that advice. But we tell our brains what's up, too. If you spruce yourself up, get out, and talk to people, your brain gets the message: "Oh, she's all right after all. Let's funnel her some energy and optimism." This is simply acting yourself into a better frame of mind. You're already doing verbal and written affirmations. This turns your life into an affirmation.

REVITALIZE YOUR LIFE WITH WORDS: *I refuse to sacrifice a day of my life. I extract the joy from each day I live.*

SEPTEMBER 28

Delve into the Spiritual Classics

There are books that contain within them truths about life that make sense of it all. When these truths become our truth, we can grow older without being afraid, and we can live today with a sense of purpose that consecrates the ordinary. These books are the spiritual classics: scriptures of all the world's religions; the works of mystical poets such as Rumi, Tagore, and Walt Whitman; and commentaries on the spiritual life from people who lived it. We do ourselves a disservice to think we're not up to such reading. These books don't exist to challenge the intellect; they're here to touch the soul.

When I worked in a library in my early twenties, I read them voraciously, but when I was feeling my age a few years ago, I never thought that reading Tagore could be as helpful as reading about antioxidants. Then I remembered how I'd felt all those years before when I could hide away for an afternoon with Evelyn Underhill's *The Ways of the Spirit*, Patanjali's *Yoga Sutras*, and a compelling collection of poetry, *The Oxford Book of English Mystical Verse*.

I realized that over time, even though I was a writer, I had become a lazy reader. I had grown used to sound bites and quotable quips and felt satisfied by them, but a sound bite had never carried me away like those afternoons in the company of musty volumes filled with big ideas. I believe that the time you spend carried away, whether reading or being in nature or meditating or creating something, you get to subtract from your age. This is time spent with your soul, and it doesn't seem at all farfetched to me that it would give your body a reprieve from aging.

I know you have a lot on both your mind and your plate, so give yourself all the time and leeway you need for this. Just pick up a book that you consider a spiritual classic—the Bible or the Bhagavad Gita or a compilation of Emerson's essays—and put it on your bedside table. Read a little, even just a verse or a paragraph, every night or every morning. When something you read speaks to you in a special way, write what it means to you in your journal. Look into other spiritual classics when you're at the library or the bookstore. Make friends of some of them. Let them carry you away.

REJUVENATE YOURSELF WITH ACTION: *Find space in your calendar sometime this month when you can give yourself two hours alone in a bookstore or library to look into some spiritual classics. You'll find them in "Religion," "Philosophy," "Mysticism," "Psychology," "Poetry"—and don't forget "Children's Literature." The Velveteen Rabbit, Alice's Adventures in Wonderland, and many of the classic fairy tales have layers of meaning to help you live happily ever after.*

SEPTEMBER 29

Added Sugar

The best way to deal with added sugar is not to add it. This can be challenging, because sugar is found in so many processed foods, leading to a daily consumption that's making too many of us tired, pudgy, and old. A constant barrage of sugar depresses immunity, lowers HDL (good cholesterol), elevates triglycerides (a risk factor in heart disease), and causes oxidation damage—i.e., free radicals on the rampage. Consumption of saturated fat, which accompanies sugar in such favorites as baked goods and ice cream, intensifies these effects.

In addition, the sugar we're eating is often the worst of the worst. Refined table sugar (sucrose) is bad enough, providing no nutrients besides calories, but most of the sugar we consume these days is high-fructose corn syrup. In the United States, we're ingesting a whopping 4000 percent more of it than we did in the 1970s. This stuff raises serum triglycerides more than ordinary sugar does. It also appears to interfere with the heart's ability to utilize minerals, it may disrupt metabolism, and there is some conjecture that it's better at making people fat than plain old sugar ever was.

Fight back:

- *Eat whole foods.* These include whole fruits, whole grains, *real* food. Over time, this will reeducate your palate so that refined sugars and other refined foods won't taste good any longer.

- *Read labels.* If sugar by any name (sugar, brown sugar, dextrose, glucose, lactose, maltose, sorbitol, or high-fructose corn syrup) is in the first four ingredients, don't buy the product. Also watch for sneaky labeling that includes two forms of sugar, each lower down on the list than they would have been if a single sugar source had been used.

- *Use natural sweeteners.* Artificial sweeteners are questionable and certainly not something any body needs. Aspartame has been implicated as a factor in migraines, mood swings, and insomnia. Alternatives include the sweet herb stevia, available at health food stores, and sweeteners like dark honey, pure maple syrup, blended dates, date sugar (powdered, dried dates), and Sucanat (dehydrated cane juice). With the exception of stevia, these are still sugars, but they come with nutrients and antioxidants so the body can use them. Besides, these sweeteners don't make their way into everything from bacon to ketchup to salad dressing, so you're not likely to consume enough of them to cause trouble.

- *Resurrect the notion of the "treat."* Most people can eat some sugar on holidays and special occasions and be fine. It's the 365-day sugar binge that's doing us in. If you don't wish to cut out sugar 100 percent, resurrect the idea of the treat. Then when you have one, it will be delectable.

REJUVENATE YOURSELF WITH ACTION: *Be aware of the added sugar in your diet. Conscientiously read labels. Choose the unsweetened variety of every manufactured food you buy. When you do eat something made with sugar, be sure it's good enough to be worth it.*

SEPTEMBER 30

Play Day!

October

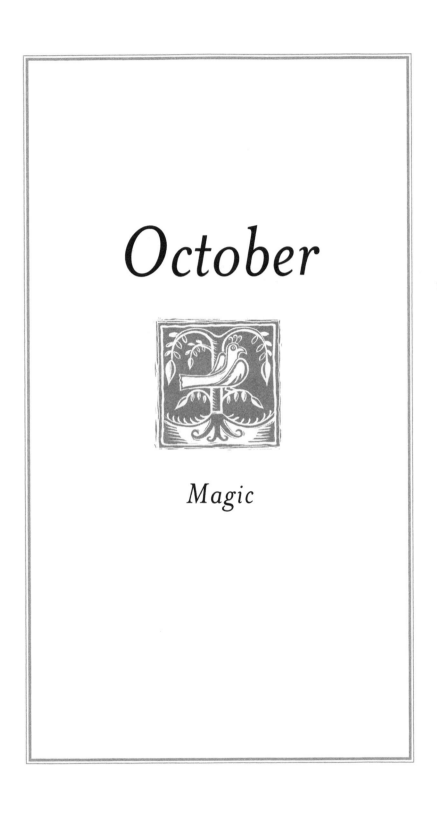

Magic

OCTOBER 1

Living Magically

The magic I'd like for you to keep in mind this month, the magic that will get you back a birthday or two or several, has to do with feeling so alive that it revolutionizes the way you perceive the world and the way it perceives you. Living with this kind of aliveness is enchanting and energizing. It's also hard work. Magical lives are uncommon, because we have the misconception that they are whimsically granted only to a chosen few. In fact, anybody can have one. Most people don't care to venture forth on such an uncharted course. You do, or else you'd be reading a different book.

Like the ancient alchemists who sought to turn dross into gold, you're seeking to turn the often downward spiral of growing older into a magical adventure instead. Some people will tell you you'd have better luck trying to get pure gold out of your costume jewelry. These are the cynics. Cynics and magicians never see eye-to-eye. Besides, the magic we're after doesn't call for spells and potions, just courage and grit and the willingness to go where few have gone before. You need to realize what makes you feel alive, and what takes that liveliness away. Be as specific as you can. For example:

A part of me dies when I . . .

- Travel for business more than twice a month

- Focus on what I want more than on what I have

- Spend time in ugly, soulless places (unless I'm there to bring some light or do some good)

I feel extraordinarily alive when I . . .

- Get up early and decide to make it a fabulous day

- Am part of a rich, deep discussion

- Know I've touched someone in a positive way

The clearer you are on what creates magic in your life, the more able you'll be to see that the magic gets there. This is necessary, because living magically doesn't just make your body younger and your life happier; it's an offering you give the rest of us. Then you're both invigorating yourself and convincing a weary world that liveliness and possibility and hope and change and beauty and magic are every bit as real as the work and worry that take up so much of so many people's time.

REVITALIZE YOUR LIFE WITH WORDS: *I put magic in my life by coming alive every single day.*

OCTOBER 2

You Look Lovely by Candlelight

One of the simplest things you can do to look radiant, a little mysterious, and years younger is put yourself in candlelight. With fall in the air and evening coming earlier, this is a great time to start lighting candles. Light some at dusk for ambience—there can be soft electric lighting, too. Have a candle or two in your bedroom to light when you meditate. Bathe by candlelight. And by all means have candlelit dinners, even when there is no company.

I heard about a little boy who, at a friend's house for dinner the first time, sat there not picking up his fork. "What's the matter?" the friend's mother asked him. "Where are the candles?" he wanted to know. At his house, candles were a nightly occurrence and this kindergartner couldn't conceive of having dinner in a hundred-watt glare. Good for him.

When you buy candles, don't go for a bargain. You want a nice flame and no smoke. You get your value from a candle that burns long and well. According to Michael Halpern of Creative Candles, a twelve-inch taper should burn eight hours—that's quite a few dinners. Unlike a taper, which can burn for a few minutes, be extinguished, and be lit again with no ill effects, a pillar candle needs to stay lit two to four hours so it burns within an eighth-inch of the rim. Otherwise you get a flame buried in an indentation and a candle that needs to be replaced too soon. Drafts, an uneven table, or being moved while lit can cause any candle to burn unevenly or succumb to what in the trade they call "forced smoking."

Scented candles, like candles in general, are to set a mood, not deodorize a room. Go for a subtle fragrance. And for safety's sake, always place candles on a noncombustible surface; keep them away from children's fingers, cats' paws, and dogs' tails; and, number-one rule, never leave a burning candle unattended. Besides, a candle can make you beautiful only when you're in the same room.

REJUVENATE YOURSELF WITH ACTION: *How is your stock of candles? Can you dine by candlelight tonight?*

OCTOBER 3

Recognize the Patterns of Your Life

Pop psychology has given the word "patterns" an unsavory reputation in emphasizing the negative habit patterns that can rob us of enjoyment and productivity. But there are positive patterns, too—your good habits, certainly, but also deeper patterns, the ones your life follows for bringing good things in.

For example, I have a pattern in which the hardest times are invariably followed by the best ones. Many of the greatest gifts of my life have come out of experiences I wouldn't wish on even the kid who called me "Fatty" in the third grade. I don't have to have darkness before something great happens, but when I'm in a place I'd prefer to be out of, I can at least remember that, based on fifty years' precedent, something splendid is coming.

Another pattern I've seen has to do with meddling in my own affairs. I did an inventory of my professional life to see what I had done to bring about past successes. I listed on one side of a page the best things that have happened in my work, and on the other side what I had done to bring these about. To my amazement, my part in these various coups was either nothing at all or just showing up in the right place at the right time. Of course, I work hard to write valuable books and give helpful presentations, but hard work by itself has never been the direct precursor of the successes I've enjoyed. This exercise taught me that my preferred pattern is "do the work and get out of the way." If I push and push, I can push myself right out of the running.

Get to know your patterns by scanning your life history in your head or on paper, looking for those motifs that show up time and again. Or take a specific aspect of your life as I did—work or relationships, health or finances—and see what you did to bring about the best that's happened yet. Then you can do it again.

REJUVENATE YOURSELF WITH ACTION: *Take a look at your life (or some part of it) and pull out one or two of the patterns apparent there. Once you recognize them, you can work with them to your advantage.*

OCTOBER 4

Consider the Guidance That May Come Through Dreams

Some dreams tell you only that you ate too much or too late, or that you have no business watching horror movies. Others are just subconscious replays of the events of the day, a sort of mental metabolism. A few dreams, however, give you insights into yourself. These special ones tend to be more vivid than the others, and they give you a sense that there is a message attached.

Experts in this field suggest giving yourself permission before bed to remember what you dreamed. They also recommend keeping a pad and pencil by your bed for jotting down the gist of a dream before it gets away. These are probably good ideas, because the more dreams you're able to bring to mind, the better you'll be able to discern which ones have something to tell you.

There are various schools of dream interpretation, the most highly respected being Jungian psychology, with its notions that every character in your dreams represents yourself, and that archetypal images (mythological impressions known to the collective mind of humanity) appear in your dreams as symbolic teachers. You can read books about dream symbolism or even consult a Jungian analyst, or simply tell yourself that if you need to understand a message from a dream, you will.

Before I moved to New York, I dreamed that I set a trapped bird free in Manhattan. Instead of taking refuge in the nearby park, this bird flew gleefully into the bustle of Times Square. In the dream, I asked a seasoned New Yorker why a bird wouldn't choose the natural setting. "Because," my dream guide told me, "she just isn't that kind of bird." My unconscious was telling me where I needed to be. Our inner selves want to communicate with us, about the things that matter anyway. You don't need to make something out of every dream, every night, but when you get one like this, listen. It's just one more way to take care of yourself.

REJUVENATE YOURSELF WITH ACTION: *Give yourself the suggestion tonight and every night through the rest of October that if a dream is worth remembering and understanding, you will remember and understand it.*

OCTOBER 5

The Inner Change of Life

Less sensational perhaps but every bit as life-altering as the physical symptoms that may accompany menopause is the inner transformation a woman undergoes at this time, a transfiguration that has more to do with her mind than her body. It is inevitable, whether you fight it or welcome it and whether you take hormones or not. You'll recognize it as a shift in your priorities. Your outlook will seem to come from a different vantage point, as if you'd spent your life in a valley and then moved to a nearby hillside. Even if you didn't go far, your view of the world now comes from another angle, another direction.

After this transformation, much that recently seemed important no longer does, but it takes awhile for new preoccupations to rise up and fill in the blank spaces. This calls for patience and poise and every scrap of dignity you've collected in living half a century or so. A woman I know was at this point in her life at the same time that she was making a name for herself in her career. Her rueful comment: "The dreams of my former life are coming true." This happens a lot in middle age. We reap the fruits of our labors and realize that these are no longer our favorite fruits. We have to get to know ourselves anew, the way our child selves had to become acquainted with our maturing selves at puberty. There are losses at both junctures, but there are gains, too. Society tends to see what time gives to children and what it takes from women. It's up to us to unearth the benefactions of this transitional time.

When you can no longer give birth to a baby, you have the uncommon opportunity to give birth to an adult: yourself—your consummate, connected self. Maybe you were once a bright, inquisitive eleven-year-old who shelved her stamp collection and her plans to study chimps in the wild when, at twelve, her interests turned to makeup and boys. Congratulations: you're about to get that eleven-year-old back. If you've given so much of yourself to other people that you've lost chunks of you, it's time to reclaim them. If you've derived the bulk of your identity from the way you look, you can finally relax, exhale, and acknowledge the tremendous beauty inside you that isn't going anywhere. Ever.

Wherever you find yourself in relation to this Really Big Change in physiology and consciousness, frame it as a blessing, even when the blessing seems well disguised. It takes every stage of life to comprise us and complete us—this one, too.

REVITALIZE YOUR LIFE WITH WORDS: *I am eager to grow into all that I can be.*

OCTOBER 6

Blender Soups

Blender soups are healthy fast food for fall and winter. They fill in for salty canned soups, and blending any vegetable or bean soup turns it into cream-of-whatever without adding cream or flour. You can put together a creamy pea soup by blending cooked peas, water, curry powder, and sea salt to taste. It's velvety smooth and ready in about a minute. If you have a dental problem or can't eat salad for some other reason, blend salad vegetables, season them with your favorite spices, serve chilled, and call it gazpacho. My guests love Jennifer Raymond's exotic pumpkin soup. (Don't let the long list of spices concern you; this is really quick and easy.)

Spicy Pumpkin Soup

1 tablespoon olive oil
1 onion, chopped
2 cloves garlic, minced
$^1/_2$ teaspoon mustard seeds
$^1/_2$ teaspoon turmeric
$^1/_2$ teaspoon ginger
$^1/_2$ teaspoon cumin
$^1/_2$ teaspoon cinnamon
$^1/_8$ teaspoon cayenne
$^3/_4$ teaspoon salt
2 cups water or vegetable stock
1 15-ounce can pumpkin
2 tablespoons maple syrup or other sweetener
1 tablespoon lemon juice
2 cups soy milk
fresh cilantro, chopped (optional)

Heat the oil in a large pot. Add the onion and garlic and cook over medium heat until the onion is soft, about five minutes. Add the mustard seeds, turmeric, ginger, cumin, cinnamon, cayenne, and salt. Cook over medium heat for two minutes, stirring constantly. Whisk in the water or vegetable stock, pumpkin, maple syrup, and lemon juice. Simmer fifteen minutes. Stir in the soy milk, then purée the soup in a blender in two or three batches until very smooth. Return it to the pan and heat over a medium flame until hot and steamy (do not let it boil), about ten minutes. Serve with a sprinkling of fresh cilantro if desired. Serves six (106 calories, 2 grams protein, 18 grams carbohydrate, and 3 grams fat per serving).

OCTOBER 7

Learn About, but Don't Decide On, Cosmetic Surgery

Cosmetic surgery is a fact of life today, although still a topic of controversy. In some circles, anyone who has it is considered self-centered or lacking in self-esteem. In another social stratum, a woman who doesn't get it is seen as lackadaisical. Other than the obvious—the implication that radical reconstruction is necessary because we're faulty the way we are or the way we age—my biggest problem with cosmetic surgery is the economic disparity it brings up. I don't like to think that we're heading for a society in which the jawline becomes yet one more divide between rich and poor. "It will be like the cell phone," I've been told. "Before long it will be so popular almost anyone who wants it can have it." Time will tell on that one.

The reason I suggest you learn about cosmetic surgery is that, even if you never get any, your sister might, or a co-worker, or the friend you thought would be the last person on earth to do it. The rationale behind not deciding on it right away is that this year of growing younger will change you inside and out; you'll make a wiser decision after you've completed this process. Besides, we're talking about surgery, which always carries risk, and you want to be sure you understand exactly what it will do for you and what risks you're taking before you start counting backwards with a mask over your face. You also want to be absolutely certain about why you're doing this. If you start with unrealistic expectations, even the best results will be disappointing.

By cosmetic surgery, I'm not speaking here of injections you can get in a dermatologist's office (May 27) to fill in lines or temporarily paralyze muscles that contract in ways that cause wrinkling of the skin. Surgical procedures can change structures (a nose, a chin), resurface areas of the skin, remove fat deposits, or lift sagging parts (e.g., breasts, eye area, or slack flesh beneath the jaw). A full facelift is major surgery, involving sizable incisions. A promising alternative is the short-scar or mini-lift. Although it's no cheaper than a traditional lift (it actually takes even more skill on the part of the surgeon), there is only half the cutting, so you can get it with local anesthesia, a shorter recovery period, and a less dramatic change so "only her doctor knows for sure." A mini-lift focuses on the mid-face, the area roughly to the front of the ears. It will help a slightly sagging chin but not full-fledged jowls, and it doesn't do much for the eyes, although another procedure just to deal with droopy eyes or puffy lids could be done at the same time.

I think cosmetic surgery, prudently considered, can be a useful tool. I had laser resurfacing for acne scars in my mid-forties. Those were the days before we got to see post-surgical patients on TV, so the extent of the temporary disfigurement—my dog yelped and wouldn't come near me—and the discomfort of recovery came as a shock. In my case, the improvement was gratifying; but I was lucky: so many people did poorly with the procedure that it has fallen out of favor and most doctors no longer do it. There are no guarantees. Still, with the right surgeon and the money saved up, I would go for a little lift, as long as I was clear that I was looking only to improve my appearance, not elevate my worth.

REJUVENATE YOURSELF WITH ACTION: *How do you feel about cosmetic surgery and people who get it? Writing about this in your journal can be a useful exercise in getting to know yourself better.*

OCTOBER 8

Osmotic Rejuvenation

Osmotic rejuvenation may sound like an expensive new spa treatment. Rather, it is a do-it-yourself proposition and it doesn't cost a cent. It's growing younger via osmosis, soaking up youthfulness by being in the presence of it. You take advantage of osmotic rejuvenation when you're around youthful people, whether they're ten, twenty, or seventy-eight. These are people who laugh easily and who are fascinated by myriad things. They model living life lightly by taking seriously only those matters that truly are.

You rejuvenate by osmosis when you put yourself in youthful places and do youthful things—e.g., going to a playground and using the equipment, seeing an animated movie (even if you don't have a child in tow), or visiting an amusement park and actually riding the rides. You do it when you take yourself on a field trip to a museum or the library or anyplace that has tour guides. Osmotic rejuvenation comes from wishing on stars, walking in the rain, and eating dessert first. (Some study suggested that eating dessert first could mean eating less overall because you'd feel safe in knowing you'd gotten what you really wanted.)

You don't have to do a thing to get osmotic rejuvenation other than allow yourself to experience wonder. Do it often.

REVITALIZE YOUR LIFE WITH WORDS: *Youthfulness, vitality, and fun are all around me. I soak them up today and make them mine.*

OCTOBER 9

Aromatherapy

The distinctive aromas of volatile plant oils have been used therapeutically since the days of the pharaohs, and contemporary studies have shown them to be top-flight stress-reducers, useful in lowering blood pressure, relieving muscular tension, and stabilizing heart rate.

Essential oils, the compelling scents used in aromatherapy, are potent, so much so that they should never be applied undiluted to your skin. The list of essential oils pregnant women should not be inhaling is long enough that part of prudence is to simply skip this if you're expecting. These caveats duly noted, start your aromatic adventure by purchasing pure essential oils singly or as blends. Some scents to try:

- *For calmness, relaxation, and stress relief:* lavender, vetiver, petitgrain, frankincense

- *For waking up and increasing energy:* eucalyptus, ylang-ylang, lemon, tangerine

- *For happier spirits:* basil, geranium, patchouli, neroli

- *For increasing confidence:* grapefruit, ginger, bergamot

- *For a romantic mood:* jasmine, sandalwood, rose, cedarwood

Using essential oils to scent a room can elevate the mood of everyone present. The easiest way to do this is to purchase an inexpensive "lamp ring," a little circle of fired clay onto which you can sprinkle a few drops of your chosen oil. Set it on a lightbulb and allow the heat from the bulb to send the delicate scent into the air.

To enjoy aromatherapy in your bath, put six to ten drops of essential oil in a tablespoon of vegetable oil (essential oils don't diffuse properly without a bland oil as a carrier) and swirl the mixture into a fully drawn bath. Adjust the temperature so you can comfortably soak for twenty minutes. Using a few drops of lavender oil in a bedtime bath and following up with a couple of drops applied directly to your pillow is like having the sandman at your beck and call.

REJUVENATE YOURSELF WITH ACTION: *Choose one essential oil or one blend that smells to you like something fresh from Shangri-la. Use it this week to scent your home or enhance your bath.*

OCTOBER 10

The Willow Effect

You experience the willow effect when your body is flexible, stretchable, when it can reach and bend with fluidity and ease. This idyllic state comes gratis with youth. You can get a goodly measure of it back, but now there is a price: the slow, careful, repeated stretching of tight muscles, always working within the current limits of your joints and spine. The stereotypical aches and pains of later life are largely a result of stiffness. When you're limber and loose, you'll feel freer in your body and appear more graceful as you move through your day. Being flexible will also improve your posture, give you greater range of motion, work out some of the tension trapped in your muscles, and help prevent exercise soreness and possible injury. Like the willow tree, your body will be able to bend instead of break under pressure.

Include easy stretches before and after your aerobic and weight training sessions—even four or five minutes can accomplish a lot. Don't stretch cold muscles; that could cause an injury instead of preventing one. Go easy. Don't strain. Hold each stretch twenty seconds or so. As you do, heed this recommendation from Wyatt Townley's book *Yoganetics:* "All stretches are rests. Ballistic bouncing is illegal here. . . . Your job is to surrender and let gravity do the work."

You can gently stretch when you awaken in the morning, even right in bed while you're still warm. Do it while watching TV: sit on the floor and do slow forward and side bends with nice long holds. Take breaks at work and stretch a little at your desk or in the ladies' room: stretch and flex your feet; reach your arms overhead; clasp your hands for a careful stretch behind your back; do wrist, ankle, and neck circles. Think of this as lubricating your moving parts. Unlike weight training, which requires a day off to let your muscles rest, stretching can be done as often as you like, and it feels so good you'll want to.

Many people gain cardiovascular endurance and muscular strength more rapidly than they increase their flexibility, but this will happen, too; just give it time and don't push. Bodies differ, and some will always be more flexible than others. You're not in competition with anyone else, or with yourself at some earlier time of your life. It is impossible to force flexibility. You're allowing yourself to become younger. Allow your body to become lithe and agile as well.

REJUVENATE YOURSELF WITH ACTION: *Gently stretch today. Do it in the morning, on your breaks at the office, and before and after you exercise. Make note of how good it feels so you'll want to keep it up.*

Speaking the Language of Transformation

Remember "magic words" and how enticing they were when you were a child? *Abracadabra! Open Sesame!* They're as enticing as ever. It's just that the magic words themselves are different: now they're the positive words that support your growth and nurture your dreams. There are words and phrases that support transformation and those that block it. When someone says, "I'm not as young as I used to be," "I guess I'll have to get used to all these aches and pains," or "It's too late now," she issues an open invitation to aches, pains, and expired opportunities. *Your brain believes what you tell it, and so does your body.*

Transformative language is both positive and precise. It speaks the truth and offers a way for any facts that aren't so hot to redeem themselves. "Well, I'm not really sure, but I think maybe I might be able to do that" is tentative; "Of course I can do it" is transformative. Some people worry that in using transformative language they aren't being honest. Not so. Of course you need to tell the doctor where it hurts, but you don't have to reiterate how much it hurts to everyone who innocently asks, "How are you?" Answering "Just fine" is usually just fine. Work up to "Great!" "Wonderful!" and "Things couldn't be better!"

Bring transformative language to the dining room as well. Avoid the insufferable phrase "I can't eat . . ." You *can* eat anything you like; you may *choose* not to eat certain things or not eat them today. In fact, it's a captivating gesture when you're passing on cocktails or dessert to say, "None today, thank you." That way you aren't indicting someone else's choices as wrong; you're simply making a choice of your own.

Did your mom ever tell you, "If you can't say something nice, don't say anything"? She was right—and talking nicely also applies when you're talking to yourself, even inside your head.

REVITALIZE YOUR LIFE WITH WORDS: *I invite transformation with my words, thoughts, and actions.*

The Hair Color Conundrum

Many women can take off a decade, visually anyway, with the careful application of a well-chosen, translucent color. Still, starting to color your hair is a big decision. (For that matter, so is stopping if you've colored for a long time and you're considering letting nature take its course.) If you color now, or if you intend to start, research the products and their formulations. Look for plant-based colors with fewer harsh chemicals than you'd be getting with another brand. There is longstanding, although unproven, concern about the possible relationship between hair color, specifically the paraphenylenediamine dyes in permanent black and dark brown hues, and certain kinds of cancer. I personally choose to use the most natural line of color I can find, and I'm gradually going from my once-natural dark brown to a luscious—and potentially safer—auburn.

It is becoming to go a shade or two lighter than your original hue, or get some delicate, well-placed highlights. Especially if your original color was dark, this little bit of brightening can do wonders for the look of your skin, which over time may have lost some of its color and firmness. If you have a lot of gray, highlighting will make the contrast between your naked roots and your colored hair less noticeable. This buys time when it comes to touching up.

Even so, coloring your hair is a commitment and an investment. Although highlights can be good for three to four months, you'll need to touch up your roots every three and a half to six weeks, depending on how fast your hair grows and how different your adopted shade is from the one growing out of your head. If you go too long between touch-ups, you'll be as two-toned as a '57 Chevy. You can save money by doing the touch-ups yourself, although when I try it, the results of my amateur endeavor are, well, amateurish. If you want to color your hair and keep it up, figure out before you do it how to fit this into your household economy. (Beauty schools are great for saving money. I also like the idea of using money no longer being spent on bad habits to implement good ones.)

All this talk of color is not to imply that gray hair can't be lovely. It can, in fact, be absolutely beautiful. Just as your genes determine how soon you'll get gray hair, they also have substantial say in how that gray will look. Hair grays, or more accurately, "whites"—i.e., loses its color pigment—differently. You might be lucky and get lustrous silver, or a blend that on someone else might be drab salt-and-pepper, but on you is flattering and striking. The less fortunate and more numerous among us get dingy yellow-gray or a mix of dark and light strands that doesn't enhance our skin tones. (Hint: if you look fabulous in your gray suit, or if platinum and silver look better on you than yellow gold, you'll probably look good with silver hair, too.)

If you can carry off the gray you get, if you have a political commitment to not hiding this sign of maturity, or if using even the best hair color is at odds with your natural lifestyle, wear it proudly. Keep it superbly conditioned, and once or twice a week use a violet-blue shampoo that will keep the yellow tones down and make your gray as radiant as can be. Above all, respect yourself for your choice and be tolerant of those who make a different one. As a society, we need to get lots more flexible about what constitutes beauty. It isn't a particular hair color or a particular body type; it's the woman who grew the hair and lives in the body. Keeping this in mind can only make things better.

REJUVENATE YOURSELF WITH ACTION: *Write in your journal about what gray hair means to you and what it means to cover it up. Write about women in general and yourself in particular. Expect to be enlightened.*

OCTOBER 13

The Longevity Recipe

Some scientists believe that a substantial decrease in caloric intake could increase life expectancy a whopping 40 percent. There are no human studies to show this definitively, and even if there were, making that "substantial decrease" in one of life's great pleasures would not appeal to most of us. Still, keeping our caloric intake modest rather than excessive may give us more time on this enticing planet.

Keep your calories in check by eating whole foods, especially salads and steamed or roasted vegetables, and eliminating or markedly cutting down on fats, sweets, and processed foods. The other salient factor is portion size. Dinner, unless you're making a meal of an oversized salad, should fit on a plate—one plate. Drinks other than water need be thought of in ounces, not quarts.

When you eat out, you don't have to finish everything. Eat until you're satisfied, of course—going slowly will help you get to that point without overeating—but restaurant portions have ballooned in the recent past. They're often plentiful enough to share, or to yield leftovers for tomorrow. Unless you're eating Japanese, where petite portions cunningly arranged are an art form, one course is probably plenty. When my mother, my daughter, and I are able to get together for a three-generational lunch, Adair, being young and dancing every day, often gets an appetizer and an entrée. The main dish is enough for me, and Mom many times orders the appetizer as her meal. Knowing yourself means knowing your needs and your capacity.

This can be difficult if you're still obeying voices from the past that said, "Clean your plate." (Funny, those same voices said, "Don't have sex," and "Never take a drink," but we got past those all right.) Change the voice. Give yourself the message that cleaning your plate is no longer called for. Sometimes routinely leaving just a little something can help break a food addiction, since it's proof that what is on the plate has no more power than we give it.

If you're healthy, have no history of eating disorders, and don't feel anxious about missing meals, consider fasting one day a week, either on pure water or fresh vegetable juice and herbal tea. In his book *Ayurveda*, Scott Gerson, MD, says, "Fasting is recommended for the normal, healthy individual. It is an effective initial treatment for many diseases because it both rids the body of toxins and enlivens *Agni*, the digestive fire."

Many people—beautiful, age-defying women among them—welcome a short fast as a freeing experience, lengthening the day, and providing a sense of lightness and mild euphoria. Those who enjoy it and feel that they benefit from it often do a longer fast of three days' duration over a weekend, perhaps at the change of seasons. Regular, brief fasts are a way to cut down on overall calorie consumption. The practice could conceivably lengthen your life. It will definitely help you see things from a different perspective.

REVITALIZE YOUR LIFE WITH WORDS: *Moderation tastes delicious.*

Nature's Schedule

As little girls, we were "good" when we went to bed on time. Most of us now pronounce ourselves "good" if we're up at midnight finishing a project for work or scrubbing gunk out of the fridge with baking soda and a sponge. The work ethic has a place, but it also has a time, and unless you're a midwife or an ambulance driver, midnight isn't it. You need your sleep now for growing younger as much as you once needed it for growing up. Being well rested erases years.

With all due respect to night people, humans are not nocturnal animals. If it weren't for Edison, night people couldn't even see where they're going. Nature expects us to keep the same hours she does: activity during the daylight, quiet when it's dark. Ayurveda affirms that health and longevity depend upon our conforming to the natural pattern. This means going to bed when the energies of the earth support repose—between nine and ten-thirty, eleven at the latest—and rising when the same energies that rouse the rooster awaken an in-tune person, too. This is early—six o'clock, give or take an hour.

If your work schedule makes it impossible to sleep on this timetable, focus on sleeping enough and sleeping well in the time you've got. Eat early. Otherwise digesting food can interfere with your sleep or trouble your dreams. (Two hours should be the minimum lapse between dinner and bedtime.) Refrain from caffeine after tea time—earlier if you're sensitive to it. If alcohol or sweets disrupt your sleep, skip those at dinner, too. Complex carbohydrates are relaxing, but refined sugar and alcohol hit the system quickly, causing a rapid spike and subsequent drop in blood sugar. When it rebounds several hours later (in the middle of the night), it can wake you up. As a constant pattern, this can age you, since your body releases youth-retaining growth hormone while you sleep.

I also suggest that you refrain from watching the late-night news. You needn't be informed in your dreams, and they'll likely be more pleasant if you're not. In fact, Ayurveda advises against watching any TV an hour before bed, using this time instead for winding down, your nightly ritual, quiet joys, a little pillow talk. Then know in the spirit of Scarlett O'Hara that tomorrow really is another day. Days are for work and achievement and getting Rhett back. Nights are for letting all of it go.

REJUVENATE YOURSELF WITH ACTION: *Look at the way your schedule stands up against nature's schedule. What can you do to bring it into closer alignment?*

OCTOBER 15

Play Day!

OCTOBER 16

What's That You're Breathing?

Those of us who are concerned about the quality of the food we eat need to be equally interested in the quality of the air we breathe. Air is, after all, our primary food.

We think of pollution as an outdoor problem, the result of auto exhaust and industrial effluent sullying the air. Surprisingly, outdoor air, even in cities, is almost always cleaner than indoor air. The reason: nature itself is a first-rate air purifier and works on cleanup 'round the clock. When we seal ourselves into houses and office buildings, we don't get the benefit of those cleanup efforts. The newer the building, the worse things are: those leaks that make old houses drafty and expensive to heat are also letting in fresh air. Energy-efficient structures, as sensible as they are in other ways, keep us breathing the same stale air.

Some ways to breathe better air more of the time include the following:

- *Open a window.* Let some of that fresh air in. This is especially important when you sleep, or if you are using a chemical like paint or chlorine bleach. Even in winter, have the window open a bit. (An exception to this is allergy season if you're allergic to pollens or grasses.)

- *When the windows are closed, have an air-cleaner running.* A good air-cleaner can largely do away with allergens like dust, mold, and animal dander; outgassing from paint, plyboard, carpeting, and cleaning products; and unpleasant odors. By "good" I mean an air-cleaner that is a fairly major purchase, one with a five-year filter or new technology that requires no filter at all.

- *When it's time to replace your vacuum cleaner, get one with a real HEPA filter.* This way, when you vacuum, you aren't sending tiny dirt particles back out into the air. As long as you're using an ordinary vac, at least open the windows when it's running and for several minutes afterwards.

- *Don't join the polluters.* We think of polluters as captains of industry or oil tankers, when in fact most of us pollute our own air every day. If you confine your household purchases to truly natural products—real wood instead of particle board, organic cotton bedding instead of chemically treated synthetics, natural cleaning products instead of harsh chemicals—you'll be breathing grade A air in no time.

REJUVENATE YOURSELF WITH ACTION: *Start today on the road to cleaner indoor air by changing how you clean house. You can have a sparkling and sanitary home without a chemical plant under the kitchen sink by choosing gentle products from nature. They work well and require little more elbow grease than you use now. As you run out of your various cleaning products, replace them with brands such as Ecover or Seventh Generation, available in natural food stores or online. You can also clean nearly everything with baking soda, club soda, borax, lemon juice, and vinegar, alone or in combination. A "recipe book" for do-it-yourself cleaning products is* Better Basics for the Home, *by Amy Berthold Bond.*

A Dazzling Smile

If you want whiter teeth, first understand that teeth come in shades. Some people's natural hue is not bright white. All teeth can get whiter, but not having teeth the color of your first communion dress is nothing to be ashamed of. The advantage of white teeth is primarily cultural. In ancient Japan, people darkened their teeth because that met their esthetic criteria. Our culture favors pearly whites, especially now that they're easier than ever to get.

You can whiten at home with products from the drugstore; or have the dentist fit you with bleaching trays and prescribe a solution keyed to the state of your teeth and gums; or go for in-office laser whitening. The results are similar, although home bleaching can take days or weeks while laser whitening is done in an hour. All these appear to be safe, although pregnant women are advised to wait to whiten until after the birth. Any whitening method can exacerbate sensitive teeth. If you have them, let your dentist know and he can steer you toward the best system for you. Unfortunately, no whitening method will prevent your teeth from yellowing again or picking up stain. Whatever will stain a white shirt will stain your teeth. Coffee, tea, and red wine are notorious for it, and cigarettes are even worse.

Using nonabrasive whitening toothpaste can remove stains between professional cleanings. If whitening is your aim, select a toothpaste that concentrates on that. If it claims to do half a dozen other things, it probably won't whiten as well as you'd like. I personally prefer a natural whitening toothpaste that does not contain saccharine or other added chemicals I'd rather not have in my mouth.

Should you be looking for a greater change than whitening alone, esthetic dentistry has become increasingly affordable. Problems such as misaligned teeth, trauma to your front teeth or lots of fillings there, or teeth that don't fit your face (maybe you got genes for Mom's mouth and Dad's teeth) can be remedied. Porcelain laminate veneers aren't just for movie stars anymore, and braces—some are invisible even—are no longer just for kids.

So much is possible in the smile department. Once you have great teeth, or even when improvements are just in the planning stages, go ahead and smile. It will make you feel happier and put other people at ease. The fact that it shows off your dazzling teeth—well, that's nice, too.

REJUVENATE YOURSELF WITH ACTION: *If you've never whitened your teeth, try it. It will make you look younger, brighter, and better groomed. If your teeth are prone to stain, limit your coffee intake or switch from black tea to green tea or an herbal blend.*

OCTOBER 18

Overdo on Inspiration

Inspiration can get a bad rap. It's seen as lightweight when compared to the action it might precede. Sometimes people describe inspirational books, poems, and movies as if they were talking about the menu choices at a snack bar: "cheesy," "corny," "sickeningly sweet." These are people who would rather feel urbane than serene, even though the two are not mutually exclusive.

The inspiration that comes from words or music, a sermon or a sunset, gives you a soul lift. That's a facelift on the inside. You take on some energy that wasn't there before. Dread becomes determination. The impossible starts looking like a piece of your favorite cake. When you do inspirational reading, for instance, it won't be the first time you've heard that you're part of all life, or that the good you do comes back to you, or that the beautiful memory you make today could be with you on your deathbed and in stories your grandchildren will tell their grandchildren. It's just that being reminded of it one more time will give you another dose of energy and magic.

Indulge in inspiration by collecting quotations, old and new, from the famous, the not famous, and the anonymous. Write them in your journal. Stick them to your fridge. Embed them in your memory. Listen to the lyrics of inspiring songs. Musical theater is great for this. Every good show has at least one song that's about achieving something incredible, or overcoming insurmountable odds. See films that make you cry, read stories that make you laugh, and send greeting cards that do one or the other. It's okay to overdo on inspiration. It will make you younger than you think.

REVITALIZE YOUR LIFE WITH WORDS: *I am open to inspiration, and it comes to me in myriad forms.*

OCTOBER 19

Attend a Costume Party

Break free from a limited conception of how you're supposed to be by spending some time as somebody else. The power of the costume party lies in how it can distance us from the way we think we're supposed to look. We get invested in how we look in the morning, how we look for work, how we look for special occasions, and how all these compare to the way we used to look. When you go out into the world as something or somebody who isn't you at all, it breaks through those mental bonds.

If you're willing to go as someone plain or even ugly, or as someone years and years older than you are, it loosens the grip of vanity. Being an animal or an inanimate object gives your ego an evening off. If you go as a woman who is more glamorous than you see yourself, you're showing yourself that this is an option for you—an option you may choose to take only on Halloween, but one that exists nonetheless. Finally, going in costume is a way to play, let loose, and give your creativity and your mischievousness a night out.

Play dress-up!—for a party, for opening the door to the trick-or-treaters, or, if your office is open to a bit of late October frivolity, to give your coworkers a little fun. You don't have to look the same way all the time or even be the same person 365 days a year. Take advantage of the day coming up when going in costume is the thing to do.

REJUVENATE YOURSELF WITH ACTION: *'Tis the season that you may be invited to a costume party. Start thinking now about what you'll be for Halloween. If you haven't received an invitation that gives you a chance for masquerade, maybe you could host the party.*

Dry Skin Brushing

For instant invigoration, as well as smoother skin, do dry skin brushing before your shower or prior to warm oil massage. Ideally, you'll use a special dry body brush for this process (find them at pharmacies and natural food stores), but a rough towel can substitute in a pinch. Start with your feet and rub them briskly, moving upward until you've given a quick brush-massage to your entire body with the exception of your head. (Facial skin is too delicate for this kind of treatment.) You can be vigorous, almost forceful, as you brush your limbs and buttocks, always heading in the direction of your heart. Go gently when brushing your abdomen and around your breasts, using circular motions.

The ways your body benefits from investing ninety seconds in dry skin brushing include:

- Exfoliation of body skin, sending dead cells packing and revealing the softer layer of skin underneath

- Increased circulation of both blood and lymph throughout the body

- Assistance in the elimination of excess fluid that might otherwise pool in your legs and feet at the end of the day

- A surge of energy that comes from your own reserves, no caffeine required

In Europe, dry skin brushing is also prescribed as first-line defense against cellulite. You already brush your hair and brush your teeth; assist your rejuvenation by brushing your body, too. It's quick, easy, and invigorating.

REJUVENATE YOURSELF WITH ACTION: *Do dry skin brushing every morning for a week. If you like what it does for you, keep it up.*

Yoga for Youthfulness

Yoga means *union:* body with soul, thought with action, human with divine. Just because you can take it at the same gym where you could also sign up for "Butt Busting" and "Smooth Moves" does not negate the majesty of this ancient discipline. Yoga can address a variety of ills: excess weight or slack muscles, a painful back or sloppy posture, an agitated mind or a restless spirit.

When I discovered yoga at seventeen, I loved it right off. It promised strength and flexibility with a soul attached, and you didn't have to be thin or fit or even young to start it. Had I stayed with yoga as a daily practice, I'm certain I would have enjoyed greater physical health and emotional well-being in every decade, and I'd probably have fared better through menopause. Instead I would let go of yoga for years at a time and pick it up every now and again. I figured that since it had been around four thousand years, it would be there the next time it struck my fancy. It always was.

Yoga is easy enough to find these days. The trick is finding the type that appeals to you. When I started, classic *hatha yoga* was all there was. It's slow and focused, an internal practice done with closed eyes in a darkened room. It still seems like "real" yoga to me, but now there are infinite variations, one of which may be more attractive to you. If you're in an area where a variety of classes are offered, try several, or at least observe them, and select the one that speaks to you. Start with one class a week and commit to practicing at home once a week as well. Read a book about yoga to give you some background and allow its precepts to mingle with the wisdom you already have.

Yoga has become sufficiently mainstream that it is subject to the flipside of popularity: becoming passé. When that happens, stay with it anyway. Nothing has more time on its youth-promoting side than this very first body/mind/spirit discipline. Yoga will always be transformational, even when it stops being cool.

REJUVENATE YOURSELF WITH ACTION: *Whether you're a current or former yoga student, or if you've not looked into it before, read*

something about yoga this week. Books I recommend include Yoga
Mind and Body *from the Sivananda Yoga Center;* Yoganetics *by
Wyatt Townley; and Jess Stern's* Yoga, Youth & Reincarnation,
originally published in the 1960s but still a worthwhile read.

OCTOBER 22

Mystics Grow Wise While Others Grow Old

Of all states of human consciousness, the one most fascinating to
me is the mystical experience. It has many names: beatific vision,
cosmic consciousness, *samadhi*. By whatever name, it is a state of
being in which separation ceases to exist and the person understands, in a way beyond intellect or explanation, that he or she is
one with all that is or ever will be. And all that is or ever will be is
good in a way beyond what we ordinarily know as good. And all
that is or ever will be is woven from a love beyond comprehension.

I have never had this experience in the fullness described here,
but I have spoken with people who have and I've read of many others. These people are given two lives in one body: the limited life
they had before their experience, and an enhanced life after it in
which they're less subject to forces we think of as immutable. Some
maintain a surprisingly youthful appearance, even into old age.
Others are indefatigable in their work or their mission, or they
overcome diseases, or they simply have an aura about them that
makes other people feel calm and safe.

A bona fide mystical experience is the spiritual equivalent of
winning the lottery; it doesn't happen often. Still, just as we've all
had strokes of good luck—I mean, I won a portable TV once—
we've all had brushes with the divine, times in nature or meditation, or with a child or a lover, when earth logic gave way to something else, if only for an instant. These encounters exist outside
space and time, and they are the most revivifying experiences we'll
ever get. Remarkably, remembering them is rejuvenating as well.
Simply recalling that you ever existed outside the ordinary is, to my
mind, as good as an injection of whatever the anti-aging doctors are
shooting into people this week—and safe and affordable, yours for
the cost of a thought.

OCTOBER 23

Zinc

Another youth-promoting nutrient, zinc is found in almost every cell of your body. It is involved in metabolizing both carbohydrates and vitamins, and helps with insulin synthesis and maintenance of bone density. An adequate intake of zinc promotes mental alertness, keeps your sense of taste acute, and may decrease cholesterol deposits. Its most exciting quality, however, is its ability to revitalize the thymus gland, essential for immune functioning.

With all that zinc has going for it, it is unfortunate that half of people over fifty-five are zinc-deficient, and conditions we often write off to age—hair loss, slow wound healing, reduced night vision—can be a direct result of too little zinc. Its absorption wanes as we mature, and all that healthy fiber we're eating further blocks absorption. The richest dietary source of zinc is oysters. It is also found in other seafood and in meat, nuts, and seeds, especially pumpkin seeds. Unless you're a big fan of oysters, though, a supplement of 15 to 30 milligrams a day is recommended.

REJUVENATE YOURSELF WITH ACTION: *Consider a zinc supplement. (Your multi may provide enough; check the label.) Also, keep some zinc lozenges on hand as we enter the cold and flu season. They've been proven to decrease a cold's duration. Whether you're popping a tablet or sucking a lozenge, always have a little food in your stomach when you take supplemental zinc. Otherwise you could experience some nausea.*

Have Your Picture Taken

"Oh, don't take my picture!"—the lament of a woman who fears documentation of the way she looks today. Certainly you don't have to be fodder for every eager amateur with a camera, but it's good to get your picture taken. It tells the world that you're happy with yourself, that you belong in the album every bit as much as the pets and the babies.

There are things you can do to look more attractive in a photo: clearly defining your lips with lipstick, wearing more eye makeup than usual and a bit more blush, and having a light matte finish of loose powder on your face. If you know you have a "good side," turn slightly so that's the side that's emphasized. If your jawline is crêpey, lift your face just a little as you look into the camera, or go for one of those fist-beneath-the-chin shots.

More important than cosmetic tricks, though, are mental ones that can turn you and the camera into best buds. Whether you're sitting for a formal photograph or your brother-in-law just shouts "Say cheese!" at a family gathering, stare down the camera like a supermodel. Look right at the lens and silently say to it (and yourself), "I am uniquely beautiful and always photogenic." You don't have to believe it at first; just think it. I swear to you, after awhile you will start looking better in pictures.

And when you see a photo of yourself, refrain from criticisms. Just say, "Nice picture," and get on with things. Don't be shy about having some photographs of yourself around either. It's not vain: if you have pictures of other people in your life displayed for all to see, you should be there, too. And if you need photos in your work— maybe you're a Realtor and use a photo on your business cards, or you're an author and use a photo on your book jackets—keep them up to date. After five years, retire the picture. When you meet someone who's seen your picture before seeing your face, you don't want to be compared to the way you looked in your high school yearbook.

REVITALIZE YOUR LIFE WITH WORDS: *I am uniquely beautiful and always photogenic.*

The Bath as Therapy

Bathing is classic therapy:

- *If you've had a rough day,* "Take a hot bath and forget it."

- *If you overworked at the gym,* "Take a hot bath; you'll feel better."

- *If you're feeling agitated and keyed up,* "Take a hot bath: you'll sleep like a baby."

The components of therapeutic bathing are scrubbing and soaking. Scrubbing with a wet, soapy loofah, a washcloth, or a powdered scrub invigorates, removes dead cells, brings blood to the surface, warms your body, and imparts a rosy glow. In cultures where the use of scrubs is common, women are less plagued by cellulite.

Whereas scrubbing stimulates, soaking soothes. It allows your skin to benefit from whatever you've added to your bath, while convincing your tight shoulders and hips and calves that letting go is both safe and plausible. You get to be, in old hippie slang, "blissed out, man," as you enter a state in which time (as it relates to aging, in any case) can stand still.

Here are some extras to make your bathing therapeutic and youth-restoring:

- *Epsom salts.* You can pour two pounds of Epsom salts into a warm-to-hot bath even when you didn't overdo on the tennis court. This creates a magnesium soak that will warm you all over, lull you to sleep, and, according to time-honored naturopathic teachings, help draw toxins you're holding inside out through your skin. Soak ten or fifteen minutes; then wrap yourself in towels (or in your terrycloth robe) and get under the covers.

- *Sea salt.* Creating a miniature ocean in your tub can relax and invigorate concurrently, and is said to help tone sagging skin. For an average tub, use four cups of coarse kosher salt, available at most supermarkets. Enhance the seaside experience by letting some nutrient-rich seaweed soak in the tub with you. Put dulse or kelp (two cups whole or one cup powdered, from a natural food store) into a cheesecloth bag or some old pantyhose fabric you've made into a pouch and secured with string or a rubber band; place it in the tub at the start of filling and let it stay there while you soak.

- *Oatmeal.* Put two cups of rolled oats in a cheesecloth or pantyhose pouch. Either affix the packet so that the water runs over it as the tub fills, or simply have it with you in the water and squeeze it every so often to infuse your bath with oatmeal's skin-soothing and skin-softening effects. You can also rub the pouch over your body as a gentle substitute for soap. Oatmeal bathing is recommended for itchy, sensitive skin and eczema.

- *Wine.* Rice wine (sake) was the geisha's secret for soft, smooth skin. The European substitution, believed to detoxify the body and rev up the circulation, is white wine. (If it comes from the sale bin, who's the wiser?) Shower off first and then soak half an hour or more in a hot bath enriched by a bottle of your chosen wine.

After any soak, apply a rich, natural lotion, concentrating on any parts of your damp self that aren't yet baby-soft. Then drink some water, don your PJs, and spend the evening in bed with a movie or a book, or give yourself an hour's refuge there before you go out on the town.

REJUVENATE YOURSELF WITH ACTION: *Tonight, or sometime this week, do a scrub-and-soak. Then schedule at least one a week for the rest of the year.*

Sunny Side Up

The research is mounting that cheerful people live longer. If for no other reason than an aversion to predeceasing the Pollyanna types, start looking on the bright side about life in general and aging in particular. A twenty-three-year-long study in Ohio determined that people who saw growing older as something positive lived a whopping seven and a half years longer than those who didn't. Statistically speaking, you can't get seven and a half extra years for any lifestyle change, so this is nothing to pooh-pooh.

The verdict is still out on whether or not optimism is inborn or can be acquired. Other than in cases of systemic depression, I have to believe that it's learnable—and that even depressives, once their biochemical imbalance is corrected, can learn it, too. I've seen too many people get over addictions that had them by the throat to believe that going from chronically hopeless to generally happy is an impossible feat. If you're not congenitally chipper, take heart: I'm not either. I was one of those teenagers who read the existentialists and thought despair was mysterious and alluring. No more. If I can't change a foul mood by force of will, I call somebody who's not afraid to say, "Snap out of it, Scrooge," or even, "You'd better read one of your own books."

Of course I despise being told to snap out of my mood, but I do know how to do it: smiling at people, making pleasant small talk, doing some little kindness, or ordering a ticket for a funny movie so I have to either go or be out ten bucks. Sometimes I force myself to play old songs like "Put on a Happy Face," "Let a Smile Be Your Umbrella," and "On the Sunny Side of the Street."

Another technique that works really well is giving the sullen situation to a Higher Power. I visualize packing the thing up like a parcel for FedEx and handing it over. Then, when the thought of it crops up during the day, I remember that I gave it away; it's not my worry any longer.

For length of days and joy of them, too, find ways to get yourself out of the depths, so when life starts to serve you the usual, it knows that your usual is sunny side up.

OCTOBER 27

Sometimes You Just Have to Walk in the Park

There will always be something to clean or file or answer or pay or decide on or worry about. Sometimes you just have to walk in the park anyway. If you wait until everything has been cleaned, filed, answered, paid, decided upon, and worried over, you may never get to the park, or it could be the dead of winter and you won't want to go.

Some people routinely walk in parks, go for bike rides, visit museums, and find time for parades and festivals and exhibitions that seem to leave town before the rest of us get around to them. If you're one of these people, you're younger than someone else your age. If not, you can become one if you're willing to learn by doing: walking in the park when you could be doing something more practical.

I was reminded of this one afternoon when I went to a dental appointment across the street from Washington Square Park in Greenwich Village, the park with the arch and the fountain they showed on the sitcom *Friends*. I had never gone there after a visit to the dentist. I am not one of those natural park-walkers and I always had something else to do, something to clean or file or answer or whatever. But this particular October day, I went. In the company of squirrels and skateboarders, toddlers and Scrabble players, students and lovers, the arch and the fountain, I walked through the park. I read a plaque about Garibaldi, bought water from a guy with a cart, and then sat on a bench and watched and listened. I felt more alive than I had in a really long time.

Sometimes, then, to remember when you're old and revel in right this minute, walk in the park—or something on that order. Do it before the winter comes. Once you get in the habit, you just might want to do it then, too.

REVITALIZE YOUR LIFE WITH WORDS: *I walk in parks. I smell flowers. I feel breezes. I am as alive as I have ever been.*

Updating Your Face

A woman's makeup often tells her age more readily than her face itself does. Trends come and go, and without being a victim of the whims of the season, you'll look younger and feel better if you change a little with them. Generally speaking, subtle colors look younger than glaring ones, and careful blending—blush to no-blush, face to neck—is imperative. Heavy makeup exaggerates the lines from which you're trying to deflect attention. For instance, while a little loose powder deftly applied can take the shine off and give a finished look, too much can settle into the creases around eyes or mouth and add half a decade.

One way to know what's current is to book an hour with a cosmetic counter's makeup artist every spring and fall. A makeup artist can match a foundation to the shade your skin is today, not what it used be, so you'll look less made up in your makeup. Although a professional is apt to use a wider variety of products on you than you would ordinarily wear (or care to purchase), this will at least give you an idea of whether the look of the moment focuses more on eyes or lips, if colors are bright or muted, or if a matte finish or a bit of gloss keynotes fashionable faces right now. Paying attention to the pro's application techniques can also be helpful since, as a rule, updating takes a light hand and the right tools. It's easier to learn to wield sponges and brushes after you've seen it done.

The person who does your face might suggest that you buy everything she used on you, and of course you're supposed to buy *some* things: there's no free lunch and no free makeover. Don't feel that you have to say yes to everything, though. Even purchasing a few new items—one eye shadow, one blush, one lipstick—can fast-forward your face to day after tomorrow.

REJUVENATE YOURSELF WITH ACTION: *Unless you've found your true self in the makeup-free life, make an appointment at your favorite cosmetic shop or counter and let a professional do wonders with your skin and eyes and bone structure.*

The Most Important To-Do List of Your Life

This morning you probably wrote in your planner or keyed into your Pilot, "Pick up dry-cleaning. Drop off jumble sale donations. Make chiropractic appointment. Meet with clients at 11, 2, and 4." If such details deserve a list, why not the yearnings of your deepest self? This is the list of what you wish to accomplish, see, and experience before you die.

Everybody says, "I wish I could . . ." and "It sure would be nice if . . ." but most dreams don't come true because they're only dreams, not intentions. When you write them down, they take on shape and substance. The act of writing them gives them reality in your own mind and in the energy field around you that acts as the bridge between what could be and what actually manifests. When you make the most important to-do list of your life, you're making an appointment with destiny.

I suggest that you write down every dream, every goal, and every simple curiosity you can come up with. One hundred is a reasonable number. That might sound like a lot, but only a few will be major endeavors ("Get PhD"); most won't be nearly that labor-intensive, and you have the rest of your life to check them off: "Wear hats more often." "Buy a juicer." "See Ireland." "Get the violin out of the attic." "Find Judy Casey from seventh grade." Reinforce all this in your mind by reading what you've written once a month and crossing off accomplishments as you make them. You're also free to add to your list at will and delete any items that cease to be of interest. Just be sure that if you cross something off it's because you genuinely don't want to do it anymore, not because it seemed too daunting and you got scared.

My daughter made a list like this when she was seven. It had extraordinary entries: "Go to Paris. Go to China. Learn scuba-diving. Be in a movie." These seemed outrageous at the time because the two of us (and three cats) comprised a single-parent family, living simply in a cabin in the Missouri Ozarks and sharing one closet. That didn't seem to matter to the universe. By the time this child was twelve, she had gone to Paris on the frequent-flyer miles she'd earned going to China twice. She had taken diving lessons in Hawaii and appeared in her first independent film. (You didn't see it and for that you're better off, but it did count.) There is no denying that we will run into more internal opposition with this than a seven-year-old: we've had more disappointments. Even so, the same mechanism operates throughout our lives. When we can see what we want, we gravitate toward what we see.

REJUVENATE YOURSELF WITH ACTION: *On a fresh page in your journal, write the most important to-do list of your life. Add to it at will and check off accomplishments with considerable fanfare. On the first day of every month, read your list.*

OCTOBER 30

Play Day!

OCTOBER 31

Getting Mortality Out of the Way

For most of us, October 31 means Halloween. In Mexico, however, this is the first of a three-day observance, *Día de los Muertos*, Day of the Dead. It is a celebration of those who have gone before and a fitting time for us to get mortality out of the way. Make no mistake: we dread aging because we fear death—not necessarily the "we" that's you and me, but the "we" that's humanity and that we're part of.

It is an error of our linear thinking, however, that we so readily link death to old age. None of us knows how long we've got. Linear thinking sees conception, birth, growth, maturity, decline, death. Cosmic thinking sees no such straight line. When you're talking birth and death and life and wonder, you're into circles and spirals and arcs and coils. Joel Goldsmith wrote a powerful book on metaphysics called *A Parenthesis in Eternity*. That is my favorite title of any book, because it defines life on earth in a pithy, perfect phrase.

When you see that the life you're living as a woman of a certain nationality and at a certain time is simply a parenthesis in eternity, you gain much more acceptance around mortality. Even so, *you*, the whole of you, are not a parenthetical expression. You're the entire book or thesis or twenty-four-volume set.

Your astonishing—and, I believe, immortal—soul has deigned to occupy your astonishing, albeit mortal, body. You've heard of guilt by association? This is grace by association. The very fact that your body is housing your soul makes it a place worthy of great respect and tender care. The reality that your soul will move on one day does not negate the sanctity of your body-soul unit today.

It stands to reason that anyone who learns to live well will die well. The skills are the same: being present in the moment, and humble, and brave, and keeping a sense of humor. A Buddhist nun once told me that, just as falling asleep happy and at peace means that you'll likely wake up in that pleasant state, dying happy and at peace means waking up that way on the other side of life.

I had a tutor for dying, and he was a cat. Albert was old—twenty-one, we figured—and thin but not apparently unwell. He seemed excited the day Gail Grasso, a producer from *The Oprah Winfrey Show*, arrived with a camera crew to film a segment at our house in Kansas City. I didn't think he would get to be on television—he was old and skinny after all—but when Gail looked at him through the lens, she said, "Albert looks great on camera." (It must be true about the camera's adding pounds.)

Albert got to be on the program, a spry, sprightly cat showing his lovely yellow, short-haired self to the world on TV. The next day, however, he wasn't able to jump up on the furniture anymore, so we made him a bed on the floor. A few days after that, he stopped eating. The vet suggested we encourage him with whole cream and shredded cheese, but nothing appealed. It wasn't long before he wasn't drinking either. I tried giving him water with an eyedropper, but he turned his head. The following morning I sat on the floor and held him. He purred just a little. Adair held him next. And then he died, with the elegance and dignity of a being who had lived both long and well. My prayer is that when my time comes, I'll be even half as poised in the face of it as Albert.

It's all circles. There was a kitten who became a cat. He grew old, got his fifteen seconds of fame (cats aren't greedy that way), and taught me how to die. Now I'm telling you, and if it helps, Albert gets a little immortality right here on earth.

Today and every day, then, live bountifully and take it all in. Of course tend to your will and a living will and the other necessary paperwork that keeps your lawyer in billable hours. Beyond all that, though, see that you love lots of people and things, give lots of money and time, learn all you can, and create colorful memories. Be good to your body and your family and friends and this planet that has graciously agreed to be your foster mom while you're here. And rest in the assurance that this four-score-and-whatever is no more the sum of your life as a whole than that spring break in Fort Lauderdale was the sum of your life this time around. There is more to you than you're able to know, and more to this process than any of us is equipped to imagine.

REVITALIZE YOUR LIFE WITH WORDS: *I live fully, knowing my life is part of a grand design.*

November

Connection

The Best-Kept Secret

The best-kept secret about life on earth, if you'll allow me an opinion on something so lofty, is how connected we are and how connected everything is: you and I and everybody else and all life and nature. This is the message of the mystics and the quantum physicists. Within it lies the implication that everything we do affects the whole. This gives us great responsibility but also great protection, knowing that we are each a part of something splendid.

In suggesting that you keep connections and connectedness in mind this month, I'm hoping you'll forge stronger bonds with your family, your friends, and strangers, animals and plants, art and beauty, every part of yourself and everything that's around you. In doing so, you'll feel stronger and more sure of yourself. The outward signs of aging won't be cause for regret—they'll seem minuscule compared to all you are and all that you're a part of.

This month, a few times or several, whenever it comes into your consciousness, remember that you are a unique individual, yes, but also one unique aspect of a glorious whole. Because understanding is a mental activity and nobody's brain is big enough to understand something this "cosmic," don't even try to understand it. Just accept it and let that acceptance enhance your life.

REVITALIZE YOUR LIFE WITH WORDS: *I am connected to all that is.*

Recall the High Times

There is a certain wealth inherent in simply having been here awhile. Part of that wealth is the many memories we have of the high times—ah-ha moments, memorable hours with marvelous people, and various triumphs of the recent and distant past.

Bringing these to mind can do wonders for any day that doesn't seem particularly triumphant. You have to do this right, though. Conjure up glory days to remind yourself of who you are, then and now, a person capable of doing something great or experiencing something fabulous. Avoid any temptation to look longingly back on past successes and use them as weapons to turn on yourself: "I was really something then. Not anymore." Instead, use recollections of the high times as evidence of how amazing you are. You are the same person. The same spunk and spirit that created earlier distinctions are in you today, with wisdom and experience added.

A high point of my youth was going to my first Beatles press conference at fourteen. I had the proper credentials—a letter from the editor of *Teen Life* magazine and a press pass—but because of my age, the guards wouldn't let me on the elevator. Then I saw Charles Finley, owner of the (then) Kansas City Athletics baseball team and the man who had brought the Beatles to town. "Mr. Finley," I said, "here's my documentation: I need to be at that press conference." For a moment, he looked quizzically at me, an overweight high school freshman with an acne problem and an unfortunate haircut. "All right," he said. "You can come with me." In a minute's time, I was eight feet from the Fab Four, pen and notebook poised.

Not long ago, channel-surfing in the big numbers, I chanced on a sports program talking about the late Mr. Finley. "He could look in your soul," a former Oakland Athletics team member was saying, "and see that you were a winner." Tears came to my eyes and I thought, "Maybe that's what he saw in me, and if he did, that winning inner self hasn't gone anywhere; it's still at the heart of me." I was able to take a triumphal moment from long ago and use it to spur me on today.

In this way, past successes cease being historic relics and become instead evidence of your present worth. If you were a competitive athlete, you still have that will and that discipline. If you were an honor student, you still have that intelligence and that focus. If you were voted most likely to succeed, you still can. You're on the same road, even if it's had some detours.

REVITALIZE YOUR LIFE WITH WORDS: *I remember the high times and I look forward to many more.*

You Can't Open the Gifts of Maturity Until You Realize There Are Some

Life *can* just keep getting better, and today we'll turn our focus to the privileges of living now and getting an extended prime. Haul out your trusty journal: you're going to be writing about your understanding of the gifts of maturity. You can simply make a list of them:

- Grandchildren

- More confidence

- Getting to talk to younger men without looking like I'm hitting on them

and so forth. Whatever you write gets an automatic A. What is one bona fide, dyed-in-the-wool, first-class perk of being the age you are? And another? And another? Write all you can think of. Write, too, some blessings of being older than you are now, those to which you get to look forward.

Ironically, the gifts of maturity seem disproportionately distributed among those mature people who are young for their age, those who stay fit and energetic. That doesn't matter, because either you are one of those people or you're becoming one of them. Write about the gifts—those you're experiencing, those you see others experiencing, and those that will come to you later.

There. That's better.

REJUVENATE YOURSELF WITH ACTION: *Write your gifts list.*

Don't Fall

If you came of age after *Fear of Flying*, you've probably never thought about fear of falling. For women over seventy, however, studies claim that taking a fall is a major fear. We can prevent the fear, and many of the falls, by starting now to make prevention second nature.

- *Lift weights.* Weight training works on the same muscle fibers that kick in to help you right yourself if you start to fall. Stay strong, stay upright.

- *Take up tai chi.* Slow and dancelike, this graceful movement series from Chinese martial arts is a study in balance for the body and mind.

- *Do other balancing exercises.* Yoga has some great ones, or you can simply stand on one leg while you're cooking or waiting in a queue or talking on the phone. The advanced version: standing on one leg with your eyes closed (obviously, not while cooking).

- *Be a kid again.* Have fun improving your balance by walking a line or a curb, with or without pretending you're on a balance beam.

- *Do the obvious.* Hold the handrail, keep your hands out of your pockets (arms are balancers and can catch you if you trip), and pay genuine attention when there's a wet floor or icy pavement.

- *Watch out for dangerous clothing.* No kidding: a long skirt that clings needs either a slip or a pink slip. Pants with legs so wide you could trip over them have to go. Ditto for scary shoes, or even sensible ones with dangling laces.

- *Have a fall-proof environment.* Do away with cords to trip on, throw rugs that could throw you, or clutter someone could fall over.

- *Go for snow boots with major tread.* The waffling on the soles of most boots is little more than decoration. For walking on icy days, get boots that are the footwear equivalent of snow tires. If you don't find them in the shoe department, go to a camping/hiking store.

- *Take care of your skeleton* (May 4 and 5). That way if you do take a tumble, you'll come through without a break.

All this said, I wouldn't want to tell any person of any age to give up what she loves, including activities like skiing or skating that could lead to a fall. If I have to fall when I'm an old woman, I'd rather do it in my ice skates than in my orthopedic oxfords.

REVITALIZE YOUR LIFE WITH WORDS: *I walk safely today and every day of my life.*

NOVEMBER 5

Demystifying Yellow and Green

Even in grade school health class, a lot was made of "yellow and orange vegetables and dark, leafy greens" (not that I ate them much: this was the era of bologna sandwiches and creme-filled cupcakes). Green and yellow vegetables, many in season right now, are nutritional powerhouses, yet, for many people, they're culinary mysteries. The first time I cooked kale, I steamed it like spinach, stems and all, and it was virtually inedible. I knew how to cook yellow vegetables—"cut in half, remove seeds if there are seeds, and bake" is pretty much it—but my husband and daughter formed a coalition of the squash-challenged and refused to try them. If you face similar hurdles, here are a couple of foolproof, family-pleasing recipes to get you started. These were created by the eternally youthful Jennifer Raymond and found in her cookbook, *The Peaceful Palate:*

Collards and Kale

1 bunch collard greens or kale (6 to 8 cups chopped)
$^1/_2$ cup water
2 teaspoons soy sauce
2–3 garlic cloves, minced

Wash the greens, remove the stems, and chop the leaves into $^1/_2$ -inch-wide strips. Heat the water and soy sauce in a large pot or skillet. Add the garlic and cook it 1 to 2 minutes. Add the chopped greens and toss to mix. Cover and cook over medium heat until tender, about 5 minutes. Serves 2 to 4. A one-cup serving has 61 calories, 3 grams of protein, 11 grams carbohydrate, and no fat.

Yams with Cranberries and Apples

3 yams, peeled
1 large, tart green apple, peeled and diced
1 tablespoon lemon juice
$^1/_2$ cup raw cranberries or $^1/_3$ cup dried cranberries
$^1/_4$ cup raisins
$^1/_4$ cup orange juice concentrate
2 tablespoons maple syrup
1 tablespoon soy sauce

Preheat the oven to 350 degrees F. Cut the yams into 1-inch chunks and spread in a large baking dish. Toss the apple and the lemon juice and add to the yams. Sprinkle with cranberries and raisins. Mix the orange juice concentrate, maple syrup, and soy sauce with $^1/_4$ cup water. Pour over the top. Cover and bake until the yams are tender when pierced with a fork, about 1 hour. Serves 8 (138 calories, 2 grams protein, 32 grams carbohydrate, and zero fat per serving).

REJUVENATE YOURSELF WITH ACTION: *Try one of these recipes, or your own favorite recipe, for greens or a dark yellow vegetable tonight. If there is an Ethiopian restaurant near you, order gomen, collard greens spiced so exquisitely you might want them every week from now on.*

The Great Water Wars

If you read too much about the right kind of water to drink, you're apt to give up and switch to vodka. People get emotionally involved in their preference for spring water or distilled or reverse-osmosis, especially if they're selling spring water or distillers or reverse-osmosis units.

The sane stance as I see it is this: If you're reading this book, you most likely live in a part of the world that has safe drinking water right from the tap. By *safe*, I mean it doesn't contain bacteria that will make you sick. It has, however, been treated with chemicals, primarily chlorine, and has perhaps been enriched with fluoride. It is part of prudence, since you're looking to grow younger, to avoid these when you can. Chlorine kills the bacteria that cause diseases like cholera and typhoid, so it is vital to public health. Once it's done its job, however, we're better off filtering out this chemical suspected of causing cancer and birth defects. Fluoride, although its judicious use may well play a role in dentistry, is the only chemical added to public water supplies not to make the water safe to drink, but to medicate people. I prefer to drink water that does not contain an additive that has been linked to Alzheimer's disease, brittle bones and bone cancer, and kidney and neurological impairment.

Take your water purity as far as you wish. Water filters, either inexpensive pitchers with changeable filters or a filtration system you can simply attach to your faucet, are an easy alternative to drinking water straight from the tap. Or you can order bottled water, spring or distilled, delivered to your home. There are exposés every so often about bottled water being untreated tap water, but this is a rare occurrence. For one thing, you can often taste or smell chlorine; it's not the easiest thing to hide. And these businesses have their reputations to protect. An unscrupulous bottled water company gets the same media treatments as a crooked cop: the headlines focus there instead of on the overwhelming majority of ethical bottlers and devoted police officers.

You can also buy a reverse-osmosis or steam-distillation unit. Reverse osmosis removes virtually everything you don't want;

distillation distills out absolutely everything but the bare-bones H_2O. This is where opinions become heated. Some people say that drinking distilled water, because it is devoid of minerals, leeches minerals from the bones. This is not scientifically validated. There are also those who believe that distilled water is the only choice, that the minerals in spring water are inorganic and therefore unusable by the body. Again, there isn't solid science to back up this contention.

My personal bias, loosely held, is for spring water. It tastes good to me and I feel an affinity for it. That's what I buy when I'm paying for water. In my tiny New York kitchen, I simply filter water at the faucet. It seems to me that anything better than tap water is, well, better than tap water. And tap water is better than no water.

REVITALIZE YOUR LIFE WITH WORDS: *I drink good water, eat good food, and breathe good air. I love taking care of myself.*

NOVEMBER 7

Polish Your Character

Character is another word for integrity, wholeness. It's doing what you say you'll do and being the same person in company as you are when you don't think anyone is looking. With character, you live in a way you're proud of in good times and bad. When you're a person of character, an archaic-sounding phrase like, "I give you my word," doesn't sound outdated when it comes out of your mouth. It sounds true.

Developing character is easier if you had high-character role models in childhood, but you can acquire it even if you didn't. Furthermore, past transgressions are irrelevant. I don't know any flesh-and-blood person who hasn't accrued some tarnish over the years. We're talking about polishing character today and making it a present priority. Furthermore, this is a personal test and not about becoming the referee charged with evaluating other people's behavior. Judging is an unbecoming trait that invites judgment back.

Begin this venture by seeing yourself as a person of high character. Find little ways to build more of it, like giving back the extra change you might get from a clerk, or reminding the waiter if he left the appetizer off the check. Observe and admire evidence of high character in people you know and those you read about. Yours is being observed and admired as well.

REJUVENATE YOURSELF WITH ACTION: *Imagine if you can a world in which character is revered as much as beauty and money and fame are now. Picture the magazine leads: "World's Most Generous Woman," "Kindest Man Alive," "Lose Ten Ugly Character Traits in Just Ten Days!" Pretend that you live in a world like that.*

NOVEMBER 8

I Can See Clearly Now

Our eyes weren't made to look at a computer screen all day and "relax" by looking at a TV screen at night. They want to look out to the horizon and up to the heavens, down and around and to the full periphery left and right. At the very least, eyes need a change of venue at least every hour or so—looking up from the computer and out the window to the farthest point they can see. They'd appreciate getting to look around in great big circles, first to the left, then to the right. And they love "palming"—a simple yogic practice that rests and refreshes tired eyes. To do it, rub the palms of your hands together briskly until they feel hot (the yogis say you're building up pranic energy this way). Then cup your hands over your closed eyes and let them rest in the warmth and darkness until the heat dissipates.

Eye exercises like these (you can find a whole list of eye exercises at www.visionworksusa.com) help with eyestrain and may improve vision. They can even slow, although they're not likely to stop, presbyopia, farsightedness. This loss of flexibility in the lens of the eye is the first sign of aging many people notice when, sometime in their forties, they find themselves holding a postcard or restaurant check at arm's length. That can be a defining moment.

If you're dealing with this very, very common condition, your options to date are reading glasses, bifocals, or "monovision," making one eye nearsighted with a contact lens so that your two eyes act as bifocals. This is a godsend for many people, although some specialists, including Marc Grossman, OD, author of *Natural Eye Care: An Encyclopedia,* have found that monovision can affect depth perception and cause secondary neck and shoulder pain as the person tilts her head slightly to accommodate the eye with near vision. Dr. Grossman likes the option of reading glasses, especially these days when so much of what we read is ahead of us on a screen rather than beneath us in print, as it was when Benjamin Franklin invented the bifocal. Still, bifocals work for many people, especially the progressive no-line models that look like ordinary glasses.

Dry eyes are another problem that can exacerbate at midlife, especially during menopause. Drug therapy is available, and high-quality eyedrops can certainly help. One study showed that 50 milligrams daily of vitamin B_6 (pyridoxine), 1500 milligrams of vitamin C, and 1500 milligrams of omega-3 fatty acids provided substantial relief for this condition.

There is also documentation supporting nutritional therapy in the prevention of vision-threatening eye problems later in life—macular degeneration, glaucoma, and cataracts. Omega-3 fatty acids are important in warding off all three. Both vitamin C and the antioxidant alpha-lipoic acid can play a role in the prevention of cataracts and glaucoma. Beta-carotene may help forestall cataracts and macular degeneration; and as little as 6 milligrams daily of the phytochemical lutein has been shown to reduce macular degeneration risk by 43 percent. Kale is the best food source of lutein, or you can take it in a gelcap before bed (away from your multivitamin since lutein and beta-carotene compete for absorption).

REVITALIZE YOUR LIFE WITH WORDS: *I see the world around me with appreciation and awe.*

NOVEMBER 9

It's Four O'Clock: Do You Know Where Your Good Intentions Are?

I want you to pay attention to what's going on with you today around three-thirty or four o'clock. For many people, this is the time of day when good intentions go south. While morning people feel great at six A.M. and night people get a second wind after dinner, I've never heard of anyone struck with an energy surge at four in the afternoon. See how you fare in this pre-twilight zone by looking in the mirror. If you wear makeup, chances are your lipstick is gone and your nose is shiny. Your hair may need some help. Going inward, how are you feeling? Do you have a hankering for coffee or candy? Or maybe you already had some? It's common to crave a pick-me-up at this time of day. And retreating further inward still, what is the status of this morning's good intentions?

Since more people disappoint themselves between three and five than any other time of day, tag this as a check-in time for yourself. Take your break for it on the job, or give yourself a break if you are self-employed. (We who are our own bosses often report to a tyrant.) Plan to refurbish your outward self a bit: comb your hair, touch up your makeup, brush your teeth, drink some water, do some stretches, or get out for a short walk and some fresh air. If you feel the need for food, have something light but satisfying. Taking my lead from Ayurveda, I believe in not eating between meals with the exception of "tea time," an exception that is especially important for someone who feels her body and spirit sink in the late afternoon.

Give yourself an emotional boost, too, a telephone check-in with someone you love, or a snippet of meditation to check in with Someone who loves you the most.

REJUVENATE YOURSELF WITH ACTION: *Resurrect three to five o'clock. Put habits into place that make this a welcome time of day.*

NOVEMBER 10

Build Your Immunity

Your immune system's forces include your skin, a barrier against microorganisms; your respiratory system, equipped to trap any microscopic enemies and push them out; and a network of "killer cells," spy-like white blood cells that can detect ailing cells and put out of their misery. Many of the suggestions you're putting into effect this year—a high-nutrient diet, food supplements, exercise, meditation and stress management, getting enough sleep, forming a network of friends, even having the right humidity level in your rooms—will help your immune system function at its best. Here are additional ways to keep your defenses up:

- *Astragalus* and *echinacea*. These are the best documented of the immune-boosting herbs. Astragalus appears to encourage the formation and activity of immune cells. Echinacea stimulates the body's manufacture of *interferon*, a protein that can destroy viruses and cancer cells. These herbs can be taken as preventatives, but they lose their effectiveness if taken all the time. Try one month on/one month off instead.

- *Acupuncture*. First used in China, acupuncture increases immunity by balancing life energy in the body. The yogi's *prana* and the acupuncturist's *ch'i* are the same energy. Before treating you, a skilled acupuncturist will take a history, examine your tongue, eyes, and nails, and do pulse diagnosis, a technique that tells the practitioner a great deal more about you than how fast your heart is beating. Acupuncture needles are very thin. Most of the time you don't feel them at all; if you do, it's slight.

- *Oscillococcinum*. If you take this homeopathic flu remedy when you get the first hint that something isn't right, you may be able to jump-start your immunity and keep yourself from getting the full-fledged flu. Find it at natural food stores and some pharmacies.

- *Optimism*. A depressed mood can lead to a depressed immune system. Studies show that when a person is depressed, those killer cells go AWOL.

- *Better living through less chemistry*. Our species has managed to ravage a planet. You don't need to be a "tree-hugger" to appreciate that we're breathing and eating toxic chemicals our cells were not designed to understand. Lessen the load as much as possible. Avoid cigarette smoke. Eat organically grown food. Use the most natural cosmetics and household cleaners you can find. Remember counting calories? Count chemicals instead. The number to strive for is zero. Of course we won't get to that, but I've always loved Browning's line, "Ah, but a man's reach should exceed his grasp, Or what's a heaven for?"

REVITALIZE YOUR LIFE WITH WORDS: *My immune system functions perfectly, and I help it every way I can.*

NOVEMBER 11

Put Yourself in the Aura of Greatness

When you have the chance to hear music played by a master, see theater performed by actors expert at their craft, or attend a lecture by a leader who might be the next Mahatma Gandhi or Martin Luther King Jr., be there. Sit in the front if you can, but even in the top row of the third balcony, you'll be in the aura of greatness. Your life will upgrade a notch every time you do this. Because we live in a period of celebrity madness, it's easy to mistake fame for greatness. They're not the same, even though one individual may have both. The point is to be in the presence of someone whose life is making a tangible difference in the world, whether this results in fame or not.

I once mentioned to Ellen, the woman who walks my dog four days a week and is my friend all seven, that I admired UN Secretary General Kofi Annan. "Oh, he greets Aspen and me lots of mornings when we walk." I was aghast. "You mean my dog knows Kofi Annan?" "Oh, yes," she assured me, confirming that there is just one degree of canine separation between a man who could be instrumental in bringing about peace on earth, and me, a woman who wants peace on earth but can't do much more than vote and write letters and send a check every once in awhile. Even this once-removed connection to the aura of greatness reminded me to redouble my own efforts and deepen my own commitment.

When you put yourself in the aura of greatness, whether it has to do with art or scholarship or humanitarianism, let it endow your life with the makings of greatness, too. You have already done some remarkable things, and you have the potential for doing many more of them. Being in the presence of great people and great works fuels that potential.

REJUVENATE YOURSELF WITH ACTION: *Write in your journal about what greatness means to you and what it would take for you to put yourself in the aura of greatness more often than you have in the past.*

NOVEMBER 12

Organic Essentials

I used to think in terms of "organic food" and "regular food." Then it hit me that organic is regular; the other stuff is irregular. Until World War II, growing food was not a chemically enhanced process. The baby-boomer generation is the first to have consumed pesticides and herbicides, antibiotics and hormones, from the cradle to the present. Amazingly, we're still here for the Orwellian follow-up chapters, food irradiation and genetic engineering.

There is substantial evidence that an organically grown tomato or carrot or stalk of wheat is more nutritious than its conventionally grown counterpart. In addition, conventional produce often contains residues of numerous chemical compounds, including known carcinogens. Although washing fruits and vegetables is a given, a goodly portion of the residues are in the food itself and can't be washed away. Pesticides also concentrate in animal tissues, so there are proportionally more of them in meat and dairy products than in fruits and vegetables.

In the most basic terms, our physiology recognizes only two substances: food (that is, something beneficial and useful) and toxins (substances that are harmful and need to be excreted by the liver, kidneys, intestines, lungs, and skin). Having to get rid of these poisons stresses the body, and stress promotes aging.

There is also a prescient metaphor here: organic farmers take loving care of the soil, and we want to take loving care of our bodies. Each complements the other. Furthermore, organic agriculture helps ensure the land's ability to produce food in the future. When you choose organic, you're contributing to a legacy even if it looks as if you're only buying milk and apples and grapes and celery. That's important enough to take an interest in, both as a consumer and as a citizen. Organic labeling laws need to demand clarity and honesty and never bend toward the interests of big business that can conceal the big picture.

If you can choose organic for only part of your grocery list, try to make it:

- *Meat and dairy products:* danger of pesticide concentration and residues of antibiotics and hormones given to the animals

- *Soy products, corn, and canola oil:* likely to be genetically modified

- *Rice and oats:* subject to pesticides and fungicides that are sprayed on crops and absorbed from groundwater

- *Strawberries, grapes, peaches, and apples:* highly sprayed and/or commonly subject to one or more of the more questionable pesticides

In one way, this is the advanced class in quality eating. That is, you need to eat an abundance of fruits and vegetables, even if you can't get or can't afford organic ones all the time. Wash non-organic produce especially well, using a little dish soap and a lot of running water. Whenever possible, choose organic. It is a further investment in your well-being. It's also a statement about what you think you're worth.

REJUVENATE YOURSELF WITH ACTION: *The next time you go shopping, think about the relationship between your food and your body, yourself and the earth, your life and other lives.*

NOVEMBER 13

Let Compliments Register

There are a few people who are so lavish with compliments that they cease to mean much. A smattering of folks, usually those who are after something, give compliments that are outright lies. Neither of these groups is large, though, and you can see through members of either one. The majority of compliments are sincere and they have their basis in fact. They're given to make you feel good and help you recognize that something about your work or your character or your appearance has made a positive impression. Put compliments like these in your mental filing cabinet under "self-image, elevated."

Give honest compliments as well. Not long ago I noticed a woman waiting for a cab on a New York street corner. Maybe she was in her sixties, or perhaps her seventies and very well preserved. Anyway, her look was striking. Her clothes were up-to-date but so cunningly coordinated that she reminded me of a fashion plate from a more elegant era. I couldn't help myself: "Excuse me, but I have to tell you: you look fabulous. So few people really dress anymore." She smiled like the sun coming out and said, "You can't imagine how your saying that has made my day."

And you know what? We can't always imagine what a kind word might mean to another person. That's reason enough not to keep it to ourselves and, when we're on the receiving end, to take it in and let it register.

REVITALIZE YOUR LIFE WITH WORDS: *I am comfortable giving and receiving honest compliments. The ones meant for me I accept with gratitude.*

NOVEMBER 14

Get to Know Your Mother

Somehow, some way, get to know your mother. If she is alive and you can see her and talk with her, do it more than you have been. She has more to teach you now than anytime since you were a little girl. You sometimes hear the phrase, "No one will ever love you like your mother." It's true to a great extent. And since you'll always be her baby, spending time with her is one way to feel young.

If your mother has passed away, learn more about her from her letters or her diaries or from conversations with her sisters, her friends, or your father. Find ways to do this if your mother was with you well into your adulthood, or if she died when you were young—even if you never knew her. If you had two mothers—biological and adopted, perhaps—or if you knew your mother but were largely raised by *her* mother, you can choose to do this exercise on either or both of them.

In addition, get to know your mother in the context of her generation. Depending on your age and hers, your mother might have roared through the 1920s and struggled through the 1930s. She might have worked for the war effort in the '40s, only to be told to retire to her kitchen in the '50s. She could have marched for civil rights or the ERA, and even if she didn't, enough of her peers did that these events affected her, shaped her. She is part of an era, a time you can learn about but never truly fathom.

Getting to know your mother better is a way to get to know yourself better, too. She pioneered and patterned life for you. Even if you opted to take a very different path, she showed you one way and you made your choice from there.

REJUVENATE YOURSELF WITH ACTION: *Take some time today, or as soon as you can, to get to know your mother (or your "other mother") better. See yourself at the end of this process saying, "Oh—now I understand."*

NOVEMBER 15

Play Day!

NOVEMBER 16

Stay Close to a Higher Power

The philosophical framework around which you've built your worldview is personal and sacrosanct. It helps make you who you are. Longevity studies support the contention that people who make it through life with the most vitality and optimism tend to be those whose belief systems include a Power greater than themselves. Whether this concept comes from traditional religion or some sensibility unique to the individual, having it to depend on apparently lifts some of life's burden and leaves a lightness in its place, a lightness you can feel and others can see.

Just believing in God, or whatever term you use for a Power greater than yourself, is, however, different from staying close to that Power. It's like working on your laptop, believing you're plugged into a power source that won't let you down, and learning only when the warning comes on the screen that you've been using your finite battery instead.

If you have no concept of a Higher Power, don't force it; but don't force it away either. Look closely at life to see how the work of some invisible hand might reveal itself. Starry nights, sunny mornings, and children's faces can be pretty good at this. If you believe in God—according to statistics, most people do—strive to go from believing to getting close. Cultivate the relationship every day so that on the days you need it most, you'll know where to find it. Bring your Higher Power into the nuts and bolts of your day with a silent thank-you or a quiet acknowledgment that you are not, and you will never be, alone.

For support and community, seek out people who share your beliefs, people whose language in the realm of the sacred is the same as yours. Pray for people you know and those you hear about, world leaders and the world itself, the things that worry you and the things you want. Say grace at meals, or say nothing at all and make the connection within yourself. We weren't put here to sink or swim on our own. We were put here so that, with a little help from a Higher Power, we could fly.

REVITALIZE YOUR LIFE WITH WORDS: *I am not, and I will never be, alone.*

NOVEMBER 17

Elevate Your EQ

Your EQ, in today's context, is your Elegance Quotient. It becomes more valuable as time passes, because elegance is age-proof. True elegance has to do with presenting yourself in a way that allows your essence to shine through. This means knowing enough of the social graces to put others at ease instead of putting them off, dressing so that people remember what you said more readily than what you wore, and outfitting the places you live and work with the necessary, the beautiful, and not one thing more.

Elegance is inherent in choosing what is real and proven over what is tentative and untried. It's making an impression by not making one, the way a single sunflower in a vacant lot can be more memorable than the building later erected there. It has something to do with rules—decorum, taste, the strictures that hold society together—but much more to do with self-control, not venting every opinion you've got or wearing every bauble you own.

You elevate your EQ by exploring elegance as a trait and a concept. When you see a woman on the street or in the media who strikes you as elegant, ask yourself what makes you think so. What is she saying? How is she dressed? Is there something about her you could borrow? Train your eye. A woman wearing all black can look elegant or funereal, depending upon how she does it. Observe enough and you'll discover the nuances.

The quintessence of elegance is that less is indeed more. Choosing muted colors and classic styles, and minimally gilding the lily that you are, creates an elegant impact. If your style is bold and vivacious, that can be elegant, too; it's just more easily mishandled and more obvious when it is. For most women who are no longer girls, an elegant look is characterized by clean lines and minimal distractions. Your presence has a chance to show when your persona doesn't overpower it. Then the impression you give is, "I don't need to shout to let you know I'm here."

REJUVENATE YOURSELF WITH ACTION: *How does the word "elegant" strike you? Do you think it describes you now, at least some of the time? What can you do to increase your EQ? Let the upcoming holiday season be a time to elevate your Elegance Quotient as you dress, decorate, entertain, and select gifts.*

Traditions

Traditions underscore our relationship to a greater whole. Then, instead of being isolated in time and space, on our own to figure things out, we're engaged with our clan or community, even with humanity as a whole. A tradition is something expected on a certain date or in response to a certain occurrence. One tradition might come from religious doctrine that dates back to antiquity, another from family lore that dates back to your childhood. Then again, you might stumble upon a new tradition tomorrow when some simple happening is sufficiently memorable or heartwarming or just plain fun that it's worth repeating this time next year. Once an activity achieves tradition status, it's dependable. You can count on it. In a world of diminishing dependability, this is precious indeed.

For your rejuvenating action today, I'll suggest that you get out a calendar and your journal, and make a list of the traditions you observe throughout the year. The idea is to have traditions sprinkled over all the months—no long dry spells. This could call for resurrecting a neglected tradition or inventing some new ones, making a big deal out of this year's premier snowfall, perhaps, or the first ripe tomato from next summer's garden.

The more traditions you have in place, the more colorful your calendar and the more comfortable your life.

REJUVENATE YOURSELF WITH ACTION: *Grab a calendar and your journal. Month by month, list the traditions you faithfully observe. If you see a lengthy stretch with no traditions punctuating it, think about one you might insert there. If the notion of an inserted tradition seems contrived, give yourself the suggestion that you will be watching for potential traditions and adopting a few.*

The Rest Cure

Earlier generations put much stock in resting. Sick people were known to overcome serious diseases in that pre-antibiotic era by taking "the rest cure," going off for a month or longer to the mountains or the seaside and letting the body marshal its healing forces. This is an odd idea today, when we distrust resting for an hour, let alone a month. It's tough to grow younger, however, without plenty of rest. The fact is this: you can do practically anything a twenty-year-old can do, just not as many hours of the day.

The summer after high school, I had a job proofreading credit cards for an oil company on the three-to-eleven shift. I usually worked overtime and then danced till half past four at the after-hours jazz and blues clubs that made Kansas City in those days the "Paris of the plains." Breakfast, lunch, and a nap in between were all I needed to start the cycle again. If I tried that now, I'd fall asleep on the dance floor. There is a time for testing limits and a time for listening to them. Now, in the second of these stages, the inner voice tells me, "You're welcome to go dancing, but you either have to start earlier or get some serious rest before you go." When I do, the good times still roll, and I'm able to roll with them.

You know those fairy tales about the beautiful princess who could be seen only during certain hours of the day? It's like that: you get to be beautiful as long as you disappear from time to time to restore yourself. This might mean a nap, some quiet time, a little light reading, or thirty minutes of a TV show that makes you laugh for at least fifteen of them. Anything relaxing or effortlessly recreational gives you the rest cure. Take it.

REVITALIZE YOUR LIFE WITH WORDS: *I regularly rest and restore myself.*

Adopt a Companion Animal

When I was getting physical therapy for frozen shoulder, my therapist Tony confided, "When nothing else helps the pain, pet your cat or your dog." He was echoing study after study reporting that animals help people heal, and people with animals in their families stay healthier and live longer. Some research implies that any animal counts: cat, parakeet, iguana; it's the relationship that matters. Other studies, having found the longevity connection only when the pet is a dog, make the assumption that walking a dog, rather than loving one, is the deciding factor. I disagree: lots of people hire dog-walkers, or get their child to walk Rover, or let him out to run in the fenced-in yard. I'm not a scientific researcher, but I am blessed with both a dog and a cat, and I believe they both keep me younger because they are eternally young.

Now obviously, if you don't like animals, or if you're allergic to dander, this suggestion is not for you, but if your heart, your home, and your immune system are up for a non-human adoptee, saving an animal's life may be adding years to your own. Your local pound or shelter has wonderful dogs, cats, and other noble beings who, through no fault of their own, have ended up in dire straits: five days to live unless somebody like you shows up with a stay of execution.

Think about it. Pet adoption is a commitment to be sure: dogs often live fifteen years, cats twenty. By inviting one in, you are taking on a family member, someone who will need consideration and care for years to come. What you get in return is a faithful companion, lots of laughs from animal antics, admiring looks and licks even when you're feeling far from admirable, and love that is truly "until death do you part." Decreased stress and lower blood pressure are bonuses. So is the opportunity to share fine times with someone who is effortlessly innocent, someone who will model for you how to grow older with selfless indifference and absolute grace.

REJUVENATE YOURSELF WITH ACTION: *If you don't have a companion animal and would like one (or two if you're gone all day), think about how this might work in your life. If you have pets, pay extra attention to them today. If you're in neither category, just send some unspoken goodwill to the furred and feathered of this world. All blessings sent out come back multiplied.*

Emphasize Superfoods

Superfoods are the ones on the nutritional most-likely-to-succeed list. While all natural foods have something to recommend them, these dietary overachievers consistently offer a high concentration of vitamins, antioxidants, phytochemicals, and other youth-preserving elements. For example:

- *Leafy greens* (collards, kale, romaine, mustard greens, broccoli)—vitamins A and C, calcium, iron, and fiber, along with more protein per calorie than traditional "high-protein" foods

- *Yellow veggies and fruits* (yams, winter squash, carrots, pumpkin, cantaloupe, apricots, papaya, mangoes, and persimmons)—the beta-carotene all-stars, with the humble sweet potato having been called the world's healthiest vegetable

- *Tomatoes* (also tomato juice, marinara sauce, salsa)—vitamin C, vitamin A, and the phytochemical lycopene, which may protect against heart disease and cancer

- *Berries and citrus fruits*—vitamin C, phytochemicals, and not enough calories to make a dent

- *Soybeans and other legumes*—protein the way the body wants it, fiber, and (in soy) hormone-balancing isoflavones

- *Nuts, seeds, and avocados* (in reasonable quantities)—essential fatty acids, zinc, and satiety value

Try to get one or two superfoods at every meal, or—even better—create entire meals from them. You'll make your cells so happy, they can't help but rejuvenate for you.

REVITALIZE YOUR LIFE WITH WORDS: *I eat superfoods and I enjoy super health.*

Gratefully Ever After

Gratitude is a vitalizing state of mind. When you feel it, it's like getting extra oxygen. "I am so lucky," "This is so great," and "You are so kind" are healing statements. Without them, we can overlook the gifts life bestows, either anonymously or through other people. When gratitude becomes a habit, we become acutely aware of these gifts. We start feeling grateful for one of them, and all of a sudden others show up.

Ways to feel more grateful include:

- *The gratitude list.* I didn't invent it but I wouldn't be without it, the habit of listing ten things for which I'm grateful every morning or night. There are no limits on what counts—you can be grateful for a talent you've had since birth, and you can be grateful for the weather this autumn morning. When you make an A.M. gratitude list, you enter into a day already ripe with good things. A P.M. list chalks this up as a good day after all.

- *The positive twist.* When something doesn't come to you the way you'd hoped, it's easy to be disappointed. If you can, find something for which to be grateful in the circumstance as delivered.

- *The lucky dog.* In my grade school, the kid who was chosen as team captain or got to go to Disneyland or was otherwise heir to some vast good fortune often heard, "You lucky dog!" See yourself this way. The tests came back negative. "You lucky dog!" The raise came through. "You lucky dog!" Your husband surprised you with the perfect present, and you hadn't even asked. "I am one lucky dog!" Get used to it.

REJUVENATE YOURSELF WITH ACTION: *Get into the gratitude-list habit—or get back into it, as the case may be.*

Steam Baths and Saunas

Most Y's and health clubs have steams rooms and saunas, and most members ignore them. Sweating without doing any work seems like cheating. It's not. Increasing body temperature increases circulation and detoxification. A steam room (usually 110 to 160 degrees Fahrenheit) is not as hot as a sauna (160 to 210 degrees) and is better tolerated by people who are unaccustomed to these therapies. In addition to being a relaxing experience, regular steaming helps clear the skin (especially for the acne-prone), assists the body in lightening its load of toxins, and helps keep winter colds at bay (or, if one is coming on, helps "sweat it out"). Any weight lost in a steam room is just water and will be back as soon as you take a drink, but regular use of a steam room or sauna makes you *feel* fitter and trimmer, and people do tend to act the way they feel.

To safely steam or sauna, start with five minutes—less if that feels like too much for you—and work up to fifteen, as long as you're comfortable. Come out, cool off, and go in again if you're game. Traditionally, it's suggested that you alternate your time in the heat with a cold dip or shower, and do this two or three times, with a warm shower following the final cold one. Pay attention to your own reactions: this isn't an endurance trial. If you get too hot, come out. Drink water. Bring yourself easily back to your comfort level. Never steam or sauna if you're pregnant or think you might be. Also avoid heat treatments if you have a high fever. Otherwise, anyone in good health should be able to enjoy them; check with your doctor if you're not sure.

REJUVENATE YOURSELF WITH ACTION: *If you have access to a steam bath or sauna, use it this week. Otherwise, ask around and see if you can visit a friend's gym for the experience. If you're pregnant or have any serious illnesses (e.g., severe hypertension, cancer, or recent heart attack or stroke), sit this one out. Ditto if you're experiencing hot flashes: know that the time will come when they'll be gone and you can again steam at will instead of at random.*

Generosity and Benevolence

Generosity and benevolence show up in all sorts of ways: giving presents, sharing what you have, inviting people over, taking their calls. It's caring about their well-being and wishing them the best as surely as you wish it for yourself. Somehow, giving makes sense of things when nothing else does. Giving money is good. Giving time is better. Either way changes your angle of vision from self-focused to other-focused.

Giving is especially important when you think you can't, when times are hard, or when you feel tapped out. You can always give *something,* and you gain from the giving. I remember my mother telling me how her mother served meals to tramps and strangers during the Great Depression, even though money was scarce and she had seven children of her own to feed. Seeing the truth that you can always give something, and believing it, is a tonic for the psyche. If you can give when you thought you couldn't, maybe everything else is possible, too. Some people take up tithing, the practice of giving 10 percent of their income to a church or charity, at a time when they're not getting by well on 100 percent and wonder how they'll ever manage on 90. They inevitably attest that they're more prosperous from the process, and among those I know who practice it, this seems to be the case.

I'm fascinated by tithing and all the other ways people find to share. One of my friends puts a dollar in her pocket every time she goes out so that she has something to give to the first homeless person or street musician who crosses her urban path. She doesn't feel guilty about the people she can't help, because she helps somebody every day. (I asked her once about people who may not be "worthy," like the guy who'll put her dollar toward a bottle of wine. She said, "I might put a twenty toward a bottle of wine. Am I not worthy?" Touché.)

To exercise more generosity and benevolence, you might simply ask, "How can I be of service today?" It's a lovely little prayer to offer as you walk out the door or put the key in the ignition. If you truly want the answer, you'll get it. The world is crying for generosity and benevolence, and it extends certain kindnesses to those who show them.

REVITALIZE YOUR LIFE WITH WORDS: *I give generously, openly, and wisely. I make my life a gift to those around me.*

NOVEMBER 25

Finding Yourself All Over Again

You've been engaged in a self-discovery process all your life. You've undoubtedly had moments when you've felt you truly found yourself—in a line of poetry in high school, when you fell in love the first time (and the second and the third . . .), and when you held each of your babies fresh from heaven. It's time to find yourself again, now, in what has the potential to be the most substantial and self-assured time of your life. Here are a pair of techniques to help yourself do this in a way that's deep and rich and relevant:

- *Do free writing.* Take out your journal and write without rules or agenda, knowing only that you'll write what you need to read. Put no pressure on your writing or yourself. Give yourself an uninterrupted thirty minutes for free writing—perhaps early in the morning before anyone else is up, or at a coffeehouse where there is bustle all around but none of it has to do with you. You may start slowly—"I don't really know what I'm going to say . . ."—but before you know it, your pen will be racing along.

- *Think back to your little girl self—your seriously* little *girl self.* Philosopher and theorist Rudolf Steiner asserted that children under seven are in touch with their soul's design in ways that few of us ever are again. The poet Wordsworth echoed this theme when he wrote that we come to earth "trailing clouds of glory." Recall what you were like as far back as you can remember. What were your hopes and dreams, your passions and aspirations? These hold clues for finding yourself now.

Give self-exploration a priority. The work ethic that permeates our culture doesn't give much credence to contemplative pursuits, but the self-discovery you do now can make the difference between your future years being golden or not even bronze. Your mind, your temperament, the whole configuration of who you are at this time of your life is singularly suited to this endeavor. All of life and nature wants you to know who you are, because when you do, you can best do the work that brought you here.

REJUVENATE YOURSELF WITH ACTION: *Carve out a little time today to either do free writing or get in touch with your little girl self.*

NOVEMBER 26

See Your Doctor Once a Year— It Helps if You Like Her

See your doctor once a year. It helps if you like him or her. In my opinion, the best of all possible health-care worlds is when your MD is well schooled in complementary medicine, too. (My Ayurvedic doctor, for example, is also a Western internist.) I understand that many people's choice of physician is limited by a miserly HMO. Whatever choice you have, take it as far as it will stretch. And when you see this doctor that you presumably like, refuse to be shortchanged. You'll want a complete blood workup—cholesterol with HDL and LDL, homocysteine, thyroid, blood sugar (fasting or two-hour post-prandial—i.e., after a meal)—the works. Perhaps you should know your blood level of key nutrients. If you're menopausal or approaching that time, you might need your hormone levels checked. If you haven't had a bone-density test, it's time; if you have, it may be time again.

An ECG to check your heart or a lung function test may be indicated as well. Unless your dermatologist already does this, you'll need "skin mapping" at least every few years to check for dermal cancers. You'll also want a Pap (okay, you don't *want* one; you *need* one), a breast exam (even though you're doing monthly ones yourself), and a mammogram if you and your doctor agree that an annual one is indicated. (Once you're over fifty, you're due for a colonoscopy as well.)

If there are conditions in your family to which you may be susceptible, or if you had an abnormal reading on something in the past and you want it checked again, or if some odd symptom has you concerned, ask, ask, ask. Too many doctors these days are treated like meat inspectors: allowed ten seconds a carcass, ten minutes a patient. This is a crime against both physicians and those who depend on them. Don't be a victim. Demand your due.

REJUVENATE YOURSELF WITH ACTION: *When was your last checkup? Do you have an appointment for your next one? If not, make it. If you dread it, see if you can switch to a doctor you'll like.*

NOVEMBER 27

Girlfriends

Clinical findings show that women don't just enjoy the company of other women; we require it for our physical and mental health. Work at UCLA indicated that in addition to the traditional "fight or flight" response to stress, women have an additional option, "nourish and nurture," mitigating tension or fear by surrounding ourselves with other women. Those with the most friends were shown to live longer and have lower blood pressure, heart rates, and cholesterol. The Harvard Nurses' Health Study reported that women with lots of friends were less likely to develop the physical impairments that too often accompany aging. The results were marked enough that the researchers ranked lack of friends as a health risk comparable to smoking or being overweight.

When I moved to New York, I left a close-knit coterie of wonderful women. I met plenty of nice people here and found my Rolodex brimming with contacts but my evenings and weekends short on friends. I set an intention to recreate a strong, supportive group of friends like the one I'd left behind. I affirmed it and visualized it and believed it. Shortly thereafter, I received an Internet mass mailing of people who were hosting study groups for peace. I e-mailed Linda, the New York City listing, to see if her apartment was anywhere near mine. *It was across the street.* I could look out my window and look into hers. In a city of eight million people, this is some coincidence. When I met her, Linda reminded me so much of one of my Kansas City friends, it was as if the universe was responding *literally* to my request to recreate what was lacking. Other extraordinary women, and some really nice guys and couples, too, followed Linda into my life.

Whatever your friendship status at this time, be grateful for the friends you have and willing to invite more in. Think about those people who make you feel warm and safe, the ones you know you can trust with your secrets and your doubts, your dreams and your triumphs. If you've lost touch with someone like this, find her. If you simply haven't spoken to one of your special friends in awhile, call her up. If someone at work or in an organization you belong to seems interesting, approach her; she may become a special friend, and if she doesn't, there's nothing lost for trying.

REVITALIZE YOUR LIFE WITH WORDS: *I have the best friends in the world.*

NOVEMBER 28

Role Models

Everybody has opinions about diet and exercise and what color lipstick we should wear. It's not people's advice that influences us most, though; it's the way they live their lives. As kids, many of us were blatant fans of other kids and select adults who weren't dreary like the rest of them. We were routinely in awe of our best friend, our older sister's best friend, a teacher or a substitute teacher (subs were best: they had mystery). I can remember once in ninth grade gushing to a cheerleader who actually spoke to underlings, "You're my idol!"

We're way past idolatry, thank goodness, but nobody outgrows the need for role models, those friends and even celebrities (if you can separate the person from the press release) who are doing something with their lives you would like to do, too. This isn't being a copycat or denying your inimitable, individual self. It is rather learning via others' example that something you may have thought wasn't possible could be after all. It's getting the word from someone who took the path before you that there is room on it for you, too.

I love noticing the finest qualities in women I know and emulating some of those, or at least appreciating them enough that maybe some will rub off. I also have role models I've never met. The late film star Gloria Swanson is one of my favorites. She was a health enthusiast when most people thought that switching to filtered cigarettes was an extreme measure. Then there is Vanda Scaravelli, a remarkable Italian yoga instructor who was photographed in complex, advanced poses in her eighties—and she was in her mid-forties when she took her first yoga class. Women like these change what maturity looks like in my mind, replacing negative cultural images with powerful, positive ones.

No role model is superhuman. One woman might look fantastic but be self-absorbed; another could be fit and healthy but also selfish or distant. If you wait around for perfect people, you'll have quite a wait. Role models are admirable, imperfect people, just like the rest of us. Come up with yours by making a list of women, those you know personally and those you know of, who have qualities you admire. Keep one of them in mind as you proceed with your aging in reverse. There she is at forty-eight or sixty-six or ninety, with a level of strength, beauty, and vigor that people her age aren't supposed to have. Because she does, however, she breaks the impossibility barrier. It's similar to what happens in sports: as long as they've kept records, no one has ever run faster or swum farther or jumped higher than a certain point. Then somebody does it. Once the impossibility barrier is down, all sorts of athletes are running and swimming and jumping at that level and beyond it. They just needed to know it could be done.

Find some rejuvenation superstars you can admire. Set your sights on doing what they've done, and when you're there, be a willing role model for someone else.

REJUVENATE YOURSELF WITH ACTION: *Make a list of your role models and what you admire about each one.*

Reflexology

Maybe reflexology works because it's relaxing. Or because your body is so impressed that you're spending money not only on yourself but on your feet, for heaven's sake, that it up and heals something out of gratitude. The theory behind it, however, is that since the body's major energy zones end in the feet, working on these points affects the corresponding body parts, relieving tension, improving circulation, and dissolving blockages.

I credit reflexology with getting me through one of the most stressful winters of my life without succumbing to fatigue, despondency, or as much as a sniffle. I drew from a severely strained budget enough money to get reflexology every other Thursday. The reflexologist explained that stress, whether caused by illness, injury, or a garden-variety hard time, gets the body out of balance; reflexology helps bring it back. It opens channels so that life energy can flow freely. The sensitive fingers of a trained reflexologist can discern the places where the energy is stagnant and focus there. She can also work on, and work out, tiny crystalline deposits on the foot that may relate to trouble, obvious or incipient, elsewhere in the body.

My current reflexologist, Irene Angster of the Health and Beauty Connection in New York City, is a deceptively youthful woman in her sixties and truly her own best advertisement. She explains reflexology—on the feet, hands, or ears—as "a little body tune-up, totally noninvasive, that helps the body heal itself." I leave her office rested, in a positive frame of mind, and with energy for the rest of the day, even if it's three in the afternoon, when I've been known to droop.

It would take unlimited time and resources to partake regularly of all of the intriguing offerings in the alternative health-care/ self-care world. This one I do think is worth trying—maybe just an hour for the experience, maybe every other Thursday, at least until spring shows up.

REJUVENATE YOURSELF WITH ACTION: *If you can, book an appointment for a professional reflexology treatment. If this isn't possible, pay extra attention to your feet and toes when you do your* A.M. *massage (January 14).*

NOVEMBER 30

Play Day!

December

Celebration

The All 'Round Response

My thesaurus gives two synonyms for celebration: *solemnization* and *festivity*. In one sense, these are opposites, but in another they show the reach of celebration as life's all 'round response. Some form of it is appropriate in times of both sadness and joy. It expresses our relationship to both the vastness of the divine and the simplicity of the delightful. Celebrating is also all 'round good exercise. It relieves stress. It takes your mind off how you're coming across and plants you securely in the moment.

This is a fitting keynote for a month that has so much to celebrate. In addition to the obvious, the holiday season, perhaps you're completing your year of growing younger, or just beginning it; either one is a passage worthy of celebration. Whatever you celebrate this December, keep in mind what you can celebrate now and always: having a day to live.

Think this month and next year how you can celebrate everything possible. Note friends' birthdays and anniversaries and give them a call or send them a card—a real one when possible: it's hard to make downloading feel like a celebration. Celebrate winning—or if you don't win, having been in the running. Celebrate having new experiences, discovering new places, making it through a rough patch, seeing the results of what you've worked for and the boons that seem to come out of the ever-generous blue. You cannot age while celebrating, unless you do it with too much champagne.

REVITALIZE YOUR LIFE WITH WORDS: *I celebrate my life every day I live.*

Never Stop Dreaming

Midlife is more likely to precipitate its eponymous crisis if we stop dreaming. There is a widespread misconception that dreaming belongs only to the young. This is simply not so. Dreaming is anticipating a future bright enough to hang around for; the longer you live, the more you need to do it. Having dreams set to come true next year, five years from now, and ten years after that is like having certificates of deposit staggered to mature over time so you can always look forward to cashing one in.

I'm not talking about pie-in-the-sky dreams (although one or two of those can't hurt) but about desiring, planning, and working toward the best you can envision—or something better still. As long as you're able to see your desire clearly and hold the vision, even when present circumstances contradict it, you're on your way. You have to be willing to do the work, endure setbacks, take detours when necessary, and make alterations when called for, all the while keeping the goal in focus. This puts you in the best position for making your dream come true—whatever it is, whatever your age, whatever obstacles may at times block your way.

Be cautious about the people with whom you share your dreams. Some people you know are jealous of them. Others think they're unrealistic, or that you're past the time in life for dreaming such a thing. Sadly, too many men and women are chronic dream-dashers. They see dreams, their own and other people's, the way Carrie Nation saw saloons: ripe for the axing. You don't want their negative thoughts infecting your positive process.

You are entitled to your dreams and to seeing them play out in real time, real life. While you're at it, you may as well dream big.

REJUVENATE YOURSELF WITH ACTION: *Check in today with your fondest dream. What is it? What are you doing to make it come true? What can you do today—even a single, small act—to get you closer?*

Give Perfectionism the Boot

If something on earth appears to be perfect, there is something you're not seeing. Of course everything is perfect in a spiritual sense, all part of an expansive plan, unfolding on schedule and in spite of human error. That's a different "perfect." I'm talking about his perfect life, her perfect body, their perfect marriage, and "Well, it's a nice enough haircut, but I thought that since I was paying more this time, it would be perfect." There ain't no perfect in these parts. Understanding this leads to happiness, satisfaction, and peace.

Giving perfectionism the boot does not preclude setting your standards high. You can do that and you should. But don't measure yourself or your life against the impossible standard of perfection. Instead, trade perfectionism for the fullness of life that you deserve. You don't have be perfect anymore. If you've labored under the harsh taskmaster of perfectionism, this is an incredible relief. It frees you to fail and get up again. It frees you to reach for the stars and celebrate lavishly if you make it "only" to the moon.

REVITALIZE YOUR LIFE WITH WORDS: *There ain't no perfect in these parts, and I'm perfectly fine with that.*

The Vintage Paradox

When your clothes are old enough, you can look younger. This is because clothing from the 1950s and earlier, at least that of high enough quality that it's still around, was so well designed and carefully crafted that when you wear it, people see elegance, not birthdays. In those days, women strove to look like women, not girls, and the clothing reflected their desire for grown-up style rather than extended adolescence. Certainly there is contemporary clothing that does this as well—some of it copied from vintage designs—but a few choice antique pieces can do wonders for your wardrobe and your state of mind.

If your mother or your grandmother can be a source of such clothing, you'll be wearing family history. My mother gave me a 1964 Diane von Furstenberg bias-cut summer dress that is a real show-stopper. I'll keep it forever, or pass it on to my daughter or stepdaughter when one of them begs with enough ardor. The rest of my vintage I've collected at various shops and sales. Wherever it came from, each vintage piece seems to be an individual, as opposed to just one more shirt or skirt or suit in my closet. I know that if these garments could talk, they'd have a lot to say. Since they can't, I get to wear them and tell their story in a visual way.

If you've never worn vintage, pop into a shop and try something on. See how it suits you. If you feel transported, you're the vintage type. If you feel foolish, try again. If it doesn't feel right after three or four ventures, contemporary is more your style. Either way, it's the spirit of experimentation that separates those women for whom dressing is a delight from those for whom it is a burden. Growing younger is a matter of increasing delights and decreasing burdens. Loving what you wear is one of the more straightforward ways to get this done.

REJUVENATE YOURSELF WITH ACTION: *Visit a vintage shop and see if there is something there for you.*

DECEMBER 5

Having Brilliant Birthdays

One way to embrace the present, accept reality, and get a good party in the bargain is to play your birthday to the hilt. The over-forty birthday needs to be relieved of its bad rap. Your birthday is when you can flagrantly ask for jewelry and eat cake and ice cream at the same meal. Every birthday calls for a fête geared to it and to you. It warrants an entire day, and if that means taking the day off work, by all means take it. Or decree the following Saturday or Sunday as your birthday this year. If the Queen of England can put hers off until the weather is good, you can postpone yours a few days to celebrate properly.

On your birthday, whether the actual day or an altered one, you deserve to get as much of what you want as you can stand or as much as you can afford, whichever comes first. Plan it in advance so that every minute, every meal, and every detail is special. Some women like to spend the first day of their personal year in solitude and reflection; others crave the company of friends. You choose—it is your day. The past couple of birthdays, I've given myself one of those "days of beauty" (massage, facial, hair, nails, even a cute little lunch) at a salon. I think it will be a tradition that sticks. After all, it's the body's birthday, so the body should stand to benefit.

I'm also fond of birthday symbolism. I've had luncheons and invited friends who represented qualities I most admire and would like to emulate. I once attended a "giveaway party" in which the celebrant took "No Gifts Please" to a new level: she set up her living room like a tag sale, but without tags. Guests were invited to stock up free of charge on whatever they could use; the hostess received in return fewer possessions and more freedom. Another friend had a "wisdom shower." We were supposed to bring her, in lieu of a present, some snippet of wisdom we'd learned in our lives that she could add to what she'd learned in hers. Still another woman I know sent out invitations that said, "Help Make My Life Count." Inside recipients were asked to make a contribution to the charity of their choice and, at the birthday party, share with the others about the work of that charity.

If you're coming upon a big birthday, a decade or half of one, or the first birthday after a major life event—your last child's leaving home, perhaps, or the start of your business—you're looking at more than a day. This is a turning point deserving of more than dinner and a gift certificate. Would you like to go away to some spot that holds fond memories, or somewhere you've never been but have wanted to see all your life? Does this birthday beg to be marked by the ocean or in the mountains or with a view of the Eiffel Tower? Maybe you want to stay home and hold a lavish celebration, or an intimate gathering of only those people who are closest to you.

Write about your options in your journal, even if your next milestone birthday is several years away. Plan ahead so you can make nearly any birthday dream come true. The big ones don't come often. Pull out the stops for them. What you do that day can set the tone not just for a year, but for a decade or an era. Make it meaningful and filled with promise.

REJUVENATE YOURSELF WITH ACTION: *Make plans for your next birthday. Jot your ideas in your journal. While you're at it, think about your next big birthday. What will you do to mark it with sufficient fanfare?*

DECEMBER 6

Childlike Is, Like, Really Good

When you feel as if you're somewhere around eight and a half, you're in rejuvenation mode, pure and simple. This isn't heavy, psychological inner child stuff, it's just letting yourself be naive. Callow. Without guile. Easily and innocently open to entertaining any awe that might be passing by.

When it comes to specifics, your childlike self is unique to you. My friend Alysia suggests wearing overalls and putting your hair in pigtails. Judith recommends going to the playground and climbing on the jungle gym. For some women, it comes out in summer with swimming and camping and picnics. For me, childlikeness is a December phenomenon. I do believe in Santa. I expect Christmas miracles. I even get excited when it snows.

Once you identify what brings out the child in you, take part in the fun. Become accustomed to the feeling so you can conjure it up when you couldn't be farther from a playground or a holiday party. Pull it out when you're around people so stuck in grown-up-ness that they could have been cloned full-grown and dressed in business suits. See something silly in such a somber assembly and laugh, even if you have to keep it under wraps. Find something light in all the heaviness, as a child would. Appreciate simple joys: silly jokes, the fortune in the cookie, dandelions—whether they're yellow and pretty or feathery and fun.

And appreciate yourself. Not long ago I took Emily, our four-year-old neighbor, to the movies. On the bus ride there, she told me that her mom said it was okay for her to stop being Emily and go by a new name, "Princess." I loved it. Didn't we all think this well of ourselves once? Do it again. You have every right to feel highborn, or gifted, or that you're the very favorite child.

REVITALIZE YOUR LIFE WITH WORDS: *I am childlike whenever appropriate and wherever necessary—in other words, as often as I want to be.*

DECEMBER 7

Overcoming Objections

Sometimes life is like a courtroom. You try to make a point or assert yourself or grow in a new direction and the people around you, in the role of opposing counsel, keep shouting, "I object!" (Usually they don't actually shout; they imply. But they may as well be implying through a bullhorn.)

It's scary for any of us when the people we're close to change. That's one reason why the empty-nest experience can be so hard. There is a part of us that wants our grown children to take on the world, and another part that wants them home for dinner. It's not so different when we start aging in reverse, becoming more vital, more attractive, more charismatic. Every group of which we're a part—friends, office, family, and the extended family you may be seeing this holiday season—has a vested interest in maintaining the status quo. If one member makes the radical move of feeling different about herself or presenting herself in a new way, the whole group, or system, has to shift. It doesn't want to and often resists.

That resistance is behind comments like, "What's gotten into you?" "You can't be serious," and "This is just not like you." If you're not under the influence of drugs or somebody brandishing a pistol, whatever you're doing *is* like you, but perhaps like a part of you that hasn't been out in awhile.

This is a time to tread softly. Discern the essential from the window-dressing. Show compassion for the people who love you, or those whose lives are intertwined with yours and who anticipate crippling seasickness if you rock the boat. Refrain from impassioned pronouncements and extreme actions. Just keep your focus on what you intend to accomplish and resolutely head in that direction.

Some people are too afraid of their own dreams to encourage yours. Others are mourning dreams that got away. There are, however, certain extraordinary human beings who will astonish you with a degree of advocacy beyond any you could reasonably expect. When others object, your response, silent or stated, will simply be, "Overruled."

REVITALIZE YOUR LIFE WITH WORDS: *I do what is best for me. Objections only spur me on.*

DECEMBER 8
_____

Enjoy Seeing Your Friends Succeed

One of the pleasures of maturity is seeing friends succeed. I'll always remember the light in Karen's eyes as she sat across from me in a Kansas coffee bar, regaling me with her account of the inauguration party when her longtime chum was elected governor. This is great stuff, the makings of high celebration.

Admittedly, it's not always easy. More people probably choke on "I'm happy for you" than any other simple sentence. It takes magnanimity to applaud a friend's promotion if you're out of work, not to mention toasting your sister on her silver anniversary if your husband left you for a woman whose second driver's license is still valid. These are times to avow, with clenched fists and teeth if need be, "This is not about me. It's about her. I love her. I am thrilled that she's getting to shine."

Besides, no one close to you gets a victory without your having had something to do with it. If you previewed her speeches when they were rough and untried, or you watched her kids while she worked late, or you listened to her tales about rejection and setbacks, a couple of square feet of her new corner office belong to you. The same is true when you're the woman of the hour. You didn't get there without family and friends and even near-strangers who supplied the coffee and emptied the wastebaskets and believed you could do it when you weren't so sure.

DECEMBER 9

Cheers!

Numerous studies indicate that a glass of red wine lowers LDL cholesterol (the kind you want less of) and raises HDL (a good thing) as soon as you drink it. It is agreed, however, that more than one glass a day could increase your risk of breast cancer, and some research suggests that any alcohol consumption puts women at a higher risk of contracting the disease. If that sounds like a choice that's not much of a choice, you're right. It is an individual call. If you enjoy having a drink, consider making it a nice red wine, and if cholesterol is a problem for you, a glass of red wine with dinner may be a smart idea. When you have the choice, choose organic wine, as grapes tend to be a heavily sprayed crop. Most good wine merchants also stock wines free of sulfites, a preservative to which some people are highly allergic and that all of us might be better off without.

If you don't handle alcohol well, of course, or if you have risk factors for breast cancer (family history, early menstruation, no children—or none born before you were thirty—or if you're on hormone replacement therapy), you're better off keeping your cholesterol in check via other means. You can even take a supplementary form of the phytochemicals found in wine. Or just stick with juice: the cholesterol-lowering talent of red wine comes from the skins of the grape; therefore, it's not lost on ordinary grape juice. Whether it's fresh from your juicer or the familiar purple kind in the bottle, grape juice is only slightly less effective in lowering cholesterol than is red wine.

Even with the body-weight difference factored out, women do not metabolize alcohol as well as men do, and it stays in our systems longer. Knowing this, I personally drink only on reasonably special occasions. The rest of the time, something sparkling in a glass with a stem on it is festive enough.

Still, there are studies suggesting that moderate drinkers (that's one shot of liquor or one glass of wine or beer for a woman, two to three times that amount for a man) live longer than teetotalers. My own opinion is that the teetotalers they looked at may have been avoiding alcohol as part of avoiding life. It may be that high spirits, whether innate or distilled, are the deciding factor. I'm hedging my bets that living fully—that includes laughing, celebrating, and socializing as robustly as anybody with a few drinks in him—promises the best of both worlds, along with steady employment as the designated driver.

REJUVENATE YOURSELF WITH ACTION: *Whether or not you choose to drink wine, take part in the good cheer that comes from serving anything in a wineglass. Use stemware for juice and smoothies and see how celebratory life can feel.*

DECEMBER 10

Good Old-Fashioned Glamour

Glamour can be good for you. If you're saying, "Not me; I'm not the type," okay. Maybe you'll never go all out with this, but a little of it is a tonic you deserve, whatever your type.

I miss glamour myself. As a little girl, I looked forward to growing up so I could be glamorous, but before I got my chance, the '60s came and went and glamour went with them. Nowadays people go to the theater in jeans and dress for church the way we used to dress for a picnic. I think one reason for the fascination with celebrities and awards shows is that I'm not the only one who feels glamour-deprived. A great many people want to turn on the TV and gawk at those exquisite dresses we don't often get to see. Thinking back, though, my mother used to wear dresses that dressy to go out to dinner.

A great thing about glamour is that it carries no age restrictions. You can be glamorous for the charity benefit and your daughter can be glamorous for the school dance. You're both allowed. The holiday season is the ideal time to insert a little glamour into your evening look, because this is the one month when glamour comes out of the closet and orders an eggnog. So glamorize yourself this December just a bit more than you'd planned. Retrieve from the back of your closet the dress that says *Hollywood*, even if the closest you get to Tinseltown is a Christmas tree lot so named. Wear a piece of jewelry that sparkles. Let your manicurist use red for a change. Do something fancy or something fanciful with your hair.

You know how we think of the stars of Hollywood's golden era as glamorous before we think of them as old, even though they are either old or dead? Glamour transcends time and erases age. Is it important, like curing cancer or stemming global warming? Of course not. But it's one of those pleasures you can give yourself that leaves you with extra energy to take on the big things.

REVITALIZE YOUR LIFE WITH WORDS: *There is a glamorous side to me, and this season I'm playing it to the hilt.*

DECEMBER 11

Keep a Clean Calendar

Conventional wisdom says that more people get depressed this time of year than any other. It's no wonder: more people are running themselves ragged trying to create Norman Rockwell–style holidays and be all things to all people. But now and every day of every year, it is essential for your sanity, as well as for your rejuvenation, that you keep a clean calendar.

Whether you track your time electronically or on paper, get some space between the appointments and the errands. It's this space, this uncommitted time, that truly belongs to you. When your to-do list defies the twenty-four-hour day, laugh. Then cut it by half or two-thirds. Most of our "things to do" can wait a day or two or several, and some of them can wait forever. You know how good it feels to cross out things you've done? Here's a radical notion: cross out some things you haven't done. Blow them off. Let them go. Give yourself breathing space. Give yourself living space. This is how you come to find yourself, and know yourself, and be yourself. When you do, you're young again. Life lightens up. You get a little more wonderment, and each new day is more a gift to open than a chore to tackle.

REJUVENATE YOURSELF WITH ACTION: *Take a look at your calendar or planner for the rest of this month. Anything excessive, anything that dampens your spirit when you think of it, is ripe for excising. I know: some of this stuff you're obligated to do. Me too. But a lot of it we obligate ourselves to. Clean up your calendar.*

DECEMBER 12

Eye Cream

Ask Santa to put some eye cream in your stocking, and keep yourself supplied with it throughout the year. As tempting as it is to use your regular moisturizer in the eye area, too, you'll take strides toward looking younger by investing in a specially designed product for this area, often the first place a woman sees lines on her face. This is because the skin around your eyes is the thinnest on your body; it has no oil glands of its own and doesn't hold moisture well. Because of its delicacy, this skin needs a specialized moisturizer, one that it can absorb and that isn't so heavy it pulls on this fragile skin.

Promise you'll apply eye cream to the skin at the edges of your eyes and beneath them every night, so help you God. Many eye creams are fortified with modern wrinkle-fighting ingredients. There are dozens of these; it may take a little trial and error to see which one your skin likes most and which one does the best job of coming through on its claims on *your* face. Because the product will be near your eyes, you may wish to look for a hypoallergenic formulation and certainly stop using anything that causes irritation to your eyes or the skin around them.

If you choose to wear eye cream in the day as well—it's a good idea—look for one with UVA/UVB protection, ideally an oil-free formulation that won't cause your makeup to smudge. And spread the word to your daughters and other young women you know. If they start now, they'll be grateful later.

REJUVENATE YOURSELF WITH ACTION: *If you aren't currently a regular wearer of eye cream, become one. If you are, renew your supply.*

Accommodate All Your Aspects

I think women like diamonds because we are like diamonds: multi-faceted. And like a diamond, we wouldn't sparkle without all our aspects. Society likes putting us into categories ("working woman," "widow," "athlete," "mother of two"). Although we may relate to one or more of these descriptors, we're so much more than any of them or even all of them. It's probably unfair to expect the world at large, or even most other people, to see us for all we are. It is essential, however, that we see ourselves for all we are.

For example, I do a pretty good job of eating the way you've been reading about in this book. I avoid gratuitous sugar and white flour and chemical additives most of the time. But in mid-December, my daughter and I bake cookies from the recipe in a kids' Christmas book she's had since she was ten. These cookies have sugar and white flour and sprinkles colored with heaven knows what. I am both a health enthusiast and a holiday traditionalist. Those disparate aspects of myself have different needs. When I am willing to accommodate all my aspects, I can satisfy both. I'm sure you have examples in your life where you've found this to be true as well.

Focus today on accepting, appreciating, and accommodating all your aspects. You can teach English literature and read romance novels. You can be the preacher's wife and take up belly dancing. You can make half a million a year and shop in thrift stores. You can be somebody's grandmother and play in a band. All these differences and subtleties, nuances and contradictions, give you the sparkle that makes you unique and keeps you young.

REVITALIZE YOUR LIFE WITH WORDS: *I am multifaceted, like a diamond.*

Ritualize Your Moments and Your Milestones

Have you ever noticed how comfortably the word "ritual" nestles inside the word "spirituality"? Ritual is the language of the spirit, that part of us that craves ceremony, the sanctification of the events of our lives. In addition to the ritual that may be part of your religion, the milestones of your life and even the conventions of your day deserve this favor. Ritual is youth-promoting because it puts a little play and more than a little awe into the everyday.

A ritual is a celebration, ancient or improvised, majestic or minuscule. Some are for public consumption, full of pomp and circumstance, while others are quiet and private, for no eyes but yours. Barbara Biziou, author of *The Joys of Everyday Ritual*, defines ritual as "the honoring of authenticity." Some events you might honor with ritual include:

- *Your wise woman status.* Such celebrations were historically held thirteen months after a woman's last menstrual period.

- *A child's leaving.* That could be leaving home or leaving for kindergarten; some families have one of each.

- *The ending of a job or the launching of a business.* Any major change in one's work in the world qualifies.

If it's part of life, it's fuel for ritual. We're not schooled in the ceremonial these days, so flying by the seat of our jeans is fully acceptable. Lighting candles is always good; so is passing around a goblet of water or wine or Welch's. This is your celebration. Do whatever you like.

You can also insert small rituals into the warp and woof of your weekdays and weekends. For example:

- *Raising the shades in the morning.* This is a ritual that states you are consciously entering into a new day, checking in with nature to see what her pleasure is, and letting in the light of morning. Shutting the drapes at night finishes the ritual begun at daybreak, giving closure to the day and thanks for its blessings and its lessons.

- A *phone-answering ritual*. This is a conscious turning from what you were doing before and a silent benediction for the person calling. (If instead of a person, the call comes from a computer trying to sell you something, the benediction just comes back to you.)

- A *ritual for food preparation*. Stand at the entrance of your kitchen, take a deep breath, and ask that you prepare the feast or the sandwich with attention and maybe even a little reverence.

Our days pass one after the other, whether kissed with the enchantment of ritual or not. Since we get only so many of them, add some enchantment every chance you get.

REJUVENATE YOURSELF WITH ACTION: *Make a ritual today out of a task or a pleasure that would otherwise have been just something to do.*

DECEMBER 15
_____

Play Day!

DECEMBER 16
_____

Ignore Uncle Leroy

When people notice you're taking better care of your health, someone is sure to regale you with the saga of incredible Uncle Leroy. Leroy, by whatever name, lived to be ninety-eight, and he'd be here today if it weren't for that nasty skateboarding accident. Leroy, however, was no health nut. Quite the contrary: he smoked two packs a day, ate exclusively from the Basic Four Grease Groups, and if anyone were in need of whisky for medicinal purposes, Leroy could always find a bottle. The message is, of course, "Why go to all this trouble? Leroy didn't bother, and look how well things turned out for him."

It is true: there are Leroys in this world. They are phenomena. By some quirk of genetics, with perhaps a little good karma thrown in, these noteworthy specimens apparently defy every known health precept and thrive anyway. People who don't want to take care of themselves, and who are threatened when they see you taking care of yourself, pull out Leroy lore as proof that abusing oneself just might do a body good. Not on your life. Most of these tales have grown taller in the telling. Leroy may not have been as spry in his old age as the saga has spun him. Moreover, for every legendary Leroy, there are countless poor souls who went to early graves and suffered a lot before they got there.

When someone tells you about this person or that one who had deplorable health habits and outlived every jogger and greens-eater on the block, say something noncommittal like, "That's really interesting," but don't let it sway you one bit. If it happens that you are the fortunate bearer of a Leroy-esque genetic code, you'll live even longer and better if you eat well, exercise, get enough sleep, manage your stress, get regular checkups, and tend to the other etceteras that Leroys apparently ignore with impunity. And if you are a mere mortal like the rest of us, doing these things could help you to a longer and more satisfying life.

REVITALIZE YOUR LIFE WITH WORDS: *I treat myself superbly, no matter what anyone else says or does.*

DECEMBER 17

Call a Truce with Your Weight

When I was eighteen I read in a fashion magazine: "There comes a time in every woman's life when she must choose between the face and the fanny." For me, that time is here. I could stand to be firmer, but if I were much thinner, I wouldn't look skinny like a model; I'd look skinny like somebody who needs to see a doctor. Being too thin can impair immunity and make the transition of menopause more difficult. There is a point at which enough is enough—even enough thinness.

Although no one is meant to be so fat—or thin—that it jeopardizes her health, some individuals and families and ethnicities are naturally sturdier or fuller-bodied, while others are leaner and more delicate. It is essential that you accept yourself the way you are and strive to become as healthy as you, with your body and your heredity, can get.

Use your maturity to deal sanely with your weight. If overeating is a concern, get help so it won't be a concern for the rest of your life. I personally am a great fan of Overeaters Anonymous, which takes a body/mind/spirit approach and offers 'round-the-clock support. In OA, there are no fees, there are no diets, and nobody weighs you. Whatever route you take, know that when it comes to weight and midlife, there is bad news and good news. You know the bad news: Metabolism slows down. Losing weight gets harder. You have to eat fewer calories to even stay the same. Fat replaces muscle, so you can weigh what you always have but be fatter than ever. Lost muscle tone makes you look fatter still. And at menopause hormonal envoys order up a rounder stomach and thicker waist. But . . .

Here's the good news: A surprising number of women who fought overeating and overweight nearly all their lives find that when they're older, they've dealt with the issues that incited their problems with food. Either through therapy, spiritual practice, or what my mother would call the "school of hard knocks," they have matured into women who no longer need to overeat.

Also, many a woman by this time has taken command of her own ship. She no longer has to look like she just stepped off a runway or follow what the latest diet fad stipulates. She's given up jumping on bandwagons, although she may well be jumping on a mini-trampoline. She's looking at life with every delusion stripped away and wants to take care of herself in order to safeguard her health and preserve the good life she's worked so hard to build. If she loses weight, it's not to please a man, one-up a girlfriend, or give herself some temporary self-esteem. She does it, slowly and intelligently, because it's the right choice. Years of experience in making both right and wrong choices have shown her which ones come with happiness attached, and which ones come with misery.

Chronologically, This Is the Youngest Day of the Rest of Your Life

Okay, it's overused, that phrase about this being the first day of the rest of your life. It is the truth, though. This is also the *youngest* day of the rest of your life. This is a time you might one day think of and, if you temporarily forget to live in the present, say, "Wouldn't it be great to be back there?"

Listen to what women who are older than you have to say about the age you are. I can still hear the voice of Mrs. Gaylord, the designer-clad magazine editor who hired me when I was twenty-two and she was forty years my senior, saying, "Get some news on the young set, those couples in their forties who are doing everything." At twenty-two, I couldn't imagine people in their forties referred to as young, yet just weeks ago my mom was having a stretch of exceptional well-being and commented, "I feel like I'm sixty again." I could say it's all relative, but that's pretty obvious.

In terms of days and moments lived, you'll never again be as young are you are right now, so spend this day, the youth of your future, in a way that deflects regret. Invest in yourself. Have some fun. Do something important. Love somebody extra. In one sense, you're just a kid, but a kid with enough years on her to know that every day is priceless.

REJUVENATE YOURSELF WITH ACTION: *Take out into the world today the fact that chronologically this is the youngest you'll ever be. Live with this in mind. Use it on future days when you will again be as young as you'll ever get.*

Enjoy Yourself by Yourself

As rejuvenating as it is to have positive people in your life to validate you and make you laugh, it is equally important to know how to enjoy yourself when there is no one else around. Many people are uneasy with the thought of being all by themselves when, in fact, solitary time can be the most gratifying. If you've yet to perfect the art of solitude, try these suggestions:

- *Go out to dinner or to the movies by yourself on purpose.* The "on purpose" is critical. Plan your date with yourself ahead of time. If you wait until some evening when your husband has to work late, the nest is feeling woefully empty, and everyone you call has tantalizing plans that don't include you, it will be hard to have a good time in your unaccompanied state.

- *Catalog solitary at-home activities that make being home alone a real treat.* There are several ideas in this book— a therapeutic bath (October 25), a mini-retreat (April 16), a detox day (September 18), or delving into one of the spiritual classics (September 28).

- *Take a weekend trip on your own.* This is the advanced class. An easy drive from where you live, there is more than likely a town known for its antique shops, summer theater, fall foliage, stately homes, or museum of something or other. Plan your trip there and make the fact that you're taking it alone part of its allure.

The true test of what you think of yourself is how thoroughly you enjoy your own companionship. When you get really good at this, you'll never feel lonely, whether in a crowd of strangers or when there's no one in sight.

REJUVENATE YOURSELF WITH ACTION: *Catalog enticing activities that are best enjoyed by yourself. Flag the page in your journal where it's written so the next time you find yourself alone, you can go to it for ideas.*

Doing the Footwork

Feet are a pay-now-or-pay-later proposition. If you wear high heels and pointy toes, you may turn heads for thirty years or longer. I've seen young men do admiring doubletakes when a fifty-plus woman walked by wearing killer shoes. If you wear them day after day, though, your feet will start to conform to the shape of the shoes and you'll find yourself with bunions, turned-in toes, corns, and the other unwelcome accoutrements of old feet. Wearing "old lady shoes" could prevent that, but they look like they belong on, well, you know who.

To navigate the middle path, collect a wardrobe, modest or extensive, of middle-of-the-road shoes, boots, and sandals. These have some style and some heel, but a basic shape that resembles a foot more than a designer's imagination. They also come with some cushioning in the sole (those fat pads that make babies' feet so adorable have, by now, diminished to a great extent). Save your vampy shoes for evening or when you need both your feminine wiles and your MBA to get the job done. Whenever you can, though, do your feet a favor and wear supportive walking shoes, sandals with an arch and thick sole, bedroom slippers, or no shoes at all.

Every chance you get, circle your ankles, point and flex your feet, and stretch and extend your toes. Don't let a day go by without stretching the hamstring muscles in the backs of your calves, especially if you wear heels, which shorten that muscle. Get foot massages or massage your feet yourself with lots of oil or lotion. Use a pumice stone or grainy scrub on calluses in every bath. If you have foot troubles you can't address on your own, find a good podiatrist, a physician and surgeon who specializes in the foot and ankle. He can keep incipient bunions from becoming full blown; deal with heel spurs, hammer toes, ingrown nails, and other ills the foot is heir to; and offer treatment options for nail fungus. (I'm sure you've noticed by now that aging in reverse does take a team. My most stylish friend said not long ago, "The older I get the more appointments I have.")

Speaking of appointments, book one for a pedicure every month or so, all year long. Even if you do these yourself, note them on your calendar so you never get behind. The pedicure separates the meticulous from the masses. You can have fun with it, too, wearing colors on your toes you wouldn't think of having on your fingers, and kicking off your shoes and having nothing to hide.

REJUVENATE YOURSELF WITH ACTION: *Bring your feet out of hiding today and do something nice for them. Consider a massage, a pedicure, or a new pair of really comfortable shoes.*

DECEMBER 21

Trains, Planes, and Automobiles

Your plans for today may include packing to go somewhere wonderful or just somewhere different. When you go, you can take your growing-younger lifestyle along, even en route.

If I had my druthers, I'd go everywhere except across oceans by train. I feel comforted by the motion of a train, and I like the fact that when it arrives, I'm where I'm going, not thirty miles out at an airport. Train seats are roomy, the corridors wide, the views panoramic, and if there's a dining car—well, be still my beating heart. I met a woman who told me that when life gets stressful, she books a weekend sleeping compartment on Amtrak and goes from Chicago, where she lives, to Washington, D.C., and back. She gets two nights alone with herself, her books, and her music, plus a few hours for lunch and exploring in the nation's capital.

Some women get a thrill from hitting the highway in an automobile. My friend Rita says road trips are her excuse to kick back and listen to country music. Make car trips healthy by:

- Looking for restaurants that have good salads or that could at least stay in business if the deep-fryer broke.

- Choosing motels you can count on to have workout facilities.

- Never driving longer than your body would comfortably go *without* a sizable cup of truck-stop coffee. Artificially pushing physiological limits (in this case, stressing the adrenal glands with a hefty shot of caffeine) is aging, not to mention a safety hazard.

When you leave the driving to an airline pilot, your trip has different pleasures and challenges. Despite airport security checks and no-frills flights, some people still love to fly. If you're not one of them, pretend. Frequent flying is less trying when you schedule flights so you don't have to get up before dawn, sleep on a plane, or endure a layover.

To combat the dehydrating effects of air travel, pack your carry-on with a bottle of water, some rich moisturizer, and saline nasal spray; drink, slather, and squeeze often. Avoid alcohol, caffeine (coffee, black tea, cola), and anything salty; these can exacerbate the dehydration for which you're trying to compensate. Loosen your shoe laces (it's common for feet to swell in flight), walk up and down the aisle (this may even ward off the rare but serious complication of DVT, deep vein thrombosis), and do ankle circles and shoulder rolls to encourage circulation and keep you from getting stiff. If it's a long flight with meal service, you can order a special meal that best suits your needs (vegetarian, kosher, low-sodium, low-carb, etc.) when you purchase your ticket. For most flights, you'll probably be offered only pretzels and a drink, so plan ahead to eat at home or at the airport.

Should you experience a time zone change of more than two hours, jet-lag symptoms can be mitigated with the homeopathic remedy Arnica Montana, 6c potency, available at health food shops. Dissolve one tiny tablet under your tongue three times the day before you travel, once during the flight (twice on a haul to the other side of the world), and as necessary every few hours for up to two days after. In addition, adapt to the hours of the place you are by eating on the new schedule even before you're able to sleep on it. Have protein (and tea or coffee if you drink them) in the morning, carbs for dinner. Go to bed within a couple of hours of what would be reasonable in the place you find yourself. Spend time outside during the day to help your body understand what time it is.

And under all circumstances, take pictures. You didn't come this far not to capture some of it.

REVITALIZE YOUR LIFE WITH WORDS: *Wherever I am and in every circumstance, I am worth taking care of.*

DECEMBER 22

The Winter Solstice

This seasonal shift gets lost amid the Hanukkah candles and the Christmas lights, but it's a magical time, this shortest day of the year. It's the beginning of the lying-in period for Mother Earth. All the life she'll burst forth with in the spring is now pure potentiality, a latent energy beneath the surface of things.

Mark this day in a way that is meaningful for you. Some ideas to consider:

- *Think about what you hope to conceive this winter and birth in the spring.* Do you have an idea for something to make or write or paint once the holiday rush has passed? Is there something you'd like to study or learn? Is there some way you want to deepen your spiritual life in the cold, quiet months ahead?

- *Stock up on moisture in every form.* How is your supply of face cream and hand cream, cuticle oil and body lotion? You're likely to need richer versions of these now to keep up with blustery winds and drying central heat.

- *Check the winterizing around your home.* There may not be time to tend to it right now, but if there are windows left to caulk or a shovel to be brought down from the attic, make a note to get to it next week or after the first of the year.

- *Do you have an indoor exercise program in place?* Consider a martial arts class, dancing lessons (a holiday gift for you and your honey, perhaps?), or hooking up with the after-work mall walkers.

- *Snuggle up with a book tonight.* Notice how you're drawn to different genres now than you were at the beach last summer.

- *Get to bed early.* It's dark and restful and you just might get your most satisfying sleep of the year.

REVITALIZE YOUR LIFE WITH WORDS: *I love the winter; I just didn't always know it.*

DECEMBER 23

Assign Yourself a Distinctive Fragrance

I happen to get a kick out of cologne and *eau de toilette* and, on the rare occasions I spring for it, real, honest-to-golly perfume. Scents bother some people and are considered improper in certain places these days—some doctor's offices and health clubs, for instance. I've also learned to ask if applying fragrance is permissible when I'm someone's houseguest. (I once gave an allergic friend a terrible headache in her own house when I spilled cologne in her bathroom. A lesson sticks when you learn it from being mortified.)

When wearing fragrance is appropriate, make the fragrance your own. Some women choose one and it's a trademark for them. Others have a day fragrance, light and fresh, and an evening scent that's heavier, sexier. The reason for having one (or two) distinctive fragrances is that this is one more way to give an added dimension to the impression you make. When you have a look, a manner, a voice, and even a subtle fragrance, you're presenting more of yourself to other people. There is more to take in and more to remember.

REJUVENATE YOURSELF WITH ACTION: *If you enjoy wearing fragrance but don't have a special one right now, linger at the perfume counter next time you're shopping and see if anything catches your fancy. Give your nose a rest if you're testing more than three scents. Otherwise it could get confused.*

424

Favorably Envision Your Older Self

Children often think about what they want to be when they grow up, but mid-adults seldom think about how they want to be when they're certified elders. I suggest that you do—not a lot, since today is the day you've got and the one in which to live—but think about it some and think about it positively. How do want to look when you're eighty-five? You won't look twenty; you know that. You're not likely to look sixty either, but you can look fabulous. And think about other things. Where do you want to be living? What do you want to be doing?

My daughter has talked since she was a little girl about having long white braids that she'll wrap around her head and, since she's in theater, getting all the grandmother roles. "So many actors give up in their thirties," she explained, "so I'll be the first old woman the casting directors think of." I thought it was odd for a child to contemplate her old age, but she got interested in sun-block and retirement funds years earlier than I had, so perhaps she wasn't the odd one after all.

Sometime when you're in reverie, then, let your thoughts drift years into the future and favorably envision your older self. See her (you) as happy, healthy, and content. Do this every now and again. When you do, you're creating a mental image toward which your body/mind/spirit complex can steer. You'll make decisions in the near future that will favorably influence your far future. You'll lay a foundation for happiness, healthiness, and contentment. Whether or not you'll have long white braids is entirely up to you.

REJUVENATE YOURSELF WITH ACTION: *One of these days when there is some time to just sit with yourself and your tea or your cocoa, think about how you want to be some years in the future. See yourself brimming with happiness, health, contentment, and whatever else you want in your life when you're old enough to play the role of the great-great-grandmother.*

Making Merry

If you are of the Christian faith, this is a holy and happy day, and I wish you great joy in it. Whether or not you celebrate Christmas, however, you're in the midst of a season dedicated to merriment. When you can make merry with the best of them, years disappear from your face and your outlook.

Making merry is simply the seasonal wording for having fun. Though born knowing how to do this, we all too frequently lose our knack for it as time passes and life intervenes. We become invested in the dull clichés we heard as children and vowed we'd never believe: "Life is tough—you'd better get used to it," "In the real world, it's every man for himself," and "It's a jungle out there." The key to merry-making is to get out of the jungle and into the celebration. It's the ability to temporarily turn away from problems and focus on jubilation instead.

This won't work if it's phony. You sometimes see parents who are embroiled in difficulties with their marriage or work or finances putting on the good show for a child's birthday or a holiday. Sadly, they're not making merry: they're faking merry. It's obvious, especially to children for whom merriment is a natural state. To bring it back for yourself, you have to set aside the harsh and the difficult. Losses and hardships exist, but today let them exist in another dimension. You'll deal with them again when the time is appropriate, but for now, you have only two obligations: to have a wonderful time and to be part of someone else's wonderful time.

How this wonderful time presents itself differs from person to person, year to year, life stage to life stage. If you remember how to make merry—or if you commit to doing it, whether you consciously remember or not—you can have a merry Christmas, a happy Hanukkah, a joyous Kwanzaa, and a glorious New Year, regardless of where you are or whom you're with. Every moment you spend in such merriment leaves you with an imprint of lightness and youthfulness that will be with you for many a Christmas future.

DECEMBER 26

Regard Sleeping in Makeup as the Eighth Deadly Sin

It's easy to fall asleep without washing your face, especially during this overbooked time of year, when more shopping and socializing go on than during any other season. Even so, no matter how late it is, how tired you are, or how pure and natural your makeup is, regard sleeping in it as the eighth deadly sin.

When you sleep, your facial skin, like the rest of your body, is supposed to be renewing itself—i.e., growing younger. Sleeping with your face on impedes the nightly detox job your pores are programmed to perform. Besides, the treatments we depend on most to make our skin soft and dewy, prevent and reverse lines, and heal angry red splotches are *night* treatments. If you go to bed all made up, you'll miss out on fostering your own restoration. There is a discipline component, too: if you're devoted about cleansing your face, even when you're aching for sleep, you etch the concept of self-care in all its aspects into your psyche.

Turn makeup removal into a little ritual. If you like the abundant feeling of using an array of cleansers and toners and lotions and creams, find a product line that leaves no stone unturned and become a devotee. If you're more a quick-and-to-the-point gal, you can do cleanser/moisturizer/eye cream and jump under the covers. Either way, raccoon eyes in the morning will become a thing of the dimly distant past.

REVITALIZE YOUR LIFE WITH WORDS: *I cleanse my face thoroughly every night. This is the face I show the world.*

The Burning Bowl

In a few days you'll be ringing in a new year. Passages such as these make us think about the past and future. As with a birthday, you can choose to make New Year's Eve and New Year's Day joy-filled indicators of where you're going and how far you've come, or depressing reminders of a time that's not coming back. Generally speaking, maudlin comes from too much looking back, mirthful from looking forward with hopefulness and expectation.

A way to symbolically commit to this is to either attend the burning bowl rite that some churches hold on New Year's Eve, or—with extreme care—have your own. To prepare for the burning bowl, each person writes on slips of paper those negative traits or situations they would like to be rid of in the year to come. Examples might be, "Resentment toward my sister," "Being underpaid," "Eleven pounds," "Feeling tired too much of the time," "Proclivity for attracting Messrs. Wrong"—anything that needs to go in the *auld acquaintance* category and be never brought to mind.

Then choose a large flame-proof bowl—clay or metal—set in a safe spot with nothing flammable above or beneath. Have a good-sized pitcher of water nearby, and bring the fire extinguisher in from the kitchen, just in case. Put the pieces of paper in the bowl and set them alight. (Cover the bowl with a piece of window screen to keep any embers from taking flight.) Say a prayer or set an intention that this unwanted baggage disappear from your life as surely as it turns to ash in the fire. When the paper is sufficiently done away with, douse the ashes with water and affirm that the old has indeed passed away and you are a ready channel for receiving the best of the new.

REJUVENATE YOURSELF WITH ACTION: *Plan to do a burning bowl ceremony—very, very safely—or some variation on the theme in the next few days. If you'd rather not play with fire, you can still write down those situations you wish to be free of and put them through a paper-shredder or symbolically destroy them in some other way.*

Remove Everything from Your Closet That Does Not Make You Feel Smashing

With a new year coming, change is in the air. This is the perfect week for removing from your closet every item of clothing that does not make you feel smashing. Besides, your wardrobe was probably augmented with holiday presents, or is about to be with gift certificates and January sales.

Try this on your next free morning: Divide the clothes you own into two groups—those you adore and those you put up with. Then divide that second group into clothes that really need to go—get rid of them and don't look back—and those that might, with an alteration or an update, get promoted to adored status.

Clothes aren't made of stone; they ask to be changed, and those in your "maybe there's some hope here" pile could be begging to be made more compatible with you. My teenaged stepdaughter, Siân, can transform a shirt by cutting off a sleeve or fraying the bottom or adorning the front with pins and patches and slogan buttons as if she were a decorated general. Her clothes become art, living and evolving. I can't do what she does because I lack her talent and am nearly three times her age, but I can get hints from her. I won't cut off sleeves, but I can push them up, or put a French-cuffed shirt beneath a jacket and make it memorable with mismatched men's cufflinks, one bargained for at a vintage store, the other found on the floor of my husband's closet. This is a playful enterprise. Consider your closet-revamping day a play date.

I promise: you will like your life more with a wardrobe of two dresses, four shirts, and three pairs of pants that you're crazy about than with a walk-in closet you can barely walk in because it's filled with outfits that don't give you a lift.

REJUVENATE YOURSELF WITH ACTION: *Set the date for removing from your closet everything that does not make you feel smashing.*

Celebrate Late Blooming and Late Bloomers

Late blooming is an honored tradition. It's a godsend for those of us who didn't fit in early on and found ourselves relegated to the outfield for softball and the sidelines for prom. Late blooming is an option if you bloomed early, too: you get to do it again. The trick is to bloom *now*, whether this is a familiar state or brand new. Blossom in any and all of the following ways:

- *Be every ounce the person you are.* The more add-ons and ought-to's you can strip away, the more unique and admirable you'll be.

- *Have the willingness to see things differently.* Middle school is for being like everybody else; middle age is for being like yourself.

- *Take your gift out into the world and offer it where it's needed.* If it's rejected, it means it wasn't needed there enough. Offer elsewhere.

- *Believe in yourself and the future and the purpose of things,* when that purpose is apparent and when it isn't.

- *Turn your present situation into one that's advantageous.* If your children are gone and you're divorced or widowed, this solitary state can be sad and lonely, or it can free you to volunteer for hospice or teach English in Tibet.

- *Take a backseat to no one and offer a helping hand to anyone.* Use the worldly wisdom you've acquired so you can be open and generous and protect yourself at the same time.

- *See your beauty and that of other late bloomers, women your age and your mother's age.* Whether friends or strangers, these are your late-blooming colleagues. When we recognize each other and realize how many of us there are, we'll have untold power to change things for the better.

DECEMBER 30

Play Day!

DECEMBER 31

Forever and a Day

If you're doing your first read-through of this book, a wondrous year of growing more vital, more beautiful, and more fully yourself lies before you. If you're completing this year of growing younger, or if you're somewhere in the middle, you have a glorious new year ahead, full of opportunities for growth and self-discovery. Whether your plans for tonight are to dance till dawn, watch the ball drop at midnight, or get to bed by ten because you've seen how terrific that makes you look and feel, a year of limitless potential is at hand. But you know what? Every new day can be like that. And when that's how you see it, and that's how you greet it, you can live to be 102 and never get old. The secret is to remain engaged with life, enchanted by the here and now, and intrigued by the mysteries of here and hereafter.

Decide that this moment, and forever and a day, there is going to be magnificence in your life, whatever it takes. Find it in your healthy kitchen and the room where you have your daily quiet time. Look for it when you're shopping or sorting through your cleared-out closet. Get to know it in a relaxing bath, in vigorous exercise, in physical intimacy with a lover or spiritual intimacy with a love. It's there, in a steaming cup of tea and one perfect piece of chocolate, in a walk in the park or a whisper of intuition. Helen Keller said, "Life is either a thrilling adventure, or else it is nothing." Allow me to paraphrase and say, "Life is either a thrilling adventure, or else it is aging."

It is a fact that humans either grow old or die young. That can seem like a huge rock and a very hard place, but you have the opportunity to become a woman of advanced age without losing the best parts of your youthfulness. I don't mean that you'll get a facelift when you're ninety, but rather that the spirit of life will grow so strong within you that every moment you spend on this earth will be flooded to overflowing with it. And when it's your time to go wherever it is we go after this, you'll take that life with you and add more glory to heaven.

REVITALIZE YOUR LIFE WITH WORDS: *My life is a thrilling adventure, today and forever.*

Recommended Reading

THE AGING PROCESS AND GROWING YOUNGER

Allegra, Suzy. *How to Be Ageless*. Berkeley: Celestial Arts, 2002.

Amerina, Jennifer. *Aging Naturally*. New York: Hermes House, 2001.

Carper, Jean. *Stop Aging Now!* New York: Harper Perennial, 1996.

Chopra, Deepak, MD. *Ageless Body, Timeless Mind*. New York: Harmony, 1993.

Conkling, Winifred. *Stopping Time*. New York: Dell Publishing, 1997.

Fotuhi, Majid, MD, PhD. *The Memory Cure*. New York: Contemporary Books, 2003.

Haddon, Dayle. *The Five Principles of Ageless Living*. New York: Atria Books, 2003.

Hersh, Sunny. *Midlife Mamas on the Moon*. Long Valley, NJ: Fast Forward Publications, 2004.

Kelder, Peter. *Ancient Secret of the Fountain of Youth*. New York: Doubleday, 1998.

Komaiko, Leah. *Am I Old Yet?: A True Story of a Timeless Friendship*. New York: St. Martin's Griffin, 2000.

Northrup, Christiane, MD. *The Wisdom of Menopause*. New York: Bantam, 2003.

Roisen, Michael F., MD. *The Real Age Makeover*. New York: HarperResource, 2004.

Scrivner, Jane. *Stay Young Detox*. London: Judy Piatkus Publishers, 2001.

Snowdon, David. *Aging with Grace*. New York: Bantam, 2001.

DIET, NUTRITION, AND WEIGHT CONTROL

Barnard, Neal, MD. *Eat Right, Live Longer*. New York: Three Rivers Press, 1996.

Fuhrman, Joel, MD. *The Eat to Live Diet*. New York: Little, Brown, 2003.

Grout, Pam. *Jumpstart Your Metabolism*. New York: Simon & Schuster, 1998.

Hatherill, J. Robert, PhD. *Eat to Beat Cancer*. New York: Renaissance Books, 1999.

Havala, Suzanne, DrPH, RD. *Being Vegetarian for Dummies*. New York: Wiley, 2001.

Moran, Victoria. *Fit from Within*. New York: Contemporary Books, 2003.

EXERCISE

Bartocci, Barbara. *Meditation in Motion*. Notre Dame, IN: Ave Maria Press, 2004.

Nelson, Miriam, PhD, with Sarah Wernick, PhD. *Strong Women Stay Young*. Rev. ed. New York: Bantam, 2000.

Price, Joan, MA, with Lawrence Kassman, MD, FACEP. *The Anytime, Anywhere Exercise Book*. Avon, MA: Adams Media, 2003.

FASHION AND BEAUTY

Keogh, Pamela Clarke. *Audrey Style*. New York: HarperCollins, 1999.

Kinsel, Brenda Reiten. *40 Over 40: 40 Things Every Woman Over 40 Needs to Know About Getting Dressed*. Berkeley: Wildcat Canyon Press, 2000.

Leigh, Michelle Dominique. *Inner Peace, Outer Beauty*. New York: Citadel Press, 1995.

McWilliams, Tracy. *Dress to Express*. Novato, CA: New World Library, 2004.

Moran, Victoria. *Lit from Within*. San Francisco: HarperSanFrancisco, 2001.

Mulvaney, Jay. *Jackie: The Clothes of Camelot*. New York: St. Martin's Press, 2001.

GENERAL HEALTH

Altman, Nathaniel. *Healing Springs*. Rochester, VT: Healing Arts Press, 2000.

Chow, Kit, and Ione Kramer. *All the Tea in China*. San Francisco: China Books, 1990.

Grossman, Marc, OD. *Natural Eye Care: An Encyclopedia*. New York: McGraw-Hill, 1994.

Mazo, Ellen, and the editors of *Prevention* Health Books, with Keith Berndtson, MD. *The Immune Advantage*. Emmaus, PA: Rodale Books, 2002.

Rowinsky, Karen. *Come Alive! 50 Easy Ways to Have More Energy Now*. Edina, MN: Beaver's Pond Press, 2000.

HOME, LIFESTYLE, AND WELL-BEING

Berthold-Bond, Annie. *Better Basics for the Home*. New York: Three Rivers Press, 1999.

Biziou, Barbara. *The Joys of Everyday Ritual*. New York: Griffin Trade Paperbacks, 2001.

Breitman, Patti, and Connie Hatch. *How to Say No Without Feeling Guilty*. New York: Broadway Books, 2001.

Dadd, Debra Lynn. *Home Safe Home*. New York: Tarcher-Putnam, 1997.

Lazenby, Gina. *The Healing Home*. Guilford, CT: Lyons Press, 2001.

Levine, Leslie. *Ice Cream for Breakfast*. New York: Contemporary Books, 2002.

———. *Wish It, Dream It, Do It*. New York: Simon & Schuster, 2003.

Lingerman, Hal A. *The Healing Energies of Music*. Wheaton, IL: Quest Books, 1995.

Louden, Jennifer. *The Woman's Retreat Book*. San Francisco: HarperSanFrancisco, 1997.

McMeekin, Gail, MSW. *The Power of Positive Choices*. Berkeley: Conari Press, 1999.

Moran, Victoria. *Creating a Charmed Life*. San Francisco: HarperSanFrancisco, 1999.

———. *Shelter for the Spirit*. New York: HarperCollins, 1998.

Mundis, Jerrold. *How to Get Out of Debt, Stay Out of Debt, and Live Prosperously*. New York: Bantam, 2001.

Sachs, Judith, and Sandra Leiblum, MD. *Getting the Sex You Want*. Lincoln, NE: ASJA Press, 2003.

Wolverton, B. C. *How to Grow Fresh Air*. New York: Penguin, 1996.

INSPIRATION AND SPIRITUALITY

Anderson, Sherry, and Patricia Hopkins. *The Feminine Face of God*. New York: Bantam, 1991.

Carlson, Richard, PhD, and Joseph Bailey, PhD. *Slowing Down to the Speed of Life*. San Francisco: HarperSanFrancisco, 1998.

Coyne, Tami, and Karen Wasserman. *The Spiritual Chicks Question Everything*. Boston: Red Wheel/Weiser, 2003.

Flinders, Carol A. *At the Root of This Longing*. San Francisco: HarperSanFrancisco, 1999.

Goldsmith, Joel. *A Parenthesis in Eternity*. San Francisco: HarperSanFrancisco, 1986.

Horn, Sam. *ConZentrate*. New York: St. Martin's Press, 2001.

Michaels, Chris. *Your Soul's Assignment*. Kansas City, MO: Awakening World Enterprises, 2003.

Nordenson, Nancy J. *Just Think*. Grand Rapids, MI: Baker Books, 2003.

Robinson, Lynn, MEd. *Compass of the Soul*. Kansas City, MO: Andrews-McMeel, 2003.

RECIPE BOOKS

Calabro, Rose Lee. *Living in the Raw*. Santa Cruz, CA: Rose Publishing, 1998.

Raymond, Jennifer. *The Peaceful Palate*. Calistoga, CA: Heart and Soul Publishing, 1996.

Trotter, Charlie, Roxanne Klein, et al. *Raw*. Berkeley: Ten Speed Press, 2003.

YOGA AND AYURVEDIC HEALTH CARE

Chopra, Deepak, MD. *Perfect Health*. New York: Harmony Books, 1991.

Gerson, Scott, MD. *Ayurveda*. Brewster, NY: NIAM Press, 2001.

Krishan, Shubhra. *Radiant Body, Restful Mind*. Novato, CA: New World Library, 2004.

Sivananda Yoga Center. *Yoga Mind and Body*. New York: DK Publishing, 1998.

Stern, Jess. *Yoga, Youth & Reincarnation*. Virginia Beach: ARE Press, 1997.

Townley, Wyatt. *Yoganetics*. San Francisco: HarperSanFrancisco, 2003.

Index

stress and, 271–72
technology, keeping up with, 57
trading PMS for PMZ, 136–37
vicarious, 279–80
weight, calling a truce with your, 416–18
Aging with Grace (Snowdon), 97
air quality, cleaners, filters, 344–45
alcoholic beverages, benefits and drawbacks, 409–10
Alexander Technique, 286, 287
allowing, the art of, 257
All the Tea in China (Chow and Kramer), 313
almonds, blanching, 133
alpha-lipoic acid, 374
Altman, Nathaniel, 214
aluminum warning, 55
Alzheimer's disease, 55, 96–97, 128
American Society of Lymphology, website, 264
Ancient Secrets of the Fountain of Youth (Kelder), 295
Anderson, Sherry, 319
Angster, Irene, 396
Annan, Kofi, 377
Antell, Darrick, 272
antioxidants, 30, 33, 69, 86–87, 100, 102–3, 132, 223, 275, 287, 303, 322, 374, 387
Anytime, Anywhere Exercise Book, The (Price), 167
aphorisms, 302
appearance
    avoiding dowdiness, 181–82
    body, acceptance of real woman's, 178
    changing, 31–32
    compliments on, 380
    cosmetic surgery, 334–35
    EQ (Elegance Quotient), 382–83
    focusing on, 240
    glamour, 410–11
    youthful, 240, 351
    weight, calling a truce with, 416–18
aromas. *See* fragrances and aromas
aromatherapy, 336–37
art for the soul, 166–67
arthritis. *See* joints

At the Root of This Longing (Flinders), 319
Auntie Mame (Dennis), 202
authority and assertiveness, 103–4, 107–8
autumnal equinox, 314–15
Ayurveda (Gerson), 342
Ayurvedic medicine, 3, 19
    abhyanga (warm oil self-massage), 23–24, 269–70
    agni (digestive fire), 86
    almonds, 133
    ama (metabolic debris), 309–10
    four seasons of life, 19–20, 175
    meal schedule, 375
    nature's schedule and sleep, 343–44
    ojas, 133

Baird, Penny Drue, 194
balneotherapy (hot-spring or mineral bathing), 213–14
Barrington, Barbara, 151
bath
    aromatherapy, 337
    balneotherapy, 213–14
    candlelight and music, 18
    as metaphor, 17–18
    steam baths and saunas, 389
    terrycloth robe for, 18
    as therapy, 354–55
    thyme for, 53
Bau-biology, 305
beauty
    affirmation, 353
    as state of being, 151–52
    bravery and, 171–72
    favor people who see yours, 163–64
    seeing yours and others', 430
    your present, 230, 305
Being Vegetarian for Dummies (Havala), 106
Berlin, Irving, 160
beta-carotene, 287–88, 374
Better Basics for the Home (Bond), 345
biographies, 201–2
birthdays, celebrating, 80–81, 148, 401, 404–6
Biziou, Barbara, 414
body shape, changes in, 204–5
Bond, Amy Berthold, 345

relationships, *continued*
favor people who see your beauty and value, 163–64
future plans and, 253
girlfriends, 393–94
osmotic rejuvenation and, 335–36
overcoming objections to change, 407–8
romance and, 50
sex and sex drive in, 197–99
See also friendships
remedies, natural, 52–53
resiliency, 36
rest cure, 385
retreats, 130–31
Rilke, Rainer Maria, 257, 296
ritual
burning bowl, 428
celebration and, 414–15
to allay guilt, 49
Robinson, Lynn, 296
role models, 394–95
romance, 45, 50–51
Ruidant, Denise, 117
Russian Baths, 178

Sachs, Judith, 71, 199
SAD (seasonal affective disorder), 60–61, 307
samadhi, 351
saying no, 210–11
Scaravelli, Vanda, 395
seasons of life, 18–20
selenium, 303
self-acceptance, 233–24
avoiding comparisons, 230
real woman's body, 178, 417–18
weight, calling a truce with, 416–18
self-actualization, 140–41
self-care
abhyanga (warm oil self-massage), 23–24, 269–70
anxiety prevented by, 115
appearance, changing, 31–32
aromatherapy, 336–37
assessing your level of, 238
avoiding dowdiness, 181–82
balneotherapy, 213–14
bathing, 17–18

bathing, therapeutic, 354–55
Botox, 179
brush and floss, 83–85
cells, treating like "somebodies," 73–74
cosmetic surgery, 334–35
detoxification, 309–10
dressing table essentials, 146–47
dry skin brushing, 349
eyebrows, shaping, 289–90
eye cream, 412
eyes and eyesight, 373–74
facials, 204–5
financing, 246–47
four o'clock refresher, 374–75
French dietary philosophy, 284–85
fun and enjoyment, 64, 212
glamour, 410–11
grooming, 15–16
hair care, 261–62
hair color, 340–41
hair style, 35–36, 117–18
legs, 276–78
lip care, 95–96
make-up, professional, 358
massage, 192–93
motivation for, fear vs. enthusiasm, 303–4
rest and restoration, 385
skin care, 29–30, 109–10, 178–80
small action on your own behalf, 169
steam baths and saunas, 389
sun protection, 30, 152–53, 224–25
sun-exposure, needed, 306–7
teeth whitening, 346–47
water, purified, 371–72
winter, 423–24
self-esteem, 58
acceptance of a real woman's body, 178, 417–18
acknowledge your inner warrior, 99–100
comparisons with others, 229–30
memories (of past success), 366–67
size, weight, and clothing, 135–36
self-image
childhood photo and, 176
childlike self, 406–7
come into your own, 81–82

448

To print a free checklist to help chart your progress through *Younger by the Day,* contact the author, receive her online newsletter, or inquire about a speaking engagement or a series of *Younger by the Day*™ coaching sessions, please visit www.victoriamoran.com.

8-